Innovations in Microbiology

ADVANCES IN PHARMACEUTICAL MICROBIOLOGY

From Bench to Bedside

Harpreet Singh, PhD
Arun Kumar Mishra, PhD
Jeyabalan Sangeetha, PhD
Devarajan Thangadurai, PhD
Editors

AAP | APPLE ACADEMIC PRESS

First edition published 2027

Apple Academic Press Inc.
1265 Goldenrod Circle, NE,
Palm Bay, FL 32905 USA

760 Laurentian Drive, Unit 19,
Burlington, ON L7N 0A4, Canada

CRC Press
2385 NW Executive Center Drive,
Suite 320, Boca Raton FL 33431

4 Park Square, Milton Park,
Abingdon, Oxon, OX14 4RN, UK

Library and Archives Canada Cataloguing in Publication

CIP data on file with Canada Library and Archives

Library of Congress Cataloging-in-Publication Data

CIP data on file with US Library of Congress

ISBN: 978-1-77964-090-1 (hbk)
ISBN: 978-1-77964-091-8 (ebk)

DOI: 10.1201/9781779640918

About the Book Series: Innovations in Microbiology

Series Editor

Dr. Jeyabalan Sangeetha

Assistant Professor, Department of Environmental Science

Central University of Kerala, Kasaragod, South India

Pre-microbiology period is the period before the invention of microscope in the 16th century. Many researchers and physicians discussed the existence of microorganisms without any scientific research and supported data. Marcus Terentius, a Roman scholar, in his book *On Agriculture*, explained the possibility of the presence of unseen organisms. During 1020, Abū Alī ibn Sīnā, known as Avicenna in West, theorized that tuberculosis and many other diseases are contagious in his book *The Canon of Medicine*. It was proposed in 1546 by Girolamo Fracastoro, an Italian physician, that transferable seed-like materials were responsible for epidemic diseases through direct or indirect contact. In 1609, Galileo Galilei invented a device known as the microscope. After the invention of microscope with many improved lenses, Antonie van Leeuwenhoek revealed that the planet is filled with unicellular organisms through his observation of animalcule-like structures that swim and tumble in water.

From there, the field of microbiology started to receive more attention from researchers worldwide. Scientists discovered the purpose of sterilization, the nature of decontamination, microbial physiology and multiplication, microbial diversity, culturing techniques, identification methods, and so on.

During 7000 BC, the first indication of cereal grain fermentation by the microorganisms to produce alcohol was obtained from the evidence from the Neolithic village of Jiahu in China. The use of biotechnological techniques was co-founded with developments in the field of microbiology. There is much evidence on the use of yeasts to produce wine, to make bread, and to brew beer discovered from the archaeological sites dating around 2000 to 1200 BC. Later, the true cause of fermentation was explained by Louis Pasteur with scientific evidence. Pasteur's work began a new era in fermentation processes to produce various fermentation-based products in the food industries. Based on the developments and new findings in the microbial world, the field microbiology emerged as one of the major science fields.

Microbiology earned the interest of the majority of industrialists and researchers as microbial products received attention from consumers for better quality. Microbiology was needed on an industrial scale, which, in turn, triggered the development of modern microbiological techniques in various fields. The recent technology in the fields of genetics, biotechnology, and bioinformatics improves and supports modern developments in the field of microbiology as well. Study of biome of microorganisms is a very tedious task as it requires lots of energy and time and also involves money-consuming processes.

The advanced technologies in molecular biology, which paved a way to reveal the entire microbial community in the given sample in a short period, provided us many chances to unravel the secrets of the microbial community to explore the beneficial applications of microbes. In 1980s, modern technological microbiology was begun when it was scientifically proved that the *Pseudomonas putida* strain is capable of degrading the compounds present in crude oil and allowed for patenting the technology. Revolution in the field of microbial biotechnology was observed when a patent registered for genetically modified *Pseudomonas* sp. by Anand Mohan Chakrabarty gained the first ever patent for living organisms. The advent of *genetically modified organisms* (GMOs) contributed many patents to the field, and many companies emerged based on creating GMOs for the development of bioengineering microbial products as well as food crops.

There are contemporary developments seen in classical microbiology through the molecular exploration of new species from various environments, including extremophiles, which led to the selection and improvement of known traits to recover target compounds or functions.

Microbiology is a multidisciplinary area, and it connects human society in both ways—as beneficial in many fields as well as detrimental for its harmful pathogens. In the life sciences, microbiology is a developing field with more mysteries yet to be revealed in the microbial world. Hence, this book series provides a collection of books that deal with advanced microbiology and innovations in microbiology. Each volume under the series covers in depth advanced knowledge on the particular filed in microbiology with various chapters contributed by worldwide scholars in the respective fields.

The book series broadly considers the contributions from the following fields:

- Environmental Microbiology
- Food Microbiology
- Industrial Microbiology
- Agricultural Microbiology
- Pharmaceutical Microbiology
- Extremophiles
- Microbes in Drug Discovery and Therapeutics
- Host–Microbiome Interactions and Applications
- Clinical Virology
- Microbiomes
- Bioremediation of Xenobiotics
- Microbial Biofuels
- Beneficial Microbes
- Microbiome and Climate Change
- Modern Trends in Fermentation Technology

BOOKS IN THE SERIES

Advances in Pharmaceutical Microbiology: From Bench to Bedside
Editors: Harpreet Singh, PhD, Arun Kumar Mishra, PhD,
Jeyabalan Sangeetha, PhD, and Devarajan Thangadurai, PhD

About the Editors

Harpreet Singh, PhD
Professor, School of Pharmaceutical Sciences, Faculty of Pharmacy, IFTM University, Moradabad, India

Harpreet Singh, PhD, is a Professor in the School of Pharmaceutical Sciences, Faculty of Pharmacy at IFTM University, Moradabad, India. His research areas include pharmaceutical microbiology, pharmacotherapeutics, community pharmacy and management, microbial biotechnology, and environmental nanotechnology. With over 13 years of teaching experience, Dr. Singh has supervised students for their MPharm and PhD degrees. He has authored 15 books and published six Indian patents, and one German patent has been granted under his name. He has to his credit over 40 research and review articles published in various journals. In addition to his academic duties, he is also engaged in administrative work as Proctor and Convener of the IFTM University Alumni Association Page Committee and Coordinator of the IFTM University Alumni Association. He is also involved with the Online Education & Learning Management System (OELMS) at Mentoring & Counselling Cell at IFTM. Dr. Singh completed his BPharm and MPharm degrees from the Gautam Budh Technical University and Mahamaya Technical University, respectively. He completed PhD in Pharmacy in 2017.

Arun Kumar Mishra, PhD
Professor and Director, Sahu Onkar Saran School of Pharmacy, Faculty of Pharmacy, IFTM University, Moradabad, Uttar Pradesh, India

Arun Kumar Mishra, PhD, is a Professor and Director of the SOS School of Pharmacy, IFTM University, Moradabad, Uttar Pradesh, India. He has over 15 years of teaching experience and has supervised 20 MPharm students. Under his supervision, seven students have been awarded PhD, two students have submitted the PhD theses and six are working for doctoral degree. His areas of interest are pharmacotherapeutics, analytical chemistry, dermatology, synthetic medicinal chemistry, natural product chemistry, and nanotechnology-based formulations. Dr. Mishra is a recipient of a workshop grant from DBT. He has also authored three books, two book chapters, and published two Indian patents. He has to his credit 84 research and 32 review articles in various journals of high repute with cumulative impact factor 41.07 in SCI indexed journals. Apart from this, Dr. Mishra has received Bentham Brand Ambassador Award, Shikshak Shree Award, Bharat Jyoti Award, Best Researcher Award, Acharya Siromani Award, etc. In addition to academic responsibility as Professor and Head (Pharmacy), Dr. Mishra is also engaged in administrative work as Dean, Students Welfare and in charge of University Guest House. Dr. Mishra completed his BPharm and MPharm degrees at UP Technical University, Uttar Pradesh, in 2006 and 2009, respectively. He has completed his PhD in Pharmacy. After qualifying GATE 2006 and 2009, Dr. Mishra received a fellowship of Rs 120,000 from the All India Council for Technical Education (AICTE).

Jeyabalan Sangeetha, PhD
Assistant Professor, Central University of Kerala, Kasaragod, South India

Jeyabalan Sangeetha, PhD, is an Assistant Professor at Central University of Kerala, Kasaragod, South India. She earned her BSc in Microbiology and PhD in Environmental Sciences from Bharathidasan University, Tiruchirappalli, Tamil Nadu, India. She holds an MSc in Environmental Sciences from Bharathiar University, Coimbatore, Tamil Nadu, India. She is the recipient of a Junior Research Fellowship of the University Grants Commission, Government of India, for her doctoral studies. She is the recipient of a Dr. D.S. Kothari Postdoctoral Fellowship and Women Postdoctoral Fellowship under the University Grants Commission. She has also been awarded with a Fast Track Young Scientist by DST, New Delhi. She has conferred with many national and international awards for her contribution in teaching and research. She has published more than 50 research and review articles in reputed and international journals and 80 book chapters in the fields of environmental microbiology, environmental biotechnology, environmental toxicology, environmental nanotechnology, and bioresources. She has authored and edited 26 books published by international publishers such as Springer, Elsevier, CRC Press, and Apple Academic Press. She has visited eight countries to participate and give talks on various topics related to her research with funding from Government of India and funding agencies from abroad.

Devarajan Thangadurai, PhD
Professor & Chairman of Botany, Karnatak University, South India

Devarajan Thangadurai, PhD, is a Professor at Karnatak University in South India. He has authored/edited over 30 books with national and international publishers and has visited 24 countries in Asia, Europe, Africa, and the Middle East for academic visits, scientific meetings, and international collaborations. He has received his PhD in Botany from Sri Krishnadevaraya University in South India as a CSIR Senior Research Fellow with funding from the Ministry of Science and Technology, Government of India. He served as a Postdoctoral Fellow at the University of Madeira, Portugal; University of Delhi, India; and ICAR National Research Centre for Banana, India. He is the recipient of a Best Young Scientist Award with a Gold Medal from Acharya Nagarjuna University, India, and the VGST-SMYSR Young Scientist Award of the Government of Karnataka, Republic of India.

Contents

Contributors

Gurupadayya Bannimath
Department of Pharmaceutical Chemistry, JSS College of Pharmacy, JSS Academy of Higher Education and Research, Mysuru, Karnataka, India

Ayon Dutta
Department of Pharmaceutical Technology, Brainware University, Barasat, West Bengal, India

Shayeri Chatterjee Ganguly
Department of Pharmaceutical Technology, Brainware University, Barasat, West Bengal, India

Sumon Giri
Department of Pharmaceutical Technology, Brainware University, Kolkata, West Bengal, India

Komal Gupta
Galgotias College of Pharmacy, Greater Noida, Uttar Pradesh, India

Zainab Irfan
Department of Pharmaceutical Technology, Brainware University, Kolkata, West Bengal, India

Archana Kapoor
Department of Pharmaceutical Sciences, Guru Jambheshwar University of Science and Technology, Hisar, Haryana, India

Sofia Khanam
Department of Drug Design and Pharmacology, University of Copenhagen, Denmark

Manish Kumar
KIET School of Pharmacy, Krishna Institute of Engineering & Technology (KIET), Ghaziabad, Delhi-NCR, Uttar Pradesh, India

Moumita Kundu
Department of Pharmaceutical Technology, Brainware University, Barasat, West Bengal, India

Joseph William Ngunda
School of Pharmaceutical Sciences, CT University Ludhiana Punjab, India

Rashmi Pathak
Department of Pharmacy, Invertis University, Bareilly, Uttar Pradesh, India

Biraj Patra
Department of Pharmaceutical Technology, Brainware University, Barasat, West Bengal, India

Mounika Peddaguravagari
Department of Pharmaceutical Chemistry, JSS College of Pharmacy, JSS Academy of Higher Education and Research, Mysuru, Karnataka, India

Shinu Pottathil
Department of Biomedical Sciences, College of Clinical Pharmacy, King Faisal University, Al Ahsa, Saudi Arabia

Sonia Sethi
Dr. B. Lal Institute of Biotechnology, Malviya Nagar, Jaipur, Rajasthan, India

Archana Shaha
Department of Pharmacy, Vishwakarma University, Pune, Maharashtra, India

Prachi Achal Shahu
Galgotias College of Pharmacy, Greater Noida, Uttar Pradesh, India

Bharti Sharma
Department of Pharmaceutical Sciences, Guru Jambheshwar University of Science and Technology, Hisar, Haryana, India

Garima Sharma
Hind School of Pharmacy, Barabanki, Lucknow, Uttar Pradesh, India

Himanshu Sharma
Department of Pharmacology, Nims Institute of Pharmacy, Nims University Rajasthan, Jaipur, Rajasthan, India

Yogita Shinde
Department of Pharmacy, Vishwakarma University, Pune, Maharashtra, India

Tohfa Siddiqui
Galgotias College of Pharmacy, Greater Noida, Uttar Pradesh, India

Gurdeep Singh
School of Pharmaceutical Sciences, Lovely Professional University, Phagwara, Punjab, India

Mukesh Kumar Singh
School of Pharmaceutical Sciences, Faculty of Pharmacy, IFTM University, Moradabad, Uttar Pradesh, India

Dipali Talele
Department of Pharmacy, Vishwakarma University, Pune, Maharashtra, India

Vir Vikram
School of Pharmaceutical Sciences, CT University Ludhiana Punjab, India

Amrendra Pratap Yadav
Department of Pharmacy, Meerut Institute of Technology, Meerut, Uttar Pradesh, India

Preface

Pharmaceutical microbiology is an important multidisciplinary field of study that integrates the science of microbiology and pharmaceutical sciences to ensure the safety, efficacy, and quality of pharmaceutical products. It is the need of hour to be acquainted with recent advancements of the microbiology field as it is essential for the rapid evolution of the pharmaceutical industry, driven by scientific and technological progress.

This book, *Advances in Pharmaceutical Microbiology: From Bench to Bedside*, is a comprehensive information resource on pharmaceutical microbiology, presenting in-depth information of core principles, methodologies, and recent advancements that impact the pharmaceutical field. This book serves as a valuable resource for researchers, academician, clinicians, and other stakeholders who are directly or indirectly involved in the practice of core concepts of pharmaceutical microbiology and seek to expand their understanding of the dynamic field of pharmaceutical microbiology. This book is majorly divided into four parts.

Part I: Foundations of Pharmaceutical Microbiology presents the fundamental principles of pharmaceutical microbiology. This part of book provides overs an overview of the connections between microbiology and pharmaceutical sciences. It also presents an analysis of microbial pathogens and drug resistance and a clarification of the fundamental principles of quality control and good manufacturing practices (GMP) that are essential for ensuring product quality and safety.

Part II: Microbial Control in Pharmaceutical Settings offers comprehensive information related to the techniques employed to eradicate microbial contamination from pharmaceutical products. This also encompasses the utilization of sterilization techniques and validation processes. This chapter showcases the way to examine the importance of microbial biofilms and their application in the pharmaceutical industry, with an emphasis on their impact on the development and manufacturing of products.

Part III: Microbiology and Drug Development explores the intricate relationship between the human microbiome and drug reactions, which provides a valuable understanding related with the emerging field of microbiome-based therapeutics. It further explores the integration of biotechnology into the field of pharmaceutical microbiology and the advancements achieved in microbial testing methods for pharmaceutical products. It underscores the significance of these progressions in pharmaceutical development and compliance with regulatory criteria.

Part IV: Regulatory Compliance and Future Perspectives presents knowledge that addresses the increasing need for global microbial surveillance and the investigation of outbreaks. It also discusses the impact of nanotechnology on the field of pharmaceutical microbiology. Additionally, it analyzes the forthcoming patterns and obstacles that the field is presently encountering.

Our objective as the editors of this book was to compile a diverse selection of chapters authored by renowned specialists in the field. Every chapter offers valuable insights and perspectives on various facets of pharmaceutical microbiology.

The completion of this book was not the exclusive accomplishment of just four of us. We would like to extend our sincere appreciation to everyone who generously contributed and deserves special recognition for dedicating their valuable time and effort. It is anticipated that this book will serve as a catalyst for additional investigation and innovation in this ever-evolving and critical domain, ultimately leading to progress in the field of pharmaceutical science and the enhancement of worldwide public health.

PART I
Foundations of Pharmaceutical Microbiology

CHAPTER 1

Microbial Pathogens and Drug Resistance

MANISH KUMAR[1*], JOSEPH WILLIAM NGUNDA[2], VIR VIKRAM[2] and SHINU POTTATHIL[3]

[1]KIET School of Pharmacy, Krishna Institute of Engineering & Technology (KIET), Ghaziabad, Delhi-NCR, Uttar Pradesh, India

[2]School of Pharmaceutical Sciences, CT University Ludhiana Punjab, India

[3]Department of Biomedical Sciences, College of Clinical Pharmacy, King Faisal University, Al Ahsa, Saudi Arabia

*Corresponding author

ABSTRACT

Modern medicine is faced with a significant problem from antibacterial medication resistance, which puts our ability to treat bacterial illnesses at risk. This chapter explores the intricate mechanisms underlying the rise in medication resistance to antibacterial agents. Through a comprehensive analysis of various resistance strategies employed by bacteria, including alteration of drug targets, reduced drug accumulation, drug inactivation, and efflux pumps, the purpose of this chapter is to offer a comprehensive knowledge of how microorganisms evade the effects of antibiotics. Additionally, the consequences of antibiotic susceptibility on policy and the general population are examined, as well as the role that horizontal mutation plays in the propagation of genes that resist. By delving into the mechanisms that drive bacterial resistance, this chapter contributes to the broader efforts to develop effective strategies to combat this pressing global health threat.

Advances in Pharmaceutical Microbiology: From Bench to Bedside. Harpreet Singh, Arun Kumar Mishra, Jeyabalan Sangeetha, and Devarajan Thangadurai (Eds.)

DOI: 10.1201/9781779640918-2

1.1 INTRODUCTION

Antimicrobial resistance (AMR) is the propensity of microorganisms, such as bacteria, viruses, fungi, and parasites, to develop resistance to the drugs (antimicrobial agents) that were initially effective against them, and it is a worldwide health dilemma. Among such drugs are antiparasitic, antiviral, antifungal, and antibiotic medicines. The difficulty of treating infections increases as bacteria develop resistance to these medications, which can result in a rise in disease, mortality, and healthcare expenses (Dadgostar, 2019). Natural selection is the mechanism by which AMR develops. Reproduction can result in the genetic transfer or mutations between different microbes, which can confer resistance to antimicrobial medications. When these medications are present, the sensitive germs perish while the resistant ones have a survival advantage and can multiply (Morrison and Zembower, 2020). Humans' excessive and improper use of antibiotics, animals, and agriculture is among the main factors contributing to AMR. Antimicrobial usage in cattle and poultry to stimulate growth or prevent sickness, as well as the unneeded or improper prescription of antibiotics, are examples of this (Wise, 1998). Patients who do not finish their prescribed antibiotic regimens are also included in this. Microorganisms with cross-resistance have the potential to grow resistant to one antimicrobial medication and, in some situations, to additional medications with comparable modes of action. When many medications stop working to cure infections, a phenomenon known as cross-resistance increases the difficulty (Marston, 2016). Healthcare associated infections in healthcare settings, patients are often exposed to a higher concentration of antibiotic medications, which could encourage the growth of resistant strains of microorganisms. Hospital-acquired illnesses brought on by microorganisms resistant to drugs, such as multidrug-resistant tuberculosis and methicillin-resistant *Staphylococcus aureus* (MRSA), are examples of the impact of AMR (Acar and Rostel, 2001).

1.2 TYPES OF MICROBIAL RESISTANCE

There are several types of microbial resistance, and each has its own processes as well as effects. These are some of the most common types.

When bacteria learn to expand and survive in the company of drugs that were formerly efficient in opposition to them, antibiotic resistance develops. Multidrug-resistant bacterial strains can arise from this kind of opposition, which can be acquired by mutations or transverse gene transfer (Geissler et al., 2003). When viruses get resistant to antiviral medications, antiviral resistance develops, just like antibiotic resistance. Over time, antiviral medicines can become less effective due to virus mutations that make them resistant to particular therapies, such as HIV and influenza (Prins et al., 2008). After prolonged therapy or frequent exposure to antifungal medications, some fungi may develop resistance to these treatments. *Aspergillus* and *Candida* species are two instances of fungi that have the ability to become resistant (Perlin et al., 2017).

In certain areas, antiparasitic medications, such as chloroquine, can cause parasites, including the *Plasmodium* species that causes malaria, to develop resistance. This makes therapy less effective (Hennessy, 1994). Resistance to one antimicrobial drug can result in resistance to another, a phenomenon known as cross-resistance. This is frequently caused by similar chemical structures or common mechanisms of action. This may reduce available treatments (Sparks et al., 2012). Multidrug resistance or MDR, is the term used to describe a microorganism's resistance to many antimicrobial medications. In healthcare environments, microorganisms that are immune to many antibiotic classes are a major concern (Tanwar et al., 2014).

Even more sophisticated types of resistance include those that are extensively drug-resistant (XDR) and pan-drug-resistant (PDR). PDR bacteria have extremely few treatment choices since they are resistant to all known medicines, whereas XDR bacteria are resistant to the majority of medications (Eatemadi et al., 2021). Because of their inherent properties, such as the capacity to evacuate medications through efflux pumps or the impermeability of their cell walls, some microbes are naturally resistant to some antimicrobial medicines (Brown and Reynolds, 1980). Mutations and horizontal gene transfer from other species can cause microbes to acquire genes that resist (e.g., plasmids or transposons) (Conrath, 2006). Because the biofilm matrix creates a protective habitat, bacteria within biofilms may grow more resistant to antimicrobial treatments (Kanwar et al., 2017). Some microorganisms may not be completely immune to a medication, yet be able to withstand greater dosages of the substance, making treatment less effective and requiring higher doses (Kester and Fortune, 2014).

1.3 DYNAMICS OF MICROBIAL RESISTANCE

This problem has wide-ranging dynamics that are influenced by several variables, and it poses a serious danger to world health. Developing effective solutions to address AMR requires an understanding of its dynamics. The following are some essential elements of the dynamics of antimicrobial opposition:

1.3.1 NATURAL SELECTION

Biological selection is the main cause of antibiotic resistance. The microbial population is subject to selection pressure when antibiotics or other antimicrobial treatments are administered. Microorganisms having modified DNA or defense mechanisms that shield them from the medication's actions will have an edge over other bacteria in terms of survival. These features can be shared or passed down to children (Ingle et al., 2018).

1.3.2 EXCESSIVE UTILIZATION AND ABUSING OF ANTIMICROBIALS

Resistance has been hastened by the widespread and improper use of antimicrobial medications in agricultural, healthcare settings, and even for pets. Misuse of antibiotics includes overprescribing them for viral illnesses and utilizing them as growth promoters in agricultural applications (Ingle et al., 2018).

1.3.3 GENE TRANSFER HORIZONTAL

Through mechanisms including conjugation, transformation, and transduction, bacteria may exchange genetic material. This implies that resistance genes can spread horizontally, even between unrelated species, within the bacterial community. This encourages resistance to spread quickly (von Wintersdorff et al., 2016).

1.3.4 HEALTHCARE SETTINGS

Hospitals and other healthcare environments are hotspots for AMR due to the close proximity of patients, use of antibiotics, and invasive procedures.

Resistant pathogens can easily spread from patient to patient (Chen et al., 2021).

1.3.5 COMMUNITY SPREAD

AMR is not limited to healthcare settings, but resistance of pathogens can also spread within the communities driven by factors such as travel, close contact, and environmental changes (Chen et al., 2021).

1.3.6 ENVIRONMENTAL FACTORS

The antibiotic resistance in environmental microorganisms can be transferred to people by the application of antimicrobials in agriculture and their discharge into the environment through sewage and waste disposal (Bengtsson-Palme et al., 2018).

1.3.7 LACK OF NOVEL ANTIMICROBIALS

The creation of novel antibiotics has significantly decreased, in part because these drugs are less profitable than treatments for chronic illnesses and come with higher R&D expenses. This makes the issue worse by making the current medications less effective (Freire-Moran et al., 2011).

1.3.8 GLOBALIZATION

Increased travel and trade facilitate the global spread of resistant microbes. An antibiotic-resistant strain that emerges in one part of the world can quickly spread to other regions (Berndtson, 2020).

1.3.9 COMMON HEALTH PERSPECTIVE

Recognizing that AMR has an impact on people, animals, and the environment, a common health approach is essential. Collaborative efforts between human health, veterinary medicine, and environmental science are needed to combat AMR effectively (Van Puyvelde, 2018).

1.3.10 PUBLIC AWARENESS AND EDUCATION

Delaying the emergence and spread of resistance requires educating the public, legislators, and healthcare professionals about the responsible use of antibiotics (World Health Organization, 2015a).

1.3.11 REGULATION AND POLICY

Governments and international organizations are implementing laws and guidelines into place to limit the use of antibiotics in healthcare, agriculture, and the environment. These policies aim to promote responsible use and reduce selective pressure (Hobæk and Lie, 2019).

1.3.12 RESEARCH AND SURVEILLANCE

Continuous monitoring and research into the evolution and growth of resistance, the creation of novel antibacterial substances, and alternative therapies are vital components of addressing AMR (Koontz, 1992).

1.4 OVERVIEW OF ANTIBIOTIC CLASSES

A wide class of medications known as antibiotics is used to treat bacterial infections. They function by selectively attacking particular bacterial cell constituents or obstructing vital bacterial functions. Antibiotics come in a variety of classes, each with a distinctive range of activity and mode of action. Amoxicillin and ampicillin are examples of penicillin antibiotics that prevent bacteria from synthesizing their cell walls. They work well against certain Gram-negative and a variety of Gram-positive bacteria (Kadri, 2020). Cephalosporin antibiotics, like ceftriaxone and cephalexin, also target bacterial cell walls. They are effective against a broader spectrum of bacteria compared to penicillins (Rahal et al., 1998). Tetracycline antibiotics, such as doxycycline and minocycline, inhibit protein synthesis in bacteria. They work well against a variety of bacteria, including Gram-positive and Gram-negative (Grossman, 2016). Macrolide antibiotics, including erythromycin and azithromycin, also interfere with bacterial protein synthesis. They are often employed to treat infections of the soft tissues and lungs (Srinivasan and Yeo, 2005).

Fluoroquinolones like ciprofloxacin and levofloxacin target bacterial DNA replication and repair. They work well against a variety of bacteria, even many species that are Gram-negative (Walker, 1999). Aminoglycoside antibiotics, such as gentamicin and neomycin, disrupt protein production through attachment to the ribosome of bacteria. They are often used in serious infections but can have toxic side effects (Krause, 2016). These antibiotics, such as sulfamethoxazole and trimethoprim, interfere with bacterial metabolism by inhibiting folic acid synthesis. They are mostly utilized in the treatment of urinary tract and lung infections (Mathews et al., 2015).

Glycopeptide antibiotics, like vancomycin, are used for treating serious infections, especially those resulted from MRSA. They disrupt cell wall synthesis (Rezvani et al., 2022). Clindamycin is an example of a lincosamide antibiotic that inhibits protein synthesis in bacteria and is used for a variety of infections. Linezolid is one of an oxazolidinone antibiotic that prevents protein production and is effective against certain drug-resistant bacteria.

Carbapenem antibiotics like imipenem and meropenem, are wide range-spectrum antibiotics used for serious infections, including those caused by bacteria that are immune to multiple drugs (Shah et al., 2016). Aztreonam is a monobactam antibiotic that targets cell wall synthesis. It is often used in individuals with penicillin allergies (Cattaneo et al., 2022).

It is paramount to use antimicrobials responsibly and correctly as the excess use and abuse of antimicrobials can result in opposition, which is a significant health concern in society. Always follow your healthcare provider's instructions when taking antibiotics and complete the full course/dose of treatment to ensure the most effective and safe outcome.

1.5 TYPES OF ANTIBACTERIAL DRUG RESISTANCE

The global concern over antibacterial antibiotic resistance is developing, and it manifests in various forms. Biofilms, which are populations of microorganisms encased in a self-produced matrix, can be formed by bacteria. Bacteria are shielded from the antibiotics' actions by the solid barrier that biofilms create (Mah and O'Toole, 2001). Bacteria can obtain resistance by naturally occurring changes in their genetic makeup, leading to changes in the target sites of antibiotics (Andersson and Hughes, 2014). Resistance genes can be horizontally transferred by bacteria via conjugation, transformation, and transduction. This makes it possible for resistance genes to proliferate quickly throughout bacterial populations (Ventola, 2015). Bacteria may produce enzymes that modify or degrade antibiotics, rendering them ineffective. For example, β-lactamase enzymes can break down beta-lactam antibiotics (Bush et al., 1995). Bacteria can have efflux pumps that actively pump out antibiotics from the bacterial cell, reducing their concentration within the cell. This reduces the effectiveness of antibiotics (Li, 1995). Antibiotics' target sites can be altered by bacteria, which stops the medications from binding and working as intended (Alekshun and Levy, 2007). It is important to note that antibiotic resistance is a complex and multifaceted issue, and these mechanisms often interact and contribute to the overall resistance of bacterial populations. Research on antibiotic resistance is ongoing, and new findings may have emerged.

1.6 ALTERATION OF DRUG TARGETS

The alteration of drug targets through structural modifications is a common strategy in drug development. This approach involves making changes to the molecular structure of a drug to optimize its interactions with specific targets in the body, such as proteins or enzymes. This can enhance the drug's effectiveness, selectivity, and safety profile. However, it is important to note that structural modifications can also lead to the development of resistance in some cases.

1.7 ALTERATION OF DRUG TARGETS THROUGH STRUCTURAL MODIFICATIONS

1.7.1 ANTIBIOTICS AND β-LACTAMASE INHIBITORS

The creation of β-lactam antibiotics has been shown to be essential in the fight against bacterial illnesses. Resistance has been brought about by the development of β-lactamase enzymes. Resistance has been successfully overcome by developing β-lactamase inhibitors in addition to structural alterations of β-lactam antibiotics. For instance, amoxicillin and clavulanic acid together work well against bacteria that produce β-lactamases (Livermore, 1995).

1.7.2 ANTIRETROVIRAL DRUGS IN HIV TREATMENT

Antiretroviral medication resistance frequently results from the ongoing evolution of the human immunodeficiency virus (HIV). The goal of developing new classes of antiretrovirals or altering the structural makeup of current medications is to combat resistance. For example, the introduction of protease inhibitors with modified structures has been effective in managing drug-resistant strains of HIV (Wainberg and Zaharatos, 1992).

1.7.3 ANTIBIOTIC RESISTANCE IN METHICILLIN-RESISTANT STAPHYLOCOCCUS AUREUS (MRSA)

Structural modifications in antibiotics, such as methicillin, have led to the emergence of MRSA. The altered penicillin-binding protein in MRSA confers resistance to methicillin and related drugs. Understanding the structural changes in the target protein is crucial in developing new strategies to combat MRSA (Chambers and DeLeo, 2009).

1.7.4 ANTICANCER DRUG RESISTANCE IN TYROSINE KINASE INHIBITORS

Resistance to tyrosine kinase inhibitors (TKIs) in cancer treatment, such as imatinib in chronic myeloid leukemia, can arise due to structural modifications in the target kinase. Mutations in the BCR-ABL kinase domain may lead to reduced drug binding affinity. Ongoing research focuses on developing next-generation TKIs with improved target specificity (O'Hare and Deininger, 2007). Understanding the interplay between structural modifications of drugs and the development of resistance is crucial for advancing drug development strategies. Continuous research and innovation are needed to stay ahead of evolving resistance mechanisms.

1.8 EFFLUX PUMPS AND MULTIDRUG RESISTANCE

Efflux pumps are protein-based transporters that play a crucial role in bacterial resistance to antibiotics and other toxic compounds. These pumps actively extract or extrude a variety of materials, including medications, from the bacterial cell, lowering the levels of those compounds inside the cell and decreasing their potency. The mechanism of efflux pump action involves several steps, and it can vary among different pump types, such as:

1.8.1 MECHANISM OF EFFLUX PUMP ACTION

Efflux pumps typically recognize a broad range of substrates, including antibiotics and other toxic compounds. The binding of substrates to the efflux pump occurs in the cytoplasm or at specific binding sites within the bacterial cell (Piddock, 2006). Efflux pumps require energy to actively transport substrates out of the cell. Most efflux pumps use the proton motive force (PMF) or ATP hydrolysis as an energy source (Li et al., 1995). The binding of substrates triggers conformational changes in the efflux pump protein. These changes lead to the formation of an open channel or tunnel through which the substrates are moved across the cell membrane (Blair et al., 2015). Substrates are actively transported across the cell membrane by the efflux pump. The direction of transport is typically from the cytoplasm to the extracellular environment (Darby et al., 2023). Substrates are expelled outside the bacterial cell, leading to a decrease in intracellular concentration. This extrusion reduces the effectiveness of antibiotics and other toxic compounds, contributing to bacterial resistance (Christaki et al., 2020).

1.8.2 TYPES AND FUNCTIONS OF EFFLUX PUMPS

Membrane transport proteins called efflux pumps are essential for the extrusion of a variety of materials from bacterial cells, including toxins, antibiotics, and other chemicals. These pumps lower the intracellular concentration of medications, which leads to the emergence of antibiotic resistance in bacteria. There are several types of efflux pumps, classified based on their structure, energy source, and substrate specificity. ABC transporters move a variety of substrates across the cell membrane by using energy produced by the hydrolysis of ATP. They have a role in the excretion of harmful substances such as antibiotics (Higgins, 1992). MFS pumps are secondary active transporters that use the PMF to extrude substrates. They contribute to the outflow of detergents, antibiotics, and other substances (Pao et al., 1998). RND pumps are involved in the efflux of a broad range of substrates, including antibiotics and detergents. They often span both the inner and outer membranes of Gram-negative bacteria (Nikaido and Pagès, 2012). SMR proteins are small membrane transporters that use the PMF for substrate efflux. They are involved in the resistance to quaternary ammonium compounds and other drugs (Bay et al., 2008). MATE transporters use ion gradients for the efflux of substrates and are involved in the resistance to a variety of drugs, including antibiotics (Bay et al., 2008).

1.9 STRATEGIES TO COMBAT ANTIBACTERIAL RESISTANCE

The rational use of antibiotics is crucial to combat antibiotic resistance to ensure effective treatment and minimize adverse effects.

1.9.1 KEY PRINCIPLES FOR THE RATIONAL USE OF ANTIBIOTICS

1.9.1.1 PRESCRIPTION GUIDELINES

Follow established clinical guidelines for antibiotic prescription. Organizations like the Infectious Diseases Society of America and the World Health Organization provide comprehensive guidelines for various infections (https://www.idsociety.org/practice-guideline).

1.9.1.2 TARGETED THERAPY

Prescribe antibiotics based on the specific pathogen causing the infection. Utilize diagnostic tests when necessary to identify the causative agent (Dellit et al., 2007).

1.9.1.3 EMPIRICAL THERAPY

When waiting for test results, choose antibiotics with a broad spectrum that covers likely pathogens. Narrow down the spectrum once results are available (Mandell et al., 2007).

1.9.1.4 DURATION OF THERAPY

Prescribe the shortest effective duration of antibiotic therapy. Avoid unnecessarily prolonged courses (Spellberg et al., 2013).

1.9.1.5 COMBINATION THERAPY

Reserve combination therapy for specific indications, such as severe infections or polymicrobial infections (Tamma et al., 2017).

1.9.1.6 ANTIBIOTIC STEWARDSHIP PROGRAMS

Implement and participate in antibiotic stewardship programs to optimize the use of antibiotics in healthcare settings (Barlam et al., 2016).

1.9.1.7 EDUCATION AND COMMUNICATION

Educate healthcare professionals, patients, and the public on the appropriate use of antibiotics to reduce unnecessary demand and misuse (World Health Organization, 2015b).

1.9.2 INNOVATIONS IN ANTIBIOTIC DEVELOPMENT

- Bacteriophages are viruses that infect and kill bacteria. Phage therapy involves using these viruses to target and eliminate specific bacterial strains (Dąbrowska et al., 2019).
- CRISPR technology has been employed to create synthetic bacteriophages that selectively target antibiotic-resistant bacteria (Bikard et al., 2014).

- Adjuvants are compounds that enhance the effectiveness of antibiotics. They can help overcome resistance mechanisms and lower the required antibiotic dosage (Brown and Wright, 2016).
- Rediscovering and modifying existing natural compounds or combining them with other drugs to enhance their efficacy and combat resistance (Ling et al., 2015).
- Utilizing machine learning algorithms to analyze large datasets and predict potential antibiotic candidates (Stokes et al., 2020).
- Implementing strategies where different antibiotics are used in rotation to reduce the emergence of resistance (Bergstrom et al., 2004).

1.9.3 OVERCOMING ANTIMICROBIAL RESISTANCE MECHANISMS STRATEGICALLY

Overcoming AMR requires a multifaceted and strategic approach that addresses the various mechanisms through which bacteria and other micro-organisms develop resistance to antibiotics. New antibiotic discovery is crucial to combat resistance. R&D efforts should focus on identifying and developing new classes of antibiotics (Ventola, 2015). Using a combination of antibiotics can help prevent the emergence of resistance. This approach is effective because it targets bacteria through multiple mechanisms (Bollenbach, 2015). Implementing antibiotic stewardship programs to ensure proper and rational use of antibiotics helps prevent the development of resistance (Dellit et al., 2007). Vaccines can prevent infections, reducing the need for antibiotics. This can indirectly contribute to reducing the selective pressure for the development of resistance (O'Neill, 2016).

Bacteriophages, viruses that infect bacteria, can be used to target and kill specific bacterial strains. Phage therapy is being explored as an alternative to traditional antibiotics (Golkar et al., 2014). Investigating alternative therapies, such as antimicrobial peptides or nanoparticles, can provide new options for treating infections (Hancock et al., 2006). Rapid and accurate diagnostic tools can help identify infections and determine the most effective treatment, reducing unnecessary antibiotic use (Murray et al., 2021).

International collaboration and the implementation of policies to regulate antibiotic use are essential to address the global nature of AMR (World Health Organization, 2015a). These strategies, when implemented collectively, can contribute to overcoming AMR and ensuring the continued effectiveness of antibiotics in the treatment of bacterial infections.

1.9.4 PROSPECTS FOR FUTURE ANTIBACTERIAL DRUG DESIGN

The prospects for future antibacterial drug design are promising yet challenging, as bacterial resistance to existing antibiotics continues to rise. Researchers are exploring various strategies to develop novel antibacterial agents that are effective, selective, and less prone to resistance.

Identification and validation of new bacterial targets can lead to the development of drugs with unique mechanisms of action. For example, targeting essential enzymes involved in bacterial cell wall synthesis or bacterial-specific metabolic pathways (Davies and Davies, 2010). Developing combination therapies that target multiple bacterial components or pathways can enhance efficacy and reduce the likelihood of resistance development. Combining antibiotics with synergistic mechanisms of action can be particularly effective (Lewis, 2020).

Nanoparticles and nanomaterials can be engineered to deliver antibiotics more effectively, improve drug stability, and overcome bacterial resistance mechanisms. Nanoparticles can enhance drug penetration into bacterial cells and biofilms (Rai et al., 2012). Developing immunotherapeutic approaches, such as vaccines or immune system modulators, to enhance the body's natural defense against bacterial infections. Vaccines can prevent infections, reducing the need for antibiotics (Plotkin, 2014). Bacteriophages, viruses that infect bacteria, are being investigated as potential therapeutic agents. Using particular bacteriophages to isolate and eradicate bacterial infections specifically is known as phage treatment (Oechslin, 2018). Creating substances that can stop or interfere with the formation of bacterial biofilms, since these structures are frequently more resistant to antibiotics. Therapies for bacterial infections that are recurrent and chronic may benefit from this (Flemming et al., 2016).

Investigating existing drugs for their potential antibacterial properties. Drug repurposing can expedite the drug development process and may lead to the discovery of new uses for existing drugs (Ashburn and Thor, 2004). Employing synthetic biology to engineer bacteria with altered susceptibility to antibiotics or to design synthetic antimicrobial peptides with enhanced efficacy (Moe-Behrens et al., 2013).

It is essential to note that the field of antibacterial drug design is an evolving and continuous study is likely to uncover new strategies and targets. The references provided are examples, and researchers should consult the latest literature for the most current developments in antibacterial drug design.

1.10 CONCLUSION

Microbial pathogens and drug resistance pose significant challenges to global public health. Drug-resistant strains of bacteria, viruses, fungi, and other microbes are emerging and spreading, which reduces the efficacy of current treatment approaches and raises morbidity, mortality, and healthcare expenses. The global incidence of drug-resistant microbial infections has been steadily increasing. Overprescription of antibiotics, incomplete treatment courses, and inappropriate use in both human and animal health care aid in the emergence of resistant strains. This alarming trend necessitates urgent and coordinated efforts to address the misuse of antimicrobial agents.

Drug-resistant infections significantly impact public health outcomes. Common infections that were before manageable become harder to control, resulting in longer hospital stays, greater death rates, and more severe infections. Particularly vulnerable groups include the elderly, those with impaired immune systems, and people suffering from long-term illnesses. The economic burden associated with microbial pathogens and drug resistance is substantial. The costs associated with prolonged treatments, hospitalizations, and the development of new drugs to combat resistance strain healthcare systems and national economies. The loss of productivity due to illness and the expense of implementing control measures further exacerbate the economic impact.

Antibiotic stewardship programs are crucial for addressing the issue of drug resistance. These programs promote responsible use of antibiotics, emphasizing appropriate prescribing practices, patient education, and surveillance of resistance patterns. Continued efforts are required to implement and enforce such programs globally. To properly address antibiotic resistance, new antimicrobial agents must be developed. It is essential to invest in R&D for new antivirals, antifungal drugs, and antibiotics. To solve this worldwide issue, it is essential to support the pharmaceutical sector innovation and offer incentives for the creation of new medications. Given the transboundary nature of infectious diseases, global cooperation is paramount. Collaborative efforts among nations, international organizations, and the private sector are essential for surveillance, information sharing, and coordinated responses to emerging microbial threats. A common health approach that considers people, animals, and environmental factors is integral to tackling the root causes of drug resistance.

In conclusion, addressing microbial pathogens and drug resistance requires a multifaceted approach that includes improved antibiotic stewardship, increased R&D efforts, and enhanced global cooperation. Failure to act decisively on this issue presents a serious risk to the general population's health, and concerted efforts are necessary to safeguard the efficacy of existing antimicrobial treatments and ensure a sustainable future for healthcare.

KEYWORDS

- **antibacterial resistance**
- **infection**
- **efflux pump**

REFERENCES

Acar, J., Rostel, B. (2001). Antimicrobial resistance: An overview. *Revue Scientifique et Technique-Office International des Epizooties*, *20*(3), 797–810.

Alekshun, M. N., Levy, S. B. (2007). Molecular mechanisms of antibacterial multidrug resistance. *Cell*, *128*(6), 1037–1050.

Andersson, D. I., Hughes, D. (2014). Microbiological effects of sublethal levels of antibiotics. *Nature Reviews Microbiology*, *12*(7), 465–478.

Ashburn, T. T., Thor, K. B. (2004). Drug repositioning: Identifying and developing new uses for existing drugs. *Nature Reviews Drug Discovery*, *3*(8), 673–683.

Barlam T.F., et al. (2016). Implementing an antibiotic stewardship program: Guidelines by the infectious diseases society of America and the society for healthcare epidemiology of America. *Clinical Infectious Diseases,* 62(10), e51–e77.

Bay, D. C., Rommens, K. L., Turner, R. J. (2008). Small multidrug resistance proteins: A multidrug transporter family that continues to grow. *Biochimica et Biophysica Acta (BBA)-Biomembranes*, *1778*(9), 1814–1838.

Bengtsson-Palme, J., Kristiansson, E., and Larsson, D. J. (2018). Environmental factors influencing the development and spread of antibiotic resistance. *FEMS Microbiology Reviews*, *42*(1), fux053.

Bergstrom, C. T., Lo, M., Lipsitch, M. (2004). Ecological theory suggests that antimicrobial cycling will not reduce antimicrobial resistance in hospitals. *Proceedings of the National Academy of Sciences*, *101*(36), 13285–13290.

Berndtson, A. E. (2020). Increasing globalization and the movement of antimicrobial resistance between countries. *Surgical Infections*, *21*(7), 579–585.

Bikard, D., Euler, C. W., Jiang, W., Nussenzweig, P. M., Goldberg, G. W., Duportet, X., and Fischetti, V. A. (2014). Exploiting CRISPR-Cas nucleases to produce sequence-specific antimicrobials. *Nature Biotechnology*, *32*(11), 1146–1150.

Blair, J. M. A., Webber, M. A., Baylay, A. J., Ogbolu, D. O., Piddock, L. J. V. (2015). Molecular mechanisms of antibiotic resistance. *Nature Reviews Microbiology*, *13*(1), 42–51.

Bollenbach, T. (2015). Antimicrobial interactions: Mechanisms and implications for drug discovery and resistance evolution. *Current Opinion in Microbiology*, *27*, 1–9.

Brown, D. F., Reynolds, P. E. (1980). Intrinsic resistance to β-lactam antibiotics in staphylococcus aureus. *FEBS Letters*, *122*(2), 275–278.

Brown, D., Wright, G. D. (2016). Antibacterial drug discovery in the resistance era. *Nature*, *529*(7586), 336–343.

Bush, K., Jacoby, G. A., Medeiros, A. A. (1995). A functional classification scheme for beta-lactamases and its correlation with molecular structure. *Antimicrobial Agents and Chemotherapy*, *39*(6), 1211–1233.

Cattaneo, D., Gervasoni, C., Corona, A. (2022). The issue of pharmacokinetic-driven drug-drug interactions of antibiotics: A narrative review. *Antibiotics*, *11*(10), 1410.

Chambers, H. F., DeLeo, F. R. (2009). Waves of resistance: Staphylococcus aureus in the antibiotic era. *Nature Reviews Microbiology*, *7*(9), 629–641.

Chen, Q., Li, D., Beiersmann, C., Neuhann, F., Moazen, B., Lu, G., Müller, O. (2021). Risk factors for antibiotic resistance development in healthcare settings in China: A systematic review. *Epidemiology and Infection*, *149*, e141.

Christaki, E., Marcou, M., Tofarides, A. (2020). Antimicrobial resistance in bacteria: mechanisms, evolution, and persistence. *Journal of Molecular Evolution*, *88*, 26–40.

Conrath, U. (2006). Systemic acquired resistance. *Plant Signaling and Behavior*, *1*(4), 179–184.

Dąbrowska, K., Abedon, S. T., Winkel, A. (2019). Bacteriophage therapy: Advances in formulation strategies and human clinical trials. *Annual Review of Virology*, *6*, 49–69.

Dadgostar, P. (2019). Antimicrobial resistance: Implications and costs. *Infection and Drug Resistance*, 12, 3903–3910.

Darby, E. M., Trampari, E., Siasat, P., Gaya, M. S., Alav, I., Webber, M. A., Blair, J. M. (2023). Molecular mechanisms of antibiotic resistance revisited. *Nature Reviews Microbiology*, *21*(5), 280–295.

Davies, J., Davies, D. (2010). Origins and evolution of antibiotic resistance. *Microbiology and Molecular Biology Reviews*, *74*(3), 417–433.

Dellit, T. H., et al. (2007). Infectious diseases society of America and the society for healthcare epidemiology of America guidelines for developing an institutional program to enhance antimicrobial stewardship. *Clinical Infectious Diseases*, *44*(2), 159–177.

Eatemadi, A., Al Risi, E., Kasliwal, A., Al Za'abi, A., Moradzadegan, H., Aslani, Z. (2021). A proposed evidence-based local guideline for definition of multidrug-resistant (MDR), extensively drug-resistant (XDR) and pan drug-resistant (PDR) bacteria by the microbiology laboratory. *International Journal of Current Science Research and Review*, *4*(3), 146–153.

Flemming, H. C., Wingender, J., Szewzyk, U., Steinberg, P., Rice, S. A., and Kjelleberg, S. (2016). Biofilms: An emergent form of bacterial life. *Nature Reviews Microbiology*, 14(9), 563–575.

Freire-Moran, L., Aronsson, B., Manz, C., Gyssens, I. C., So, A. D., Monnet, D. L., ECDC-EMA Working Group. (2011). Critical shortage of new antibiotics in development against multidrug-resistant bacteria—time to react is now. *Drug Resistance Updates*, *14*(2), 118–124.

Geissler, A., Gerbeaux, P., Granier, I., Blanc, P., Facon, K., Durand-Gasselin, J. (2003). Rational use of antibiotics in the intensive care unit: Impact on microbial resistance and costs. *Intensive Care Medicine*, *29*, 49–54.

Golkar, Z., Bagasra, O., Pace, D. G. (2014). Bacteriophage therapy: A potential solution for the antibiotic resistance crisis. *Journal of Infection in Developing Countries*, *8*(2), 129–136.

Grossman, T. H. (2016). Tetracycline antibiotics and resistance. *Cold Spring Harbor Perspectives in Medicine*, *6*(4), a025387.

Hancock, R. E. W., Sahl, H.-G. (2006). Antimicrobial and host-defense peptides as new anti-infective therapeutic strategies. *Nature Biotechnology*, *24*(12), 1551–1557.

Hennessy, D. R. (1994). The disposition of antiparasitic drugs in relation to the development of resistance by parasites of livestock. *Acta Tropica*, *56*(2–3), 125–141.

Higgins, C. F. (1992). ABC transporters: From microorganisms to man. *Annual Reviews of Cell Biology*, *8*(1), 67–113.

Hobæk, B., Lie, A. K. (2019). Less is more: Norwegian drug regulation, antibiotic policy, and the "need clause". *The Milbank Quarterly*, *97*(3), 762–795.

Ingle, D. J., Levine, M. M., Kotloff, K. L., Holt, K. E., Robins-Browne, R. M. (2018). Dynamics of antimicrobial resistance in intestinal *Escherichia coli* from children in community settings in South Asia and sub-Saharan Africa. *Nature Microbiology*, *3*(9), 1063–1073.

Kadri, S. S. (2020). Key takeaways from the US CDC's 2019 antibiotic resistance threats report for frontline providers. *Critical Care Medicine*, *48*(7), 939–945.

Kanwar, I., K Sah, A., K Suresh, P. (2017). Biofilm-mediated antibiotic-resistant oral bacterial infections: mechanism and combat strategies. *Current Pharmaceutical Design*, *23*(14), 2084–2095.

Kester, J. C., Fortune, S. M. (2014). Persisters and beyond: Mechanisms of phenotypic drug resistance and drug tolerance in bacteria. *Critical Reviews in Biochemistry and Molecular Biology*, *49*(2), 91–101.

Koontz, F. P. (1992). Microbial resistance surveillance techniques. Blood culture versus multiple body site monitoring. *Diagnostic Microbiology and Infectious Disease*, *15*(2S), 31S–35S.

Krause, K. M., Serio, A. W., Kane, T. R., Connolly, L. E. (2016). Aminoglycosides: An overview. *Cold Spring Harbor Perspectives in Medicine*, *6*(6), a027029.

Lewis, K. (2020). The science of antibiotic discovery. *Cell*, *181*(1), 29–45.

Li, X.-Z., Nikaido, H., Poole, K. (1995). Role of mexA-mexB-oprM in antibiotic efflux in *Pseudomonas aeruginosa. Antimicrobial Agents and Chemotherapy*, *39*(9), 1948–1953.

Ling, L. L., Schneider, T., Peoples, A. J., Spoering, A. L., Engels, I., Conlon, B. P., Anna Mueller, A., Schäberle, T. F., Hughes, D. E., Epstein, S., Jones, M., Lazarides, L., Steadman, V. A., Cohen, D. R., Felix, C. R., Ashley Fetterman, K., Millett, W. P., Nitti, A. G., Zullo, A. M., Chen, C. Lewis, K. (2015). A new antibiotic kills pathogen without detectable resistance. *Nature*, *517*(7535), 455–459.

Livermore, D. M. (1995). Beta-Lactamases in laboratory and clinical resistance. *Clinical Microbiology Reviews*, *8*(4), 557–584.

Mah, T.-F. C., O'Toole, G. A. (2001). Mechanisms of biofilm resistance to antimicrobial agents. *Trends in Microbiology*, *9*(1), 34–39.

Mandell, L.A., et al. (2007). Infectious diseases society of America/American thoracic society consensus guidelines on the management of community-acquired pneumonia in adults. *Clinical Infectious Diseases,* 44(S2), S27–S72.

Marston, H. D., Dixon, D. M., Knisely, J. M., Palmore, T. N., Fauci, A. S. (2016). Antimicrobial resistance. *JAMA*, *316*(11), 1193–1204.

Mathews, S. M., Jiju, V., Thomas, I., Panicker, J. T., Kuriakose, L. S. (2015). Sulfa drugs and the skin. *World Journal of Pharmaceutical Research*, *4*(10), 382–390.

Moe-Behrens, G. H., Davis, R., and Haynes, K. A. (2013). Preparing synthetic biology for the world. *Frontiers in Microbiology*, *4*, 5.

Morrison, L., Zembower, T. R. (2020). Antimicrobial resistance. *Gastrointestinal Endoscopy Clinics*, *30*(4), 619–635.

Murray, P. R., et al. (2021). *Manual of Clinical Microbiology*, 12th edn. ASM Press.

Nikaido, H., Pagès, J. M. (2012). Broad-specificity efflux pumps and their role in multidrug resistance of Gram-negative bacteria. *FEMS Microbiology Reviews*, 36(2), 340–363.

O'Neill, J. (2016). Tackling drug-resistant infections globally: Final report and recommendations. The Review on Antimicrobial Resistance.

Oechslin, F. (2018). Resistance development to bacteriophages occurring during bacteriophage therapy. *Viruses*, *10*(8), 351.

O'Hare, T., Deininger, M. W. (2007). Tyrosine kinase inhibitors in chronic myeloid leukemia: A phase II study of imatinib plus hydroxyurea in patients failing interferon-alpha. *Blood*, *100*(13), 229a–229a.

Pao, S. S., Paulsen, I. T., and Saier Jr, M. H. (1998). Major facilitator superfamily. *Microbiology and Molecular Biology Reviews*, *62*(1), 1–34.

Perlin, D. S., Rautemaa-Richardson, R., Alastruey-Izquierdo, A. (2017). The global problem of antifungal resistance: Prevalence, mechanisms, and management. *The Lancet Infectious Diseases*, *17*(12), e383–e392.

Piddock, L. J. (2006). Clinically relevant chromosomally encoded multidrug resistance efflux pumps in bacteria. *Clinical Microbiology Reviews*, *19*(2), 382–402.

Plotkin, S. A. (2014). Vaccines: Correlates of vaccine-induced immunity. *Clinical Infectious Diseases*, *47*(3), 401–409.

Prins, M., Laimer, M., Noris, E., Schubert, J., Wassenegger, M., Tepfer, M. (2008). Strategies for antiviral resistance in transgenic plants. *Molecular Plant Pathology*, *9*(1), 73–83.

Rahal, J. J., Urban, C., Horn, D., Freeman, K., Segal-Maurer, S., Maurer, J., Mariano, N., Marks, S., Burns, J. M., Dominick, D., Lim, M. (1998). Class restriction of cephalosporin use to control total cephalosporin resistance in nosocomial *Klebsiella. JAMA*, *280*(14), 1233–1237.

Rai, M., Deshmukh, S. D., Ingle, A. P., Gade, A. K. (2012). Silver nanoparticles: The powerful nanoweapon against multidrug-resistant bacteria. *Journal of Applied Microbiology*, *112*(5), 841–852.

Rezvani, M., Kharazmkia, A., Amiri, A., Sherkatolabbasieh, H. R., Birjandi, M. (2022). Drug utilization evaluation (DUE) of vancomycin: A cross-sectional study. *Annals of Medicine and Surgery*, *80*, 104169.

Shah, P. J., Hanson, C., Larson, P., Patel, J. (2016). Carbapenem-resistant *Escherichia coli* resistant to ceftazidime–avibactam: The need for a commercially available testing product. *American Journal of Health-System Pharmacy*, *73*(14), 1029–1030.

Sparks, T. C., Dripps, J. E., Watson, G. B., Paroonagian, D. (2012). Resistance and cross-resistance to the spinosyns—a review and analysis. *Pesticide Biochemistry and Physiology*, *102*(1), 1–10.

Spellberg, B, Bartlett, JG, Gilbert, DN. (2013). The future of antibiotics and resistance. *New England Journal of Medicine*, 368(4),299–302.

Srinivasan, R., Yeo, T. H. (2005). Are newer macrolides effective in eradicating carriage of pertussis? *Archives of Disease in Childhood*, *90*(3), 322–324.

Stokes, J. M., Yang, K., Swanson, K., Jin, W., Cubillos-Ruiz, A., Donghia, N. M., MacNair, C. R., French, S., Carfrae, L. A., Bloom-Ackermann, Z., Tran, V. M., Chiappino-Pepe, A., Badran, A. H., Andrews, I. W., Chory, Emma J., Church, G. M., Brown, E. D., Jaakkola, T. S., Barzilay, R., Collins, J. J. (2020). A deep learning approach to antibiotic discovery. *Cell*, 180(4), 688–702.

Tamma, P. D. et al. (2017). The use of combination antibiotic therapy for the treatment of critically ill patients with gram-negative infections: A systematic review and meta-analysis. *Critical Care Medicine, 45*(11), 1772–1779.

Tanwar, J., Das, S., Fatima, Z., Hameed, S. (2014). Multidrug resistance: An emerging crisis. *Interdisciplinary Perspectives on Infectious Diseases*, 2014, 541340.

Van Puyvelde, S., Deborggraeve, S., Jacobs, J. (2018). Why the antibiotic resistance crisis requires a one health approach. *The Lancet Infectious Diseases*, *18*(2), 132–134.

Ventola, C. L. (2015). The Antibiotic resistance crisis: Part 1: Causes and threats. *Pharmacy & Therapeutics: A Peer-Reviewed Journal for Formulary Management*, *40*(4), 277–283.

Von Wintersdorff, C. J., Penders, J., Van Niekerk, J. M., Mills, N. D., Majumder, S., Van Alphen, L. B., Savelkoul, P. H. M., Wolffs, P. F. (2016). Dissemination of antimicrobial resistance in microbial ecosystems through horizontal gene transfer. *Frontiers in Microbiology*, *7*, 173.

Wainberg, M. A., Zaharatos, G. J. (1992). Development of antiretroviral drug resistance. *New England Journal of Medicine*, 327(6), 388–391.

Walker, R. C. (1999). The fluoroquinolones. In *Mayo Clinic Proceedings* (Vol. 74, No. 10, pp. 1030–1037). Elsevier.

Wise, R., Hart, T., Cars, O., Streulens, M., Helmuth, R., Huovinen, P., Sprenger, M. (1998). Antimicrobial resistance. *British Medical Journal*, *317*(7159), 609–610.

World Health Organization (2015a). Global Action Plan on Antimicrobial Resistance.

World Health Organization (2015b). Antibiotic Resistance: Multi-Country Public Awareness Survey.

CHAPTER 2

Quality Control and Good Manufacturing Practices in Pharmaceutical Microbiology

GURUPADAYYA BANNIMATH* and MOUNIKA PEDDAGURAVAGARI

Department of Pharmaceutical Chemistry, JSS College of Pharmacy, JSS Academy of Higher Education and Research, Mysuru, Karnataka, India

*Corresponding author

ABSTRACT

Pharmaceutical microbiology plays a major role in quality control (QC) as well as manufacturing processes to assure safety, productivity, and reliability of the pharmaceutical compounds. The importance of QC and production methods ensures microbiological integrity in the entire manufacturing process. Microbial contamination leads to the degradation of pharmaceutical products, which results in major health consequences in patients. So, there is a necessity for strict revision of QC measures for identification and prevention of microbial growth in pharmaceutical compounds. Good manufacturing practices have a set of regulations specifically for production, facility, and documentation of pharmaceutical products. Early detection technologies and risk restriction of undesirable microbiological contamination have to be implemented to avoid recall of products for public health concerns. Furtherly, this chapter mainly focuses on QC guidelines of regulatory authorities such as the World Health Organization, implemented standards for restriction of microbial contamination while manufacturing of pharmaceutical products by pharma industries.

Advances in Pharmaceutical Microbiology: From Bench to Bedside. Harpreet Singh, Arun Kumar Mishra, Jeyabalan Sangeetha, and Devarajan Thangadurai (Eds.)

DOI: 10.1201/9781779640918-3

Pharmaceutical companies should stick to the latest advancements for microbial testing to maintain high quality standards to build trust in the public for the well-being of patients.

2.1 INTRODUCTION

The pharmaceutical market has high standards for quality, safety, and efficacy on quality control (QC) and good manufacturing practices (GMP). In pharmaceutical microbiology, where microbes have reached their effects has to be restricted with strict QC measures and strictly adhere to the GMP guidelines are essential (MacLeod et al., 1969; Conn et al., 1975). This provides an overview of crucial areas in pharmaceutical microbiology, is QC and GMP. It reveals the importance of these topics and their principles along with their relationship between manufacturing standards and testing in the production of pharmaceuticals by pharmaceutical companies (Ukuku et al., 2001; Cross-Smiecinski, 2002; FDA, 2004).

2.2 QUALITY CONTROL IN PHARMACEUTICAL MICROBIOLOGY

Pharmaceutical microbiology revolves around QC, a sophisticated system of checks and balances designed to monitor, evaluate, and maintain the microbiological purity of pharmaceutical products. Pharmaceutical microbiology QC uses cutting-edge testing techniques to comb through the world of microorganisms in order to find even the tiniest contamination remnants. These tests are the protectors for human safety, ensuring that every prescription is free of potentially dangerous microorganisms. They are more than just figures and facts (Taylor, 1987; FDA, 1994, 2002).

2.2.1 MICROBIAL CONTAMINATION CONTROL

Pharmaceutical goods' microbiological quality is affected by a number of variables, including the formulation and environment, raw materials, equipment, atmosphere, personnel using the product, and the end container. The kind of formulation being made dictates the microbiological standard and level of danger of the necessary air supply. For instance, in the case of injectable and ophthalmic medications, the sterility test may miss the accidental contamination of a few containers due to an inadequate air count. UV radiation, chemical disinfection, and filtration can all lower the number of microorganisms in the air. For the majority of aseptic operations, particles larger than 0.1 μm must be removed. However, a standard of fewer than 100 particles of 0.5 μm or bigger per 3.5 l is sufficient for many procedures. The distribution infrastructure and the raw water's quality, together with any necessary processing, are the two key factors at play. There are not as many deep-water sources like springs or wells since the water is filtered away. Any method used to stop growth or ensure life during the pharmaceutical production process—whether it is chemical or in-process should be considered crucial and managed appropriately. Natural sources of raw materials that have not been processed typically harbor a wide variety of microorganisms. For liquid or semi-solid goods, closure liners made of pulpboard or cork are frequently a source of mold contamination unless they are specifically treated with a preservative, foil coating, or wax coating. Procedures for handling samples, including the application of aseptic methods, are recorded. This contains information on the participants, the tools used, and any anomalies found during testing. Pharmaceutical microbiologists make sure that their testing procedures are dependable, accurate, and free from contamination by putting these strict QC methods into place. Adherence to these protocols not only ensures the excellence of pharmaceutical items but also fosters confidence between regulatory bodies and customers.

2.2.2 TESTING AND ANALYSIS

The many types of microbiological tests used for pharmaceuticals include the microbial limit test, sterility test, growth promotion test, bacterial endotoxin test, water microbiological analysis, and microbial identification.

- **Microbial limits test:** It is also known as Bioburden testing. The test counts the total number of microorganisms that are viable. The product's microbiological content comprises the total yeast and mold count, as well as the total bacterial count.
- **Sterility testing:** The test is mainly used to test the sterile products, such as injectables and ophthalmic solutions. It is mainly used to confirm the absence of growth of microorganisms in pharmaceutical products.

- **Bacterial endotoxin test:** Using limulus amoebocyte lysate, the bacterial endotoxin test is used to identify or measure endotoxins. Testing for and managing endotoxins is crucial because they can have major negative consequences on people.
- The growth promotion test evaluates any medium's capacity to promote growth in the presence of a limited number of microorganisms in the inoculum.
- The total viable count is examined for microbiological contamination during water testing.
- Microbial identification can be done by using various tests for *E. coli*, *Salmonella* sp., *Pseudomonas aeruginosa*, and *Staphylococcus aureus*.

2.2.3 DOCUMENTATION AND RECORD KEEPING

Any communicable material used to inform about the characteristics of an object, system, or technique is considered documentation. An integral component of every system for QC and assurance is documentation. It primarily defines the production process, management, and specification for all materials. Regulations often specify how long records have to be maintained. QC laboratories must adhere to these guidelines to guarantee that records are accessible for the pertinent time period. Precise documentation and record-keeping methods are essential in pharmaceutical microbiology to ensure regulatory compliance, maintain product quality, and foster a continuous improvement culture. Pharmaceutical businesses can produce safe and effective treatments that meet the highest quality criteria because accurate and up-to-date data form the basis of their decision-making processes (Commission European, 2004; Welty, 2009; Gallant, 2014).

2.3 QUALITY ASSURANCE IN PHARMACEUTICAL MICROBIOLOGY

A systematic approach to guaranteeing that pharmaceutical items are produced consistently and up to the required standards is known as quality assurance (QA). A variety of processes and actions are included in QA with the goals of avoiding errors, ensuring legal compliance, and maintaining efficacy as well as the safety of pharmaceutical compounds. Ensuring microbiological purity for pharmaceutical commodities and preventing microbial contamination are the primary objectives of QC in the field of microbiology (ICH, 2005; 2008; EMA, 2012).

2.3.1 *REGULATORY COMPLIANCE*

The framework of pharmaceutical microbiology is adherence to GMP regulations, which guarantee the effectiveness, safety, and quality of pharmaceuticals. European Medicines Agency and USFD, national regulatory agencies, as well as other organizations, have set statutory standards and guidelines that pharmaceutical companies are required to abide by. Pharmaceutical companies may guarantee the effectiveness, safety, and quality of their products by closely adhering to certain regulatory requirements. In addition to preserving the reputation of the pharmaceutical sector and fostering patient and healthcare provider confidence, compliance also assures consumer safety (ICH, 2009; Wright, 2012a, 2012b). For a pharmaceutical manufacturing business to operate effectively and sustainably, regulatory compliance is essential.

2.4 GOOD MANUFACTURING PRACTICES

The Twentieth World Health Assembly requested that a group of specialists draft the 1st World Health Organization (WHO) document on GMP, which was regulated in 1967. After being accepted, it was submitted to the 21st World Health Assembly entitled as "Draft standards for good manufacturing practise in the manufacture and quality control of medicines and pharmaceutical specialties."

2.4.1 *OVERARCHING ASSUMPTIONS*

Certified pharmaceutical items should only be produced by licensed producers (those holding a production permit), whose operations are regularly inspected by capable national authorities (marketing authorization). This GMP guide will serve as a standard for evaluating manufacturing permit applications and as a foundation for manufacturing facility inspections. One of the elements of the WHO Certification Scheme regarding the quality of pharmaceutical goods travelling in international trade is the GMP status. It may also be utilized as training material for industry staff in manufacturing, QC, and assurance, as well as government inspectors of pharmaceuticals. The manual can be used for large-scale hospital manufacturing procedures that produce medications in completed dose forms as well as for setting up supplies needed for clinical studies. The recommended methods listed below should be viewed as broad guidelines that can be customized to fit specific requirements. It is important to verify the equivalency of various techniques to QA. The environmental protection and safety concerns for workers involved in manufacturing are not included in this chapter as a whole; these are typically covered by national laws. Furthermore, a newly proposed technique of hazard analysis that covers threats to worker safety and production issues is provided in Annexure 7 of the ICH Q9 guidelines (ICH, 2005). In addition to ensuring worker safety, the company should take the required precautions to avoid polluting the surrounding area. When available, the International Nonproprietary Names for pharmaceutical drugs authorized by the WHO should be used in addition to other recognized names.

2.5 GOOD MANUFACTURING PRACTICES FOR PHARMACEUTICAL PRODUCTS

GMP, a part of QA, ensure that products are produced and regulated to the quality standards required for their intended use and specified by the marketing license. The primary objective of GMP is to lessen the risks associated with pharmaceutical manufacturing. These hazards basically fall into two categories:

- False labeling on containers, for example, can lead to misunderstanding and cross-contamination, especially with unanticipated pollutants. Under GMP, every manufacturing process is thoroughly described, evaluated in the context of experience, and shown to be capable of producing pharmaceutical products that consistently satisfy their requirements and the required caliber; suitable materials, containers, and labels; approved protocols and guidelines; adequate space and facilities; appropriate equipment and services; appropriately qualified and trained personnel; appropriate storage and transportation; enough people, labs, and equipment for in-process controls are among the resources that can be used for validation and qualification. Operators get training on correct operation, and instructions and procedures that are particularly relevant to the provided facilities are provided in straightforward language. The complete history of a batch may be tracked thanks to the understandable and simply available format in which production and delivery data are maintained. Throughout the manufacturing process, manual and/or recording instrument records are kept to show that all processes specified in the established protocols and instructions have been followed and that the product's quantity and quality are as expected. Any notable deviations are meticulously documented and examined. The goods are distributed and stored properly to reduce any potential risks to their quality; any batch of goods may be recalled from sale or supply using the current system; complaints regarding marketed items are reviewed, the reasons for quality issues are looked into, and suitable action is taken regarding the faulty products to stop them from happening again.

- Strict cleanliness and hygiene standards should be followed at every stage of the production process for pharmaceutical products. Sanitation and hygiene cover everything from workers to buildings and machinery, supplies and containers used in production, cleaning and disinfection treatments, and everything else that might contaminate the product. To eliminate all possible sources of contamination, a comprehensive and integrated sanitation and hygiene program has to be put in place.

2.6 QUALIFICATION AND VALIDATION

It is the responsibility of each manufacturer to determine what certification and validation tasks are necessary to demonstrate that the critical components of their specific operation are handled and comply with GMP. A validation master plan should have a comprehensive definition and documentation of all the essential components of a company's certification and validation program. Construction and installation of buildings, utilities, and equipment must follow their design specifications (IQ), function in line with their design specifications (OQ), and be designed in accordance with GMP design qualification requirements. A process must also consistently yield a product that satisfies its predetermined specifications and quality attributes. Written documentation that uses qualification and validation to show these criteria is necessary (process validation or PV, also called performance qualification). All aspects of the business, including significant alterations to structures, machinery, facilities, or processes that might directly or indirectly affect the quality of the product, must be verified and validated. Validation and qualification are continuous processes that should not be disregarded. Following the first rollout, there needs to be an ongoing initiative based on an annual assessment. An agreement to maintain continuous validation status should be included in the relevant business materials, such as the quality manual or validation master plan. It is necessary to identify the individual in charge of carrying out the validation procedure. Validation studies are an essential part of GMP and have to be conducted in compliance with approved requirements. It is necessary to compile the information and draw conclusions into a written report, which must then be presented. The validation results should serve as the basis for developing new processes and procedures. Analytical test methods, cleaning techniques, and automated system validation should all get special attention (Sandle, 2010; Lynn, 2013).

Personnel includes every employee who should get both initial and ongoing training covering pertinent hygiene instructions and the GMP principles that pertain to them. It is necessary to inspire all employees to help set and uphold high standards. In case of personal hygiene, all employees should get a health examination prior to employment and whenever necessary thereafter. Workers doing visual inspections must be required to get regular eye exams. Basic personal hygiene training must be provided to all staff members. No one handling pharmaceutical items, in-process materials, packaging materials, or beginning materials should have obvious lesions that might compromise the product's quality until the condition is determined to be no longer a concern. All staff members should be advised and encouraged to report to their immediate supervisor any occurrences involving individuals, objects, or machinery that they feel might have a detrimental effect on the goods. Starting materials, bulk goods, intermediate products, and large packing materials should not come into touch with the operator's hands directly. Employees should dress in clean, suitable body covers for their jobs, including enough hair covering, to ensure that the product is shielded from contamination. Clothes that may be recycled should be kept separate and locked until they have been washed and, if needed, disinfected. Any area used for production, testing, storage, or any other area where they can have a detrimental effect on the quality of the finished product shall not allow smoking, eating, drinking, chewing, or storing plants, food, drink, smoking materials, or personal drugs. Everyone who enters a manufacturing plant—guests, senior managers, inspectors, contractors, and permanent employees should wear protective gear and practice basic personal hygiene.

2.7 GOOD MANUFACTURING PRACTICES IN PHARMACEUTICAL MICROBIOLOGY

Labs studying pharmaceutical microbiology may work on the following projects: sterility testing; assay adopting microorganisms as part of the test system; detection, isolation, enumeration, and identification of micro-organisms (bacteria, yeast, and molds); testing for bacterial endotoxins in various materials (e.g., starting materials, water), products, surfaces, clothing, and the environment.

2.7.1 PERSONNEL

Only those with a degree in microbiology or its equivalent should be qualified to conduct and oversee microbiological tests. Before being permitted to carry out tasks covered by the testing scope, staff members should possess a foundational understanding of microbiology as well as appropriate practical experience. The management of the laboratory should make sure that all staff members have obtained the necessary training to conduct tests and operate equipment competently. The appropriate protocols for containing germs inside the laboratory setting should be taught to the staff. Employees have to get training on handling germs safely.

2.7.2 ENVIRONMENT

Particularly when it comes to production areas, microbiology labs, and specific support equipment (such as autoclaves and glassware) must be kept apart and designated as separate spaces. The layout of microbiology labs should be planned to accommodate the tasks that will be performed there. Production units and laboratories should have their own air supply. Only authorized workers should have access to the microbiological laboratory. Entry and exit protocols, including gowning, should be followed, as well as the purpose of each location and the rationale behind any work limitations. Appropriate containment levels should also be considered. Cleaning, disinfection, along with hygiene include a written cleaning and disinfection schedule that ought to be in place. When relevant, the outcomes of environmental monitoring should be taken into account. A protocol ought to be established for managing spills. Facilities for completely cleaning and disinfecting hands must be easily available. Validation of test methods includes standardized testing protocols or pharmacopoeia, which are considered validated. Test protocols that are not based on reliable references or compendia ought to be checked before being employed. Determining precision, accuracy, specificity, linearity, robustness, limit of quantitation, limit of detection, and other relevant parameters should all be included in the validation process. It is important to include any possible inhibitory effects resulting from the sample while analyzing different types of samples. Using the statistical techniques outlined in regional, national, or international pharmacopoeias, the results must be assessed. Each piece of equipment, instrument, or other object used for testing, verification, and calibration has to be uniquely identified. As part of its quality system, a laboratory should have a documented program for the certification, calibration, performance verification, maintenance, and a way to monitor how its equipment is being utilized. Verification of performance, calibration, and usage monitoring has an instrument label, should prominently display the date of calibration and service, as well as the upcoming recalibration deadline. Based on the equipment's need, kind, and past performance, documented experience will be used to establish how frequently calibration and performance verification should be done. Reagents and culture media include labs need to make sure that the medium and reagents they employ are of the right quality for the particular test. Each batch of essential reagents for the test should be checked by laboratories both at the beginning and throughout its shelf life. Media can be bought partially or fully prepared, or it can be created internally. Media vendors ought to be certified and approved. Labeling has every reagent needs to be properly labeled with details about its identification, concentration, requirements for storage, date of manufacture, confirmed expiration date, and/or recommended storage durations, if any. Diluents, media, stock solutions, and other suspending fluids fall under this category. In documentation, the planning coordinator should be clearly identified. Revive an organism includes when test procedures could injure cells in a way that is not deadly; organism resuscitation is necessary. Adverse effects associated with processing encompass a variety of situations, including exposure to high or low osmotic pressure, severe pH levels, heat, antimicrobial agents, and preservatives. The following methods can be used to revive an organism: soaking it for two hours in a liquid healing medium (such as a simple room-temperature salt solution); soaking it for four to six hours in a solid healing medium (Wingate, 2014).

2.8 LITERATURE SOURCES AND CULTURAL REFERENCES

Literature sources with cultural references are often followed in microbiological laboratories for equipment qualification, verification, and calibration. These reference resources ought to be used in suitable matrices wherever feasible. For example, pharmacopoeia reference materials and international standards are used to: assess potency or content; verify procedures; allow technique comparisons; carry out growth promotion experiments; and undertake positive controls. Reference materials ought to be utilized in the proper matrices, if at all feasible.

2.9 CONCLUSION

Pharmaceutical firms rely heavily on QC and good manufacturing techniques in pharmaceutical microbiology to manufacture their goods. They preserve the integrity of the pharmaceutical sector, safeguard patients, and enforce industry standards. Consistent adherence to these standards by the pharmaceutical business guarantees not just regulatory compliance but also demonstrates the company's commitment to the global population's well-being. GMP-compliant pharmaceuticals that meet the highest quality requirements primarily concentrate on improving pharmaceutical ingredients that have a significant positive impact on public health and safety.

KEYWORDS

- **microbial contamination**
- **quality control**
- **microbial culture**
- **preventive measures**
- **endotoxin assay**
- **personal hygiene**
- **public health**

REFERENCES

Commission European. (2004). Good manufacturing practice, annex 1: Manufacture of sterile medicinal products. In: *Bruxelles, Bio Contamination Control (ISO 14698)*. International Organization for Standardization: Geneva.

Conn, R. B., Charache, P., Chappelle, E. W. (1975). Limits of applicability of the firefly luminescence ATP assay for the detection of bacteria in clinical specimens. *American Journal of Clinical Pathology, 63(4)*, 493–501.

Cross-Smiecinski, *A. J. (2002)*. Quality assurance. In: Hurst, C. J. (Ed.), *Manual of Environmental Microbiology* (pp. 158–165). ASM: Washington, DC.

Food and Drug Administration. (1994). Guidance for Industry for the Submission Documentation for Sterilization Process Validation in Applications for Human and Veterinary Drug Products. Office of Training and Communication, Division of Drug Information, CDER, FDA. http://www.fda.gov/cder/guidance/cmc2.pdf.

Food and Drug Administration. (August 21, 2002). Pharmaceutical cGMPs for the 21st Century: A Risk-Based Approach. FDA Concept Paper.

Food and Drug Administration. (2004). Guidance for Industry PAT—A Framework for Innovative Pharmaceutical Development, Manufacturing, and Quality Assurance. Office of Training and Communication, Division of Drug Information, CDER, FDA. http://www.fda.gov/cder/guidance/6419fnl.pdf.

Gallant, J. (2014). The road to a culture of quality. *Pharmaceutical Online*.

Guideline on Process Validation, EMA/ CHMP/CVMP/QP/70278, Rev 1, 29 Mar 2012.

ICH Harmonized Tripartite Guideline. (9 Nov 2005). Quality risk management, Q9, current step 4.

ICH Harmonized Tripartite Guideline. (4 June 2008). Pharmaceutical quality system, Q10, current step 4.

ICH Harmonized Tripartite Guideline. (Aug 2009). Pharmaceutical development Q8 (R2), current step 4.

Lynn, S. (2013). *Product Manufacturing and Manufacturing Practices (CGMPs)*. USFDA.

MacLeod, N. H., Chappelle, E. W., Crawford, *A. M. (1969)*. ATP assay of terrestrial soils: A test of an exobiological experiment. *Nature, 223(203), 67–268.*

Sandle, T. (2010). Best practices in microbiology laboratory training. In: Hodges. N., Hanlon, G. (Eds.), *Industrial Pharmaceutical Microbiology: Standards and Controls* (pp. S11.1–S11.16). Euromed: Basingstoke, Supplement 11.

Taylor, *J. K. (1987). Quality Assurance of Chemical Measurements. Lewis Publishers, Inc.: Chelsea, MI, USA.*

Ukuku, *D. O.*, Pilizota, V., Sapers, G. M. (2001). Bioluminescence ATP assay for estimating total plate counts of surface microflora of whole cantaloupe and determining efficacy of washing treatments *Journal of Food Protection, 64(6), 813–819.*

Welty, G. (2009). Developing a continuing CGMP training program. *Journal of GXP Compliance*, *13*(4), 86–96.

Wingate, G. (2014). Moving from quality control to quality assurance. *Pharmaceutical Engineering*, *34*, 2.

Wright, R. (2012a). How to create an innovative culture in a pharma company. *Pharmaceutical Online*.

Wright, R. (2012b). How to take charge of your manufacturing process. *Pharmaceutical Online*.

CHAPTER 3

Microbial Contamination Control in Pharmaceuticals

MOUMITA KUNDU, AYON DUTTA, BIRAJ PATRA, and SHAYERI CHATTERJEE GANGULY*

Department of Pharmaceutical Technology, Brainware University, Barasat, West Bengal, India

*Corresponding author

ABSTRACT

Microbial contamination remains a critical concern in the pharmaceutical industry due to its potential to compromise product quality, patient safety, and regulatory compliance. An overview of the principal strategies used to prevent microbial contamination in pharmaceutical production processes is presented here. It also emphasizes preserving sterile conditions throughout the production cycle and the intricate interactions between manufacturing machinery, personnel, and environmental elements. It explores the numerous preventive measures, such as aseptic techniques, facility design, sterilization procedures, staff training, and sanitation practices, which work together to reduce the risk of microbial contamination. Moreover, this chapter includes the regulatory environment and standards for microbiological contamination control, highlighting the requirement for pharmaceutical industries to follow rigorous standards established by global health organizations. It also discusses the potential implications of microbial contamination occurrences, including product recalls, monetary losses, reputational damage, and, most crucially, impaired patient well-being. The importance of establishing a thorough contamination control approach by detailing these implications has also been explained here.

Advances in Pharmaceutical Microbiology: From Bench to Bedside. Harpreet Singh, Arun Kumar Mishra, Jeyabalan Sangeetha, and Devarajan Thangadurai (Eds.)

DOI: 10.1201/9781779640918-4

The conclusion section highlights the necessity for a comprehensive strategy incorporating technology improvements, strict adherence to regulatory requirements, and a culture of knowledge and accountability among all stakeholders.

3.1 INTRODUCTION

Microbial contamination is a major concern for the pharmaceutical industry as it can threaten patient safety and public health and ultimately affect the reputation of pharmaceutical companies. Despite recent advancements in technology and production techniques, microbiological contamination poses a persistent threat in the pharmaceutical sector. The pharmaceutical industry involves drug production for the treatment, diagnosis, and prevention of various illnesses, rendering it essential to public health. Drug delivery systems, including parenteral, capsules, tablets, and ophthalmic preparations, aim to supply therapeutic ingredients for treating or curing diseases and patient health protection. Therefore, strict adherence to quality, safety, and efficacy guidelines is necessary (Mugoyela et al., 2010). Production and manufacturing of pharmaceuticals is an intricate procedure that may be contaminated by microbes (Patel et al., 2019). Microbial contamination is related to the unforeseen inclusion of viruses, bacteria, fungi, or any other microbes in medicinal products. These contaminations may be introduced during the production process, starting from raw materials to the finished product. It can lead to several adverse effects, including the risk of patient injury, regulatory penalties, and a negative impact on the reputation and sustainability of a pharmaceutical manufacturer's business (Ratajczak et al., 2015).

Deep knowledge about the contamination types and sources is vital to develop effective strategies for prevention and control. Natural pathogens like *Clostridium tetani* microbe cause infection in healthy people and illnesses. Bacterial contamination of pharmaceutical items puts patients' health at risk (Hao et al., 2021; Pollard and Bijker, 2021). Opportunistic pathogens, like *Pseudomonas aeruginosa*, usually do not harm healthy persons. However, their presence in pharmaceutical items may be very dangerous as they can lead to infections in immunocompromised individuals (Moradali et al., 2017; Pachori et al., 2019).

Pharmaceutical microbial contamination can be introduced during the production process via contaminated raw materials, including water, excipients, or active components of pharmaceutical products (Obuekwe and Eichie, 2006; de Santos et al., 2023). Human operators' unintentional introduction of contaminants in pharmaceutical production facilities highlights the importance of maintaining cleanliness and aseptic techniques (Suvikas-Peltonen et al., 2017). The final product may get contaminated if cleanroom conditions are not supported or production equipment is contaminated. Moreover, microorganisms may infect medicinal products during shipping and storage due to improper packaging and storage conditions (Tršan et al., 2019). Microbial contamination in pharmaceuticals can have several consequences, and the severity depends on different factors such as the type and quantity of contaminants, individual susceptibility, and overall patient health (Bonadonna et al., 2017). These effects can be very diverse. In addition, there will be adverse effects on the company and regulation, such as loss of market share, regulatory penalties, product recalls, and reputational harm (Cunningham-Oakes et al., 2019).

The application of strict regulatory control to the pharmaceutical business can ensure the efficacy and safety of pharmaceutical products. Different state and federal regulatory bodies have set tight standards and test procedures to control microbial contamination in medicinal products. Good Manufacturing Practices (GMP) and USP pharmacopoeial standards, microbiological limits testing, validation, and verification are key regulatory aspects (Gouveia et al., 2015). Prevention of microbiological contamination during production is also required to ensure the safety and quality of pharmaceutical products. The first line of defense in keeping low microbial levels in sterile environments is prevention, even with the availability of numerous sterilizing and decontamination techniques (Mohapatra, 2017). Moreover, adherence to GMP rules and regulations, use of aseptic techniques, maintenance of cleanroom design, quality control and testing, sterilizing procedures, raw material control, etc., are essential to prevent microbial contamination (Patel and Chotai, 2011). In spite of advanced technology and production methods, microbial contamination remains a major challenge in the pharmaceutical industry that can lead to a severe impact on patient safety, the business reputation, and regulatory compliance. This chapter discusses different types and sources of microbial contamination, microbial detection methods, preventive measures, regulatory guidelines, and recovery strategies to ensure public health and maintain the trust and reliability of the pharmaceutical industry.

3.2 TYPES AND SOURCES OF MICROBIAL CONTAMINATION

Pharmaceutical products may be of two types: sterile and nonsterile (Ratajczak et al., 2015). Sterile products, such as ophthalmic or parenteral preparations, involve the application to mucosal epithelial tissue, internal organs, or wounded body parts (Sandle, 2016). However, to ensure that nonsterile medications remain safe for consumer use and to stay medicinally active, close observation of microbial contamination is necessary. Several bacteria including *Enterococcus* sp., *Bacillus* sp., *Micrococcus* sp., *Staphylococcus aureus*, *Pseudomonas aeruginosa*, and *Salmonella* sp. and mold fungi like *Mucor* sp., *Aspergillus* sp., *Rhizopus* sp., and *Alternaria* sp. are the most common microbial contaminations observed in nonsterile drugs (Ratajczak et al., 2015). Microbes may be introduced in drugs during the manufacturing process, shipping, or patient use (Zeitoun et al., 2015). Contamination can arise from the following causes in large, medium, and small-scale pharmaceutical manufacturing.

3.2.1 WATER

The most frequently revealed type of microbial contamination of medicinal preparations is Gram-positive bacterial contamination resulting from human involvement. In contrast, pharmaceutical products have been comparatively less contaminated by Gram-negative bacteria. Common waterborne microorganisms such as *Pseudomonas*, *Achromo*, and Gram-negative bacteria can contaminate portable and filtered water (Jimenez, 2004). Water sources can affect ion exchange columns, and microorganisms may flourish there, contaminating sterilized water. If the osmosis membrane is not adequately cleaned, water that has been cleansed via reverse osmosis may also be polluted. If distilled water is kept at room temperature for a few days, it could become polluted (Roy et al., 2023).

3.2.2 RAW MATERIALS

Several components, like soil and clay minerals, which are widely employed in pharmaceutical products, are susceptible to anaerobic spores (*Clostridium* sp.) (Jimenez, 2004). Raw materials produced by microbial fermentation, chemical reaction, natural resources extraction, and recombinant DNA technology can be easily contaminated with microbes. Most pharmaceutical raw materials support different types of microbial proliferation based on their moisture content and nutritional attributes. Several herbal medicinal preparations containing natural components make the products far more vulnerable to contamination by Gram-negative bacteria, as performing an antimicrobial before treatment is unfeasible. Studies reported that numerous commercially accessible herbal dosages (pills, powders, tablets, and capsules) are tainted with *Escherichia coli* and other Gram-negative bacteria. For example, several pathogenic bacteria, *E. coli*, *Streptococcus* sp., *Erwinia* sp., *Lactobacillus* sp., *Pseudomonas* sp., *Bacillus* sp., and actinomycetes may be present in natural excipients (starch, tragacanth, gum acacia, powdered rhubarb, and agar). Moreover, animal-derived products may contain *Salmonella* sp. and *E. coli* (Ratajczak et al., 2015). Furthermore, crops used to produce herbal items may inadvertently get tainted by partially decaying organic fertilizers or bovine feces containing bacteria from the Enterobacteriaceae family, including *E. coli* (Ratajczak et al., 2015). Many of the raw materials used in herbal preparations have *Aspergillus flavus*, a fungus producing potentially toxic aflatoxin B, resulting in the probability of elevated aflatoxin contamination in unprocessed herbal materials (Benkerroum, 2020).

3.2.3 MANUFACTURING PERSONNEL, EQUIPMENT, AND ENVIRONMENT

Coliform bacteria, staphylococci, streptococci, actinobacteria, candida infections, and significant microbial contamination in pharmaceutical products may infect pharmaceutical workers. Improved health examinations, immunizations, and staff cleanliness can reduce this kind of contamination. Wearing protective gear and providing staff with adequate training can help reduce contamination (Roy et al., 2023).

Such Gram-negative bacterial contamination may be triggered by improper preparation methods and tainted/nonsterile supplies and equipment (Zeitoun et al., 2015). In the air, billions of suspended particles and microorganisms (fungal spores such as penicillium, mucor, aspergillus, and bacterial spores, such as *Bacillus* sp.) may contaminate pharmaceutical products. The practice of production in aseptic and clean rooms having a constant flow of sterile air through a high-efficiency particulate air (HEPA) filter minimizes this kind of contamination (Brągoszewska and Biedroń, 2021).

3.2.4 STORAGE PARAMETERS

In moisture-prone environments, the condensed water films may accumulate on the surface of dry pharmaceuticals (pills or bulk oils) to promote fungal growth (Dedesko and Siegel, 2015). Contrary to their intended function of shielding the formulation from microorganisms, preservatives can also act as additional sources of microbial contamination attributed to their nutritional features and aromatic characteristics at low concentrations (McDonnell and Russell, 1999). The pH of pharmaceutical preparation may vary and shift dramatically depending on basic or acidic metabolites released by microorganisms that initiate a secondary attack previously inhibited by the product's initial pH. For example, syrups having fruit juice flavors (low pH levels 3–4) are particularly vulnerable to yeast or mold growth. Since yeasts can encourage the growth of secondary bacteria by elevating pH through metabolizing organic acids. Conversely, microbes rarely ruin soap-based emulsions since their pH exceeds 8 (Sanchez and Demain, 2008). Studies in Nepal (taking 15 nonsterile multivitamins and cough syrups individually) reported comparatively less (86.67%) microbial contaminations in 13 multivitamins than 14 cough syrups (93.3%), probably attributed to the presence of antioxidants and minerals in multivitamin syrups (Gurung and Rai, 2021). Further, Hefny et al. (2022) demonstrated 79.17% and 12.78% of nonsterile pharmaceutical drops had lower ($10–10^2$ cfu/ml) bacterial and fungal populations, respectively, among 360 samples (Hefny et al., 2022). Recent Food and Drug Administration (FDA) rejected pharmaceutical preparations are listed in Table 3.1.

TABLE 3.1 Recently Recalling Pharmaceutical Preparations by the FDA

Brand Name	Drug	Identified Pathogen	Probable Risk	Date of Recalling
CVS Health Magnesium Citrate, Saline Laxative Oral Solution, Lemon Flavor	Magnesium citrate	*Gluconacetobacter liquefaciens*	Fatal to immuno-compromised patients	June 22, 2022
Allergy Bee Gone®	Ascorbic acid+Honey	*Bacillus cereus*	Pneumonia, fungal rhinosinusitis, and sepsis	July 6, 2022
Snore Stop®	*Nux vomica*, *Belladonna*, *Ephedra vulgaris*, *Hydrastis canadensis*, *Kali bichromicum*	*Providencia rettgeri*	Pneumonia, fungal rhinosinusitis, and sepsis	June 9, 2022
SyrSpend®	Oral liquid-suspending vehicles comprising food starch	*Burkholderia gladioli*	Respiratory disorders, cystic fibrosis	May 2, 2022
Taro-clobetasol	Clobetasol-propionate	*Ralstonia pickettii*	Pneumonia, meningitis, sepsis, bone marrow inflammation, joint fluid, and tissue infections	December 30, 2021

3.3 REGULATORY GUIDELINES AND DISINFECTION PROTOCOLS

The documented procedure confirming the consistent and effective cleanliness of equipment, known as pharma production equipment validation, is crucial to prevent cross-contamination and adulteration of medications (Chen, 2019; Sharma et al., 2018). Several national and international bodies such as American Society for Testing and Materials, Active Pharmaceutical Ingredients (APIs) Committee, International Society for Pharmaceutical Engineering, Parents' Drug Association, Health Canada, European Medicines Agency (EMA), Administration for Therapeutic Goods and Services, Pharmaceutical Inspection Co-operation Scheme,

World Health Organization, and US FDA develop and execute standards protocols for operating, cleaning, validating equipment and finally manufacturing and storing pharmaceuticals (Abinash, 2022).

The American Society for Testing and Materials, an international standards body, establishes and disseminates technical standardized frameworks, including cleaning, manufacturing, and quality control testing for pharmaceutical products (Bunn, 2019). The International Pharmaceutical Excipients Council group, popularly known as the APIs group, is responsible for monitoring the quality and safety of APIs through their utility advancement in the pharmaceutical business. The international standard body develops standards and guidelines for cleaning validation criteria, manufacturing, and quality control of API (Wadher, 2017; Abinash, 2022). The International Society for Pharmaceutical Engineering, a global nonprofit organization, provides services to the pharmaceutical and bio-pharmaceutical industries through instruction, training, and the creation of best practices and guidelines regarding production facilities, equipment, and systems, cleaning validation for operational and technical promotion of pharmaceutical industry (Kumar et al., 2011; Abinash, 2022). The Parenteral Drug Association represents the interests of the pharmaceutics and biopharmaceutical businesses to promote the field of pharmaceutical manufacturing science, explicitly concentrating on parenteral (injectable) products via offering industry norms and educational materials, including cleaning validation guidelines, risk assessment, approval criteria, and the creation of cleaning validation methodologies (Raposo and Barceló, 2021; Abinash, 2022). Health Canada, a national regulatory agency, is responsible for the safety and effectiveness of health products in Canada by providing guidelines for cleaning validation (including evaluation of cleaning requirements, a suitable choice of cleaning agents with definite methods and their effectiveness) in the pharmaceutical industry and inspecting to assuring the development of contamination-free pharmaceuticals. The Administration for Therapeutic Goods and Services, a national regulatory agency in Australia, provides safety guidelines (including cleaning validation and manufacturing process, fundamentals of acceptance parameters employing analytical techniques), maintains therapeutic efficiency of pharmaceuticals, and inspects to assess parameters to ensure the development of contaminant-free medications. Moreover, the Pharmaceutical Inspection Co-operation Scheme monitors the cross-contamination process of pharmaceuticals. EMA also demonstrated similar cleaning guidelines for validation and disinfection (Abinash, 2022).

The pharmaceutical manufacturing industries must follow several rules and criteria (Table 3.2) by the US FDA to ensure that the cleaning validation procedure is conducted correctly (Sharma et al., 2018).

TABLE 3.2 USFDA Guidelines for the Pharmaceutical Industry

Guidelines	Regulations
Current Good Manufacturing Practice	General specifications for the production, examination, and quality assurance of pharmaceuticals
	Specific criteria for cleaning validation, like the demand for written cleaning validation protocols, the application of suitable cleaning agents and techniques, and the documentation and maintenance of cleaning validation activity records
Guidance for Industry: Sterile Drug Products Produced by Aseptic Processing	Design and facilities of an aseptic area to prepare sterile products
	The cleaning validation process, including risk evaluation, a suitable cleaning agent, and method identification
Guidance for Industry: Inspection of Pharmaceutical Quality Control Laboratories	Information regarding inspection for quality control in pharmaceutical laboratories and the cleaning validation process
Guidance for Industry: Inspection of Manufacturing Plants	Information regarding inspection of manufacturing premises with cleaning validation protocols

3.4 FACILITY DESIGN, ENVIRONMENTAL CONTROL, AND PERSONNEL TRAINING

Proper environmental management is very crucial in the pharmaceutical field. Keeping the air pressure in aseptic rooms higher than in nearby controlled areas is essential. Reaching the designated clean room class can be governed by accurate air filtration and calibration. A unidirectional laminar airflow capable of sweeping particles away from filling/closing zones is necessary to protect essential areas during operations (Xu, 2014). In addition to air quality, suitable ranges for ambient temperature and humidity must be maintained. Specialized systems such as ventilated cabinets, restricted access barrier systems (RABS), and isolators may be used, contingent on risk evaluations, to provide complete or partial barriers against microorganisms. When dividing spaces with different risk levels, door barriers and ultraviolet airlocks should be used. It is also essential to carry out open-container processing operations for sterile items inside RABS or isolators (Gola et al., 2021). The changing room's air pressure design should be pessimistic regarding the corridor leading to the manufacturing area but optimistic regarding the adjacent outdoor regions. Impermeable walls prevent cross-contamination between zones, and ventilation components and services accessible from outside manufacturing areas are strategically positioned to enable maintenance (Xu and Zhou, 2017). Heating, ventilation, and air conditioning must be placed and constructed properly to prevent the spread of pollutants inside the space. The strict quality requirements maintained in aseptic procedures result from routinely checking rooms and surfaces for viable and nonviable particles and semiannual facility recertification (Wilson et al., 2006).

The inside surfaces of pharmaceutical facilities, such as the walls, ceilings, and floors, are given special consideration when it comes to architectural regulations. These surfaces must be flawless and crack-free to simplify cleaning procedures. Integral for observation, windows and viewing panels are made nonopening, flat with wall panels, and tightly sealed to remove dust and microbiological debris. Pipework, ventilation, and light fixtures are all thoughtfully designed to eliminate crevices that could be difficult to clean. Sinks in industrial areas are made of stainless steel, emphasizing hygienic design and longevity (National Research Council, 2011). The domain of sanitation and decontamination holds significant importance in upholding pharmaceutical production guidelines. It is essential to clean frequently and disinfect when needed. Every aspect of the production of pharmaceutical products is devoted to strict cleaning and hygienic practices. When designing the cleaning process, careful consideration is given to the chemical composition, mechanical action, temperature, contact time, application, and application to minimize health concerns. Cleaning materials are kept away from the product to protect product integrity. Validating cleaning procedures becomes essential since it shows how well they control microbiological contamination (Rutala and Weber, 2015).

In the context of utilities, water used in the production of pharmaceutical products must be suitable for the intended purpose, microbiologically controlled, and monitored. Steam is a multipurpose tool that must be additive-free and clean for cleaning, disinfecting manufacturing tools and equipment, autoclave supply, and humidification. This all-encompassing strategy for utilities, cleaning, and building design highlights the dedication to upholding strict pharmaceutical quality requirements (Miguel et al., 2022).

Adherence to GMP criteria in pharmaceutical firms necessitates effectively training workers. Personnel in manufacturing, quality control, and laboratories must get extensive training covering regulatory GMP standards, aseptic processes, safety protocols, hygiene, microbiology, and job-specific abilities (Patel and Chotai, 2011). Specifically, introductory microbiology activities aim to inform staff members about the possible risks that microbes may bring to patients and merchandise. However, a significant upgrade to training approaches is required due to the increasing focus on contamination management. Guidance on remedial steps for risk mitigation should be included with specific instructions on assessing contamination risks associated with different actions and conditions. Because of low regulation and hygiene requirements, workers with access to pharmaceutical manufacturing, packing, and transportation are considered important sources of contamination (National Research Council (US) Subcommittee on Microbiological Criteria, 1985).

Strict training regimens that emphasize hygiene standards must be implemented for all employees directly involved in the manufacturing and handling of products to address this problem. It becomes essential to standardize the usage of personal protective equipment (PPE) in production units, such as face masks, hair caps, overshoes, and hand gloves (Verbeek et al., 2020). It is critical to stress the importance of maintaining excellent personal hygiene among employees. Strict attention to appropriate and legally required clothing washing and disinfection procedures is also crucial. Careful attention to detail is necessary to avoid workers' hands from coming into close contact with any aspect of the product. Controlling access to production areas also helps significantly with contamination control efforts by guaranteeing that only workers with the necessary training can enter the manufacturing unit (National Research Council, 2011).

3.5 ASEPTIC TECHNIQUES AND EQUIPMENT DESIGN AND MAINTENANCE

3.5.1 ASEPTIC TECHNIQUES

Aseptic techniques are critical in the pharmaceutical industry to prevent microbial contamination while manufacturing, processing, and handling pharmaceutical products. Aseptic processing is the processing and packaging of a commercially sterile product into sterilized containers. Aseptic processing includes compounding, filtration, and filling. The contamination control strategy should focus on protecting the product from a microbial contamination event at the point of most significant risk. Some fundamental aseptic techniques commonly used are as follows (Bykowski and Stevenson, 2008, 2020):

1. Clean rooms are controlled areas with minimal surface and air contamination
2. Protective clothing such as PPE
3. Visual inspection
4. Cleaning and sanitization
5. Procedural manipulation
6. Disposal and cleanup
7. Sterile instruments
8. Sterile draping
9. Gloved "no touch" technique

Other aseptic techniques include:

1. Respiratory hygiene and cough etiquette
2. Safe use of sharps
3. Environmental cleaning
4. Reprocessing of medical equipment
5. Appropriate handling of linen and waste management
6. Testing the laminar-airflow workbench for leaks, airflow velocity, and airflow patterns
7. Sealing ceilings to prevent the entry of microbial contaminants

Standard tests for microbial contamination include enzyme-linked immunosorbent assay (ELISA), real-time polymerase chain reaction (PCR) tests, nutrient plates, and agar plates.

3.5.2 EQUIPMENT DESIGN AND MAINTENANCE

3.5.2.1 MATERIALS SELECTION

Using stainless steel or other corrosion-resistant materials for equipment and piping minimizes contamination risk, and implementing a rigorous maintenance schedule for equipment ensures proper functioning and cleanliness. Smooth surfaces in equipment design facilitate easy cleaning and prevent microbial build-up (Staat and Beakley, 1968). HEPA filters and air handling systems control airborne contaminants in pharmaceutical facilities. Regular validation of cleaning procedures and processes leads to effective microbial contamination control. Selecting appropriate gasket materials resistant to degradation and microbial growth is essential. Equipment with minimal dead legs or cracks is designed so that microbes cannot accumulate.

3.5.2.2 EQUIPMENT VALIDATION

Regular cleaning and maintenance of equipment are crucial for managing contamination in pharmaceuticals. Designing the equipment with surfaces with easy-to-clean features is essential to prevent microbes' build-up. Equipment validation involves testing to ensure that the equipment consistently delivers results that meet requirements. This validation process includes installation qualification, operational qualification, and performance qualification to guarantee the reliability and effectiveness of the equipment in controlling contamination (Griffith, 2016). The critical equipment in the process involves:

1. Cleanrooms: Aseptic processing facilities contain clean rooms with regulated air supply and equipment.
2. Equipment: Equipment should have smooth surfaces that facilitate cleaning.
3. Design of cleanroom: Its components should in no way aid in contamination by shedding particles or by outgassing.
4. Laminar airflow tops: Horizontal hoods or tops are able to reduce major contamination that can come from personnel.

3.5.2.3 PREVENTIVE CARE

Inspections and thorough cleaning of the equipment are done to ensure its intactness. This process is done by adherence to the manufacturer-recommended maintenance schedules and procedures. A maintenance program is established to address issues before they escalate into problems. Training is provided to staff members on cleaning and maintenance practices for the equipment, and these are recorded for reference to monitor the performance of the equipment.

3.6 MICROBIAL DETECTION METHODS

3.6.1 PLATE COUNT AGAR

This method depends on culture to assess the presence of contaminants in pharmaceutical products by utilizing agar media, which helps in microbial growth found in a sample. The number of colonies that develop on the agar plate after incubation is counted, making it possible to assess the microbial load in the sample. This method is widely employed for quantifying bacteria. Fungi are also present in pharmaceuticals. The significance of this method lies in safeguarding that pharmaceutical products follow the quality standards and remain free from microbial contamination (Elbing and Brent, 2019).

3.6.2 SABOURAUD DEXTROSE AGAR

It serves as a medium that accelerates the growth of fungi while preventing the growth of bacteria. In pharmaceuticals, this is widely utilized to isolate and determine yeast and molds, which are found in products, materials, and environments. When colonies appear on the plates, it shows the presence of contamination. Further tests can then be employed to detect and characterize these contaminants. This method plays a role in confirming the safety and quality of products as it helps to categorize potential sources of contamination (Odds, 1991).

3.6.3 MEMBRANE FILTRATION

This technique is employed in the pharmaceutical industry to detect the presence of microbes. The process involves passing the sample through a membrane filter, which traps the microorganisms, present in the sample. These captured microorganisms can then be separated and studied to determine the extent of contamination present. Membrane filtration finds applications in raw materials and finished pharmaceutical products in testing water to control microbial contamination (McKinnon and Avis, 1993).

3.6.4 RAPID MICROBIAL METHODS

Adenosine triphosphate (ATP) bioluminescence technique: It detects the light emitted when ATP, which is present in all living beings, interacts with an enzyme, namely, luciferase. This reaction is like the one observed in fireflies. As ATP serves as an indicator of activity, this method is applied to estimate cleanliness and the presence of microbial contaminants on the surfaces. This technique assesses the microbial load qualitatively, including viable and nonviable microorganisms, on the surface of a sample (Datar et al., 2021).

3.6.5 POLYMERASE CHAIN REACTION

PCR is a method that is used to identify pathogens, detect the quantification of microbial load, and separate strains; PCR, thus, is another essential method for investigating the presence of microorganisms. It comprises clinical diagnostics, food and pharmaceutical safety, environmental monitoring, along with forensic microbiology. Antibiotic resistance genes are found with this reaction, which contributes to epidemiological studies. Even with its strength, rigorous experimental planning and quality assurance are necessary; innovations like real-time PCR increase the sensitivity of microbiological detection (Waters and Shapter, 2014).

3.6.6 FLOW CYTOMETRY

This method examines particles in a liquid sample when they move through a laser beam. It detects the fluorescent light, which helps identify and count cells or particles. It also aids in counting and analyzing cells in the liquid sample with respect to cell size, texture, and fluorescence characteristics (Botes et al., 2013; Manohar et al., 2021).

3.6.7 IMMUNOLOGICAL METHODS

ELISA is mainly used in immunology which works on the interaction between antibodies and antigens. It is used to identify the presence of an antigen by employing an enzyme-linked antibody. ELISA can be implemented in determining the presence of antigens or antibodies within a given sample. It is extensively used for diagnosing diseases, detecting toxins, and detecting the points of contamination, due to microbes (Tabatabaei and Ahmed, 2022).

3.6.8 FLUORESCENT ANTIBODY TECHNIQUES

This technique utilizes dyes or markers that are associated with antibodies. When these antibodies attach to antigens, fluorescence can be observed through a microscope or flow cytometry. This method visualizes and distinguishes cells or specific elements within them. It is beneficial in identifying pathogens in samples and evaluating the extent of microbial contamination (Odell and Cook, 2013).

3.7 RISK ASSESSMENT, IMPLICATIONS, AND CONSEQUENCES

3.7.1 PRINCIPLES FOR THE RISK ASSESSMENT FROM THE MICROBIOLOGICALLY CONTAMINATED BATCH

Several fundamental components for such an analysis should be considered when evaluating the risk of infection from a pharmaceutical batch that has been microbiologically contaminated with an unfavorable microbe that has not been found in quality control testing:

The Poisson distribution is generally followed by microbial contamination (Jimenez, 2007; Gapp and Holzknecht, 2011). This trend influences the detectability of quality control tests and the microbial distribution in the final dosage forms.

Regarding product faults, the risk considers qualitative features (Oxborrow et al., 1974) (such as go/not-to-go, pass/fail, or, more appropriately, noncontaminated/contaminated).

The evaluation covers two product categories with binary results: sterile medication (sterile/not sterile) and nonsterile dosage forms, the microbiological components of which can be nonobjectionable/objectionable or nonpathogenic/pathogenic. A numerical count with an acceptability cut-off value, such as 100 CFU/g or mL of the tested product, is also used to test nonsterile products for bioburden contents.

The detectability of quality control tests and the type of product contamination are the three elements of this risk assessment. Product kind, delivery method, and contaminant type—also known as the severity term-determine the form of contamination. The number of noxious microorganisms or contamination per manufacturing batch is the second factor determining the contamination type (Oxborrow et al.,1974; Cassells, 1997).

The following method can be used to determine the risk probability index (P_{ri}):P_{ri} (Risk probability index) equals P_{det} (probability of detecting defects). [(Σ P_{inf})/*N*]...eq. 1, where *N* is the batch size, P_{inf} (*P*robability of infection) is the probability of infection for a particular microorganism from a single unit of the batch. P_{det} is the probability of passing the test (either for the pathogen in nonsterile products or sterility for sterile manufacturing), which translates to "the probability of missing contamination units from the manufactured lot."

A particular dose-response model of infection is chosen for a specific microorganism that can be employed as an indicator microbe based on the product type and the manner of delivery. In the present investigation, for instance, the injectable product-related septicemia can be treated using the Pseudomonas aeruginosa dose-response model of infection (Chandrasekaran and Jiang, 2019; Rodríguez-Gascón et al., 2021)

The term for detectability is P_{det}, and the combination of severity and frequency terms, representing the counterparts of the traditional known risk ranking equation, is (Σ P_{inf})/*N*. Severity × Frequency × Detectability equals the risk prioritization number (RPN). The upcoming sections (Ouédraogo et al., 2011; Park et al., 2018) will analyze the equation's two components.

3.7.2 MICROBIOLOGICALLY DEFECTIVE SAMPLES' DETECTABILITY (PDET)

Instead of uniform distribution, microbial contamination exhibits a Poisson-type distribution, a unique binomial distribution (Hazlett et al., 1978). A count of a characteristic (such as flaws) over a constant observation space is described by the Poisson distribution (Tim Sandle, 2016). Because the present quality control techniques are destructive, only a few samples are employed for testing, which is one of their limitations. As a result, there is little chance that tainted batches will be found through sterility testing utilizing 20 units out of a batch of, say, 50,000 units. This formula can be used to determine the probability (P_{det}) of finding flaws in a batch:

$$\text{With } e = 2.7182818,\ P_{det} = 1-(e-\lambda)n \qquad (3.1)$$

When a quality control test, such as the sterility test, is passed without any failures found, the likelihood is expressed as $(e-\lambda)n$. λ is the relationship between the sample size and the test sensitivity at various values for various contamination rates.

As Sutton showed, the following percentages of contaminated units/probabilities of failing the sterility test will apply to the current sample size ($N = 20$ units): 0.1%/0.02, 0.5%/0.1, 1%/0.2, 5%/0.6, 10%/0.9, and 50%/1 (Deutschmann et al., 2023). This means the likelihood of finding a faulty microbiological attribute reduces as the number of contaminated units in a batch drops. As such, improved detectability is not much impacted by larger sample sizes. It is noteworthy, nonetheless, that the influence of sample size starts to significantly improve the test's sensitivity at the rate of contamination (λ) = 5%. The main problem is a lower probability of detecting defects when the product's microbiological quality improves. The main problem is less probability of detecting defects when the product's microbiological quality improves. The impact of doubling the sample size at different lambda values is presented. When the defect rate is 2%, the impact of a larger sample size is more noticeable.

3.7.3 RISK ANALYSIS AND IMPLICATIONS

The risks were analyzed once the nonconformities (NCs) were found and categorized based on cGMP infractions. Following the risk assessment, an Ishikawa diagram was used to conduct a cause-and-effect analysis. An Ishikawa diagram's six categories—mother nature, labor, machinery, materials, measurements, and methods—were used to group the NCs discovered in warning letters and nonconformity reports (NCRs). This classification maps the root cause of NC and subsequently understands its effect, microbial contamination. This mapping must be done for every type of organism, disinfectant, and coupon (for surface tests only). The combination tested must show that the medium can support the growth of any viable organism. Risk identification is the step in the Quality Risk Management (QRM) process that presents the biggest obstacle. The following steps are typically successful after the risks associated with a process are fully recognized, mapped out, and understood in terms of causation. EMA and the FDA's NCRs were consulted as trustworthy sources of information for this work (Lira et al., 2017; Aust and Pons, 2021). The Ishikawa diagram is shown in Figure 3.1.

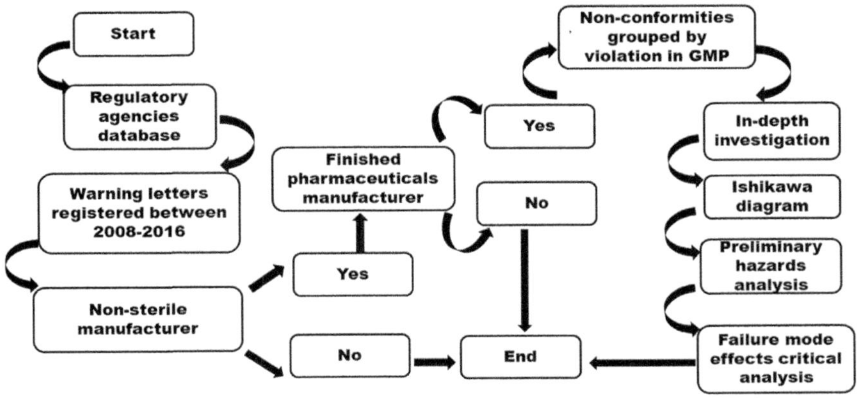

FIGURE 3.1 Ishikawa diagram.

3.8 STRATEGIES FOR RECOVERY AND IMPROVEMENT

Defining methods to manage the risks is crucial once they have been recognized and assessed. Several tactics can be used to mitigate, transfer, accept, or avoid the classified high risks. Following ICH Q9, the risk's significance should determine how much work and attention are put into risk control. Including benefit–cost analysis in the risk strategy is recommended (Charoo and Ali, 2013). The risk acceptance for microbiological contaminations is relatively low because of the potentially significant effects on patient health and drug product quality. To evaluate nonsterile medication goods' quality and specify the hazards that are tolerable, the maker should carry out a thorough and careful risk assessment process that is tailored to their specific situation and takes into account elements like (Charoo and Ali, 2013) the drug's intended use product, such as the administration method and dose form (Guilfoyle et al., 2013); the kind and characteristics of the microorganisms causing the contamination (Burgalassi et al., 2021); the product features, including formulation and makeup; and (Greenberg and Lowrie, 2009) how the therapeutic product might affect the population that receives it (Burgalassi et al., 2021; Guilfoyle et al., 2013).

Given that multiple NCs may have the same risk ranking index or RPN but differ in terms of severity, occurrence, and detection, as well as in terms of acceptability, it is wise to examine each NC separately (Greenberg and Lowrie, 2009). The most significant NCs were process control, quality agreements, deviation investigation, and personal training. The results of this study indicate that strong quality cultures must be established in organizations and that quality systems play a critical role in efficient microbial control strategies. Most NCs found in warning letters from the FDA and NCRs from the EMA are related to labor and materials, so the first preventive action that needs to be implemented is regular and more efficient training and awareness for staff members, along with more efficient methods of conducting documentation reviews (Santos et al., 2018).

A microbial control program must incorporate sanitation and disinfection techniques. Manufacturing environments for pharmaceutical goods are susceptible to microbiological contamination; hence, measures to maintain the microbial quality of the environment must be taken. Removing trash and particles containing microbial cells is possible using physical cleaning methods. Inactivating potentially harmful bacteria in the background, chemical sanitizers and disinfectants lessen microbial contamination. Sporazines, disinfectants, and sanitizers are chemical substances that kill bacteria through classification. Some essential variables to consider while selecting a disinfectant are compatibility of surfaces with disinfectants; operator safety; necessity for residual antimicrobial activity; population and types of microbial contaminants that need to be eliminated; chemical quality, sterility, and stability; disinfectant's cleaning ability; vendor support; cost and availability; and regulations. Rotating disinfectants is a typical practice in the pharmaceutical business and is required by law as a proactive measure to eradicate a wide range of bacteria that may be present in a facility. It is mentioned in another source (Tropea, 2022) that many types of disinfectants should be utilized while using them. Consistent monitoring is necessary to identify the emergence of resistant strains.

In situ testing is conducted to ascertain whether the cleaning and disinfection processes are effective. These investigations are usually performed by monitoring the manufacturing facilities over many days, both before and after routine cleaning. Because in situ studies provide real-world findings from the appropriate usage and application procedures of the chemical agents and personnel practices, they offer value to the overall cleaning/disinfection effectiveness assessment. When it comes to *in vitro* testing, all of the procedures are conducted in a laboratory because the test methods require testing the chemical agents on living cultures. Chemical cleaning is necessary before using pharmaceutical manufacturing equipment that cannot be autoclaved or steam-in-place cleaned using oxidizing, caustic, and acidic agents such as sodium hypochlorite solutions and hydrogen peroxide; chemical sanitization can be achieved. Neutralization and microbiological recovery investigations must be included in the study protocol as test controls to guarantee the validity of the findings derived from *in vitro* disinfectant qualification tests. The capacity of the medium to support the development of any live organism must be demonstrated by neutralization experiments for every type of organism, disinfectant, and a coupon for surface test—only combination examined (Shintani, 2015).

3.9 FUTURE TRENDS AND CONCLUSION

By using an Ishikawa diagram and its six categories, it was possible to determine the likely causes of the most common NCs. These QRM tools improved our understanding of the nature of noted NCs. In conclusion, producers of nonsterile pharmaceuticals ought to pay close attention to the quality agreements, mainly when acting on behalf of other parties. The quality agreements must be explicit and detailed regarding the microbiological control tactics each party is expected to implement. The prevention of microbiological contaminations depends heavily on carefully planning facilities and processes and stringent daily operating procedures. Enforcing microbiological contamination controls just through finished product testing is insufficient. Pharmaceutical businesses should review their microbial ecology, manufacturing methods, unique circumstances, and dosage form characteristics, among other things, using the data collected in such studies to enhance their understanding of particular microbiological dangers. By applying science-based techniques to risk management and enforcing a quality culture that inherently lowers risk behaviors and attitudes, an industry that is better and more resilient in decreasing risks of microbial contamination would result.

With ongoing technological breakthroughs, strict regulatory requirements, and an increasing focus on quality assurance, the prospects for microbial contamination control in the pharmaceutical business seem bright. Innovative techniques like fast microbial detection techniques, state-of-the-art cleanroom technologies, and data analytics for real-time monitoring are anticipated to become increasingly popular as pharmaceutical businesses work to fulfil ever-tougher regulations. Furthermore, by incorporating artificial intelligence and machine learning into quality control procedures, the sector may be able to identify and stop microbiological contamination even better. These advancements demonstrate a dedication to patient safety and improve pharmaceutical manufacturing's general effectiveness. Ultimately, the way microbiological contamination management is being developed in the pharmaceutical industry shows that this industry is committed to upholding the highest standards of product quality and responding proactively to new difficulties. The prospect for microbial contamination management is constant improvement and increased efficacy as long as the sector keeps adopting cutting-edge technologies and sharpening its regulatory frameworks. In addition to satisfying the strict requirements of the present, this guarantees that pharmaceutical goods will also be able to predict and handle the changing complexity of the future healthcare environment.

KEYWORDS

- **microbial contamination**
- **regulatory compliance**
- **aseptic techniques**
- **environmental elements**
- **patient well-being**

REFERENCES

Abinash, P. (2022). A brief review on cleaning validation-regulatory guidelines for pharmaceuticals. *Journal of Pharmaceutical Negative Results, 13*(8), 4795–4799.

Aust, J., Pons, D. (2021). Methodology for evaluating risk of visual inspection tasks of aircraft engine blades. *Aerospace, 8*(4), 117.

Benkerroum. (2020). Aflatoxins: Producing-molds, structure, health issues and incidence in Southeast Asian and Sub-Saharan African countries. *International Journal of Environmental Research and Public Health, 17*(4), 1215.

Bonadonna, L., Briancesco, R., Coccia, A. M. (2017). *Analysis of Microorganisms in Hospital Environments and Potential Risks* (pp. 53–62). doi: 10.1007/978-3-319-49160-8_5

Botes, M., de Kwaadsteniet, M., Cloete, T. E. (2013). Application of quantitative PCR for the detection of microorganisms in water. *Analytical and Bioanalytical Chemistry, 405*(1), 91–108.

Brągoszewska, E., Biedroń, I. (2021). Efficiency of air purifiers at removing air pollutants in educational facilities: A preliminary study. *Frontiers in Environmental Science*, *9*, 709–718.

Bunn, G. P. (Ed.). (2019). *Good Manufacturing Practices for Pharmaceuticals*. CRC Press.

Burgalassi, S., Ceccanti, S., Vecchiani, S., Leonangeli, G., Federigi, I., Carducci, A., Verani, M. (2021). Objectionable microorganisms in pharmaceutical production: Validation of a decision tree. *European Journal of Pharmaceutical Sciences*, *166*, 105984.

Bykowski, T., Stevenson, B. (2008). Aseptic technique. *Current Protocols in Microbiology*, *11*(1), e98.

Bykowski, T., Stevenson, B. (2020). Aseptic technique. *Current Protocols in Microbiology*, *56*(1), e98.

Cassells, A. C. (1997). *Pathogen and Microbial Contamination Management in Micropropagation—An Overview* (pp. 1–13). Springer Nature.

Chandrasekaran, S., Jiang, S. C. (2019). A dose response model for quantifying the infection risk of antibiotic-resistant bacteria. *Scientific Reports*, *9*(1), 17093.

Charoo, N. A., Ali, A. A. (2013). Quality risk management in pharmaceutical development. *Drug Development and Industrial Pharmacy*, *39*(7), 947–960.

Chen, Y.-L. (2019). Two-level process validation approach for medical devices. *Journal of Medical Engineering & Technology*, *43*(2), 139–149.

Cunningham-Oakes, E., Weiser, R., Pointon, T., Mahenthiralingam, E. (2019). Understanding the challenges of non-food industrial product contamination. *FEMS Microbiology Letters*, *366*(23), fnaa010.

Datar, R., Orenga, S., Pogorelcnik, R., Rochas, O., Simner, P. J., van Belkum, A. (2021). Recent advances in rapid antimicrobial susceptibility testing. *Clinical Chemistry*, *68*(1), 91–98.

de Santos, M., Oliveira de Souza, C., Marcelino, H. R. (2023). Blue technology for a sustainable pharmaceutical industry: Microalgae for bioremediation and pharmaceutical production. *Algal Research*, *69*, 102931.

Dedesko, S., Siegel, J. A. (2015). Moisture parameters and fungal communities associated with gypsum drywall in buildings. *Microbiome*, *3*(1), 71.

Deutschmann, S., Paul, M., Claassen-Willemse, M., van den Berg, J., IJzerman-Boon, P., Grunert da Fonseca, V., Brunbech, E., Johnson, L., Knutsen, C., Plourde, L., Salvas, J., Villari, P., Wysocki, L. (2023). Rapid sterility test systems in the pharmaceutical industry: Applying a structured approach to their evaluation, validation and global implementation. *PDA Journal of Pharmaceutical Science and Technology*, *77*(3), 211–235.

Elbing, K. L., Brent, R. (2019). Growth of *E. coli* on solid media. *Current Protocols in Molecular Biology*, *125*(1), e82.

Gapp, G., Holzknecht, P. (2011). Risk analysis of sterile production plants: A new and simple, workable approach. *PDA Journal of Pharmaceutical Science and Technology*, *65*(3), 217–226.

Gola, M., Caggiano, G., De Giglio, O., Napoli, C., Diella, G., Carlucci, M., Carpagnano, L. F., D'Alessandro, D., Joppolo, C. M., Capolongo, S., Montagna, M. T. (2021). SARS-CoV-2 indoor contamination: Considerations on anti-COVID-19 management of ventilation systems, and finishing materials in healthcare facilities. *Annali Di Igiene : Medicina Preventiva e Di Comunita*, *33*(4), 381–392.

Gouveia, B., Rijo, P., Gonçalo, T., Reis, C. (2015). Good manufacturing practices for medicinal products for human use. *Journal of Pharmacy and Bioallied Sciences*, *7*(2), 87.

Greenberg, M. R., Lowrie, K. W. (2009). From the editors. *Risk Analysis*, *29*(3), 315–316.

Griffith, C. (2016). Surface sampling and the detection of contamination. In: *Handbook of Hygiene Control in the Food Industry* (pp. 673–696). Elsevier.

Guilfoyle, D. E., Friedman, R. L., Hughes, P. F., Hussong, D., Rosenberg, A. S., Brorson, K. (2013). Microbial risk in pharmaceutical manufacturing and ICH Q9. *PDA Journal of Pharmaceutical Science and Technology*, *67*(2), 79–80.

Gurung, K., Rai, M. K. (2021). Assessment of microbial qualities of some cough syrups and multivitamins marketed in Pokhara, Nepal. *Prithvi Academic Journal*, *4*, 1–6.

Hao, N. Van, Huyen, N. N. M., Ny, N. T. H., Trang, V. T. N., Hoang, N. V. M., Thuy, D. B., Nguyen, N. T., Lieu, P. T., Duong, H. T. H., Thuy, T. T. D., Nhat, P. T. H., Tam, D. T. H., Boni, M. F., Yen, L. M., Tan, L. Van, Thanh, T. T., Campbell, J., Thwaites, C. L. (2021). The role of the gastrointestinal tract in toxigenic *Clostridium tetani*infection: A case-control study. *The American Journal of Tropical Medicine and Hygiene*, *105*(2), 494–497.

Hazlett, L. D., Rosen, D. D., Berk, R. S. (1978). Age-related susceptibility to *Pseudomonas aeruginosa* ocular infections in mice. *Infection and Immunity*, *20*(1), 25–29.

Hefny, M. H. M., Galal, S. E. M., Ahmed, A. A. A., Mansy, M. S., Shabayek, S. (2022). Microbial contamination of non-sterile pharmaceutical drops produced in Egypt. *Bulletin of Faculty of Pharmacy Cairo University*, *60*(1), article 5.

Jimenez, L. (Ed.). (2004). *Microbial Contamination Control in the Pharmaceutical Industry*. CRC Press.

Jimenez, L. (2007). Microbial diversity in pharmaceutical product recalls and environments. *PDA Journal of Pharmaceutical Science and Technology*, *61*(5), 383–399.

Kumar, N., Sangeetha, D., Balakrishna, P. (2011). Development and validation of a UPLC method for the determination of duloxetine hydrochloride residues on pharmaceutical manufacturing equipment surfaces. *Pharmaceutical Methods*, *2*(3), 161–166.

Lira, L. H., Hirai, F. E., Oliveira, M., Portellinha, W., Nakano, E. M. (2017). Use of the Ishikawa diagram in a case-control analysis to assess the causes of a diffuse lamellar keratitis outbreak. *Arquivos Brasileiros de Oftalmologia*, *80*(5), 281–284.

Manohar, S. M., Shah, P., Nair, A. (2021). Flow cytometry: Principles, applications and recent advances. *Bioanalysis*, *13*(3), 181–198.

McDonnell, G., Russell, A. D. (1999). Antiseptics and disinfectants: Activity, action, and resistance. *Clinical Microbiology Reviews*, *12*(1), 147–179.

McKinnon, B. T., Avis, K. E. (1993). Membrane filtration of pharmaceutical solutions. *American Journal of Hospital Pharmacy*, *50*(9), 1921–1936.

Miguel, E. A., Laranjeira, P. R., Ishii, M., Pinto, T. J. A. (2022). Analysis of water quality over non-condensable gases concentration on steam used for sterilization. *PLoS One*, *17*(9), e0274924.

Mohapatra, S. (2017). Sterilization and disinfection. In: *Essentials of Neuroanesthesia* (pp. 929–944). Elsevier.

Moradali, M. F., Ghods, S., Rehm, B. H. A. (2017). *Pseudomonas aeruginosa*lifestyle: A paradigm for adaptation, survival, and persistence. *Frontiers in Cellular and Infection Microbiology*, *7*, 39.

Mugoyela, V., Mugoyela, V., Mwambete, K. D. (2010). Microbial contamination of nonsterile pharmaceuticals in public hospital settings. *Therapeutics and Clinical Risk Management*, *6*, 443–448.

National Research Council (US) Subcommittee on Microbiological Criteria. (1985). *An Evaluation of the Role of Microbiological Criteria for Foods and Food Ingredients*. National Academies Press (US): Washington (DC). PMID: 25032416.

National Research Council. (2011). *Prudent Practices in the Laboratory*. National Academies Press.

Obuekwe, I. F., Eichie, F. (2006). The presence of microorganisms in some common excipients used in tablet formulation. *Acta Poloniae Pharmaceutica*, *63*(2), 121–125.

Odds, F. C. (1991). Sabouraud('s) agar. *Medical Mycology*, *29*(6), 355–359.

Odell, I. D., Cook, D. (2013). Immunofluorescence techniques. *Journal of Investigative Dermatology*, *133*(1), 1–4.

Ouédraogo, A., Groso, A., Meyer, T. (2011). Risk analysis in research environment – Part I: Modeling lab criticity index using improved risk priority number. *Safety Science*, *49*(6), 778–784.

Oxborrow, G. S., Roark, A. L., Fields, N. D., Puleo, J. R. (1974). Mathematical estimation of the level of microbial contamination on spacecraft surfaces by volumetric air sampling. *Applied Microbiology*, *27*(4), 706–712.

Pachori, P., Gothalwal, R., Gandhi, P. (2019). Emergence of antibiotic resistance *Pseudomonas aeruginosa* in intensive care unit; a critical review. *Genes and Diseases*, *6*(2), 109–119.

Park, J., Park, C., Ahn, S. (2018). Assessment of structural risks using the fuzzy weighted Euclidean FMEA and block diagram analysis. *The International Journal of Advanced Manufacturing Technology*, *99*(9–12), 2071–2080.

Patel, K. T., Chotai, N. P. (2011). Documentation and records: Harmonized GMP requirements. *Journal of Young Pharmacists*, *3*(2), 138–150.

Patel, M., Kumar, R., Kishor, K., Mlsna, T., Pittman, C. U., Mohan, D. (2019). Pharmaceuticals of emerging concern in aquatic systems: Chemistry, occurrence, effects, and removal methods. *Chemical Reviews*, *119*(6), 3510–3673.

Pollard, A. J., Bijker, E. M. (2021). A guide to vaccinology: From basic principles to new developments. *Nature Reviews Immunology*, *21*(2), 83–100.

Raposo, F., Barceló, D. (2021). Challenges and strategies of matrix effects using chromatography-mass spectrometry: An overview from research versus regulatory viewpoints. *TrAC Trends in Analytical Chemistry*, *134*, 116068.

Ratajczak, M., Kubicka, M. M., Kamińska, D., Sawicka, P., Długaszewska, J. (2015). Microbiological quality of non-sterile pharmaceutical products. *Saudi Pharmaceutical Journal*, *23*(3), 303–307.

Rodríguez-Gascón, A., Solinís, M. Á., Isla, A. (2021). The Role of PK/PD Analysis in the development and evaluation of antimicrobials. *Pharmaceutics*, *13*(6), 833.

Roy, S., Majumder, S., Deb, A., Choudhury, L. (2023). Microbial contamination of cosmetics and the pharmaceutical products, and their preservation strategies: A comprehensive review. *Novel Research in Microbiology Journal*, *7*(5), 2116–2137.

Rutala, W. A., Weber, D. J. (2015). Disinfection, sterilization, and control of hospital waste. In: *Mandell, Douglas, and Bennett's Principles and Practice of Infectious Diseases* (pp. 3294–3309.e4). Elsevier.

Sanchez, S., Demain, A. L. (2008). Metabolic regulation and overproduction of primary metabolites. *Microbial Biotechnology*, *1*(4), 283–319.

Sandle, T. (2016). Microbiological challenges to the pharmaceuticals and healthcare. In: *Pharmaceutical Microbiology* (pp. 281–294). Elsevier.

Santos, A. M. C., Doria, M. S., Meirinhos-Soares, L., Almeida, A. J., Menezes, J. C. (2018). A QRM discussion of microbial contamination of non-sterile drug products, using FDA and EMA warning letters recorded between 2008 and 2016. *PDA Journal of Pharmaceutical Science and Technology*, *72*(1), 62–72.

Sharma, S., Goyal, S., Chauhan, K. (2018). A review on analytical method development and validation. *International Journal of Applied Pharmaceutics*, *10*(6), 8.

Shintani, H. (2015). Validation studies for microbial contamination and control of contaminants. *Biocontrol Science*, *20*(3), 161–170.

Staat, R. H., Beakley, J. W. (1968). Evaluation of laminar flow microbiological safety cabinets. *Applied Microbiology*, *16*(10), 1478–1482.

Suvikas-Peltonen, E., Hakoinen, S., Celikkayalar, E., Laaksonen, R., Airaksinen, M. (2017). Incorrect aseptic techniques in medicine preparation and recommendations for safer practices: A systematic review. *European Journal of Hospital Pharmacy*, *24*(3), 175–181.

Tabatabaei, M. S., Ahmed, M. (2022). *Enzyme-Linked Immunosorbent Assay (ELISA), 2508,* 115–134.

Tim Sandle. (2016). *Pharmaceutical Microbiology: Essentials for Quality Assurance and Quality Control*. Elsevier.

Tropea, A. (2022). Microbial contamination and public health: An overview. *International Journal of Environmental Research and Public Health*, *19*(12), 7441.

Tršan, M., Seme, K., Srčič, S. (2019). The environmental monitoring in hospital pharmacy cleanroom and microbiota catalogue preparation. *Saudi Pharmaceutical Journal*, *27*(4), 455–462.

Verbeek, J. H., Rajamaki, B., Ijaz, S., Sauni, R., Toomey, E., Blackwood, B., Tikka, C., Ruotsalainen, J. H., Kilinc Balci, F. S. (2020). Personal protective equipment for preventing highly infectious diseases due to exposure to contaminated body fluids in healthcare staff. *Cochrane Database of Systematic Reviews*, *4*(4), CD011621.

Wadher, D. S. J. (2017). Validation: A review. *World Journal of Pharmaceutical Research*, 2228–2241.

Waters, D. L. E., Shapter, F. M. (2014). *The Polymerase Chain Reaction (PCR): General Methods* (pp. 65–75).

Wilson, S. C., Holder, H. W., Martin, J. M., Brasel, T. L., Andriychuk, L. A., Wu, C., Straus, D. C., Aguilar, R. (2006). An indoor air quality study of an alligator (*Alligator mississippiensis*) holding facility. *Journal of Zoo and Wildlife Medicine*, *37*(2), 108–115.

Xu, Z., Zhou, B. (2017). Three misunderstandings for design of negative pressure ward. In: *Dynamic Isolation Technologies in Negative Pressure Isolation Wards* (pp. 13–49). Springer: Singapore.

Xu, Z. (2014). Principle of cleanroom. In: *Fundamentals of Air Cleaning Technology and Its Application in Cleanrooms* (pp. 377–465). Springer: Berlin Heidelberg.

Zeitoun, H., Kassem, M., Raafat, D., AbouShlieb, H., Fanaki, N. (2015). Microbiological testing of pharmaceuticals and cosmetics in Egypt. *BMC Microbiology*, *15*(1), 275.

PART II

Microbial Control in Pharmaceutical Settings

CHAPTER 4

Sterilization Techniques and Their Validation with Reference to Pharmaceutical Microbiology

MUKESH KUMAR SINGH[1*], GURDEEP SINGH[2], AMRENDRA PRATAP YADAV[3], and GARIMA SHARMA[4]

[1]*School of Pharmaceutical Sciences, Faculty of Pharmacy, IFTM University, Moradabad, Uttar Pradesh, India*

[2]*School of Pharmaceutical Sciences, Lovely Professional University, Phagwara, Punjab, India*

[3]*Department of Pharmacy, Meerut Institute of Technology, Meerut, Uttar Pradesh, India*

[4]*Hind School of Pharmacy, Barabanki, Lucknow, Uttar Pradesh, India*

*Corresponding author

ABSTRACT

Sterilization is frequently used to eliminate all living germs, including bacterial, viral, and fungal ones, from a product. The goal of the sterilization process is to preserve the substance for a long time. It includes applying heat or chemicals to things like medicines, food, surgical instruments, nutraceuticals, etc. Since disease-causing germs are typically invisible to the naked eye, numerous sterilization procedures are used in microbiology. Pharmaceutical formulations designed for parenteral, ocular, implantation, or any other specialized application must be sterilized as per mandated clinical and regulatory standards. Any pharmaceutical dosage form must be free of pyrogens, meet the industry's quality requirements

Advances in Pharmaceutical Microbiology: From Bench to Bedside. Harpreet Singh, Arun Kumar Mishra, Jeyabalan Sangeetha, and Devarajan Thangadurai (Eds.)

DOI: 10.1201/9781779640918-6

as outlined in pharmacopoeias, and be secure for use as intended. The sterilization process aids in removing all pollutants, pyrogen, microorganisms, and microbial spores from the formulation. The overkill method is not preferred for all sterilization procedures. Sterilization validation technique is used for microbial inactivation processes. For the assessment of sterilization validation, bioburden-based or bioburden-biological indicator combined approaches are occasionally preferred. All sterilization processes are subject to the same validation program concepts, such as cleaning validations and the like. This chapter provides a comprehensive overview of the concept of sterilization, sterilization methods, including the factors affecting sterilization, risk assessment, sterility testing protocols, incubation, examination, and validation of sterility tests.

4.1 AN OVERVIEW OF STERILIZATION

The factual perception of sterilization emerged after the germ theory ("Infers: many diseases are caused by microorganisms"). Aseptic conditions were created in 1867 by employing carbolic acid to inactivate the bacteria. A few years later, in 1876, Charles Chamberland, a student and collaborator of Louis Pasteur, created the first pressure steam sterilizer, also known as an autoclave. English Physicist John Tyndall discovered heat-resistant microorganisms in the same year. He created the erratic (intermittent) heating technique for tyndallization. Later, in 1881, all surgical instruments, including gowns, dressings, and linens, were sterilized by boiling. Ernst von Bergmann (German Physician) used a steam sterilizer for the first time to sterilize surgical materials in 1885. In 1886, Gustav Neuber reported mercury chloride to clean an apron. The author recommended sterilizing everything that came into contact with the wounds and washing the furnishings with a disinfectant. The adoption of the sterilization procedure was intended to render the material sterile by eradicating bacteria or preventing their growth and upholding aseptic conditions (Abuhanoglu and Ozer, 2014).

4.1.1 STERILIZATION AND DISINFECTION

The state in which one is entirely free of all microorganisms capable of regenerating is called "sterility." Maintaining sterility is essential since

its loss or breakdown during application, manufacture, or packaging could have fatal consequences. "Sterilization" is the process of achieving a sterile condition. Sterilization is crucial for all kinds of dosage forms, including internal and external uses (Rutala and Weber, 2013). An object may only be either "sterile" or "nonsterile." There is no such thing as "fractional sterile." The term "microorganism" refers to any living thing that can be seen under a microscope and can have either a multicellular or unicellular structure. Microorganisms come in many forms, consisting of bacteria, fungi, parasites, and viruses (Basu et al., 2014).
Disinfection is a term used to describe a procedure on inanimate things that eliminates most pathogenic germs, except bacterial spores. Sterilization differs from disinfection in that the former focuses on eliminating all germs, including bacterial spores and endotoxins, while the latter only reduces the microbial load. To put it another way, the distinction between disinfection and sterilization is that the former involves total elimination. In contrast, the latter consists of obliterating or inactivating bacteria or microbial colonies to reduce their quantity (Rutala and Weber, 2016).

4.1.2 OBJECTIVES OF STERILIZATION

Reduction of initially existing bacteria or other potential pathogens is the primary goal of sterilization. From the pharmaceutical formulation perspective, sterilization's main goal is to eliminate all bacteria and their spores to prevent microbial growth. Sterilization is also essential to ensure that surgical and medical devices do not expose patients to infectious germs. Sterilization's primary goals are reducing the number, controlling the microbial population, and amputating undesirable or targeted microorganisms.

4.2 DRUG PERSPECTIVE ON THE SIGNIFICANCE OF STERILIZATION

Mainly, when a pharmaceutical substance is administered within the eye or ear or is directly transported into the bloodstream, it must be sterile. Since sterile items did not allow bacteria to develop, they reduced the risk of infection (Hasanain et al., 2014). Sterile products are used in pharmaceutical sterile product manufacturing units to maintain sterility throughout the whole process, from production to administration. Sterilization is necessary in order to administer clean products, such as injectable syringes and needles (Cooper et al., 2014). Bacteria, viruses, and fungi can increase and revert to viability given the right circumstances. Furthermore, the poisons these microorganisms release—endotoxins, exotoxins, or enterotoxins—are naturally very resistant. Certain environmental conditions, such as humidity, can encourage the growth of microbes. Consequently, nonsterility in sterile items is a constant problem. Only when additional parts of the product, such as the containers, processing machinery, disposable kits, packaging, syringes, or sterile, are cleaned, sterilized, and sterile, can the product's sterility be preserved. Furthermore, they are equally important and have to meet the sterility requirements. For instance, needles and packing materials are sterilized using gas sterilization, and steam sterilization can be used to sterilize stainless steel vessels (Mehmood, 2014).

Maintaining the sterility of the medication or device requires the employment of numerous integrated aspects utilized to make sterile products, such as production, processing, packing, marketing, and storage, in addition to the end user's usage of the product. Currently, there is no standard method for sterilization because it is a highly significant topic in the medical field. Several interconnected components that are used to create sterile products must be used to conserve the sterility of the medical equipment or medication. There may be differences in the technologies, techniques, and procedures used in the formulation units for sterilized product creation. The next section highlights the concepts of "sterilization and sterility" and the variables that affect sterilization (Sandle, 2013). To maintain quality and avoid tragedies caused by technical errors, sterile product manufacturing experts must understand this concept (McCrudden et al., 2015).

4.3 METHODS OF STERILIZATION

Sterilization in microbiology is achieved using a variety of chemical and physical methods. Sterilization can be classified into two categories: chemical and physical (Figure 4.1).

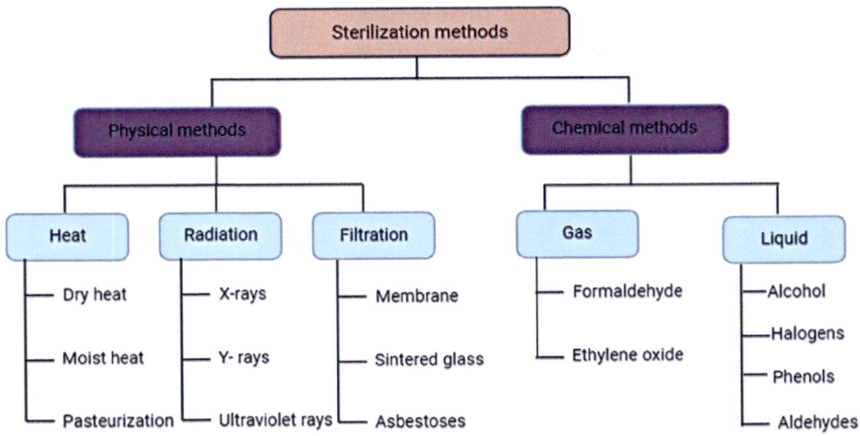

FIGURE 4.1 Classification of sterilization processes based on physical and chemical methods.

4.3.1 PHYSICAL STERILIZATION TECHNIQUES

The following techniques are included in physical sterilization.

4.3.1.1 HEAT STERILIZATION

The most efficient way of sterilization is heat sterilization, which destroys enzymes and cell components to eradicate microorganisms. The most common way of sterilization is heat. It is also a very dependable and successful procedure. Dry heat and wet heat are the two main ways that heat is used in sterilization. There is a similar idea underlying both these approaches. Because of the high concentration of electrolytes, dry heat causes oxidative damage, protein denaturation, and toxic effects. Furthermore, the microorganism's DNA may be harmed by the dry heat. Consequently, the microbe was destroyed. Through protein denaturation and coagulation, moist heat kills bacteria. Numerous variables might affect the heat-killing procedure, such as: (1) Temperature and duration—There is an inverse relationship between temperature and duration. Therefore, the temperature will decrease when heat is applied for a longer period of time for sterilization, and the duration will decrease when heat is used for a higher temperature. (2) Characteristics of microorganisms—There are two types of microorganisms: vegetative and spore. In general, spore types resist heat. As a result, the sterilization procedure will change depending on the microorganism's characteristics. In their vegetative and spore forms, microorganisms are frequently protected by organic compounds, which lessen the fatal effect of heat. In addition, the materials must be heat-stable for the compounds to be properly sterilized. There are two approaches to it.

4.3.1.1.1 Moist Heat Sterilization

This is one of the oldest approaches for sterilization. One instrument used in the moist heat sterilization process is an autoclave. The concept of pressure-induced steam generation underlies the operation of an autoclave. Wet heat sterilization is also known as steam sterilization. Water is heated to 121–134°C in an autoclave under 15 PSI of pressure. As a result, the microorganism's proteins coagulate and are essentially destroyed.

4.3.1.1.2 Dry Heat Sterilization

This technique is applied to moisture-sensitive items. Applying dry heat, or moisture-free heat, to an object's surface causes the proteins to get denatured and lyse, which causes oxidative damage and, in the end, the microbial cell burns or dies. This method includes flaming processes, incinerators, and hot air ovens (Moondra et al., 2018).

4.3.1.2 FILTRATION

In microbiology, this is a mechanical method of sterilization. This technique filters the liquid using membranous filters with tiny pores, preventing the passage of larger particles or microorganisms. Filtration involves three steps: sieving, adsorption, and trapping. Moreover, it can be used to sterilize gases and liquids and clarify them by blocking the passage of both living and dead particles. The three primary filtration methods within the filter material matrix are sieving, adsorption, and trapping.

Membranous filters are used in filtration because of their tiny holes, which allow liquid to pass through while blocking the passage of larger particles such as germs. Subsequently, the filter is more likely to avoid more objects from passing through it, the smaller the pore. Membrane filters, in particular, are useful in sterility testing because they may be used to collect and hold onto contaminated organisms in test solutions.

After that, these filters are incubated to promote growth and turbidity in a liquid nutritional medium. Sterilization-grade filters are mainly used to sterilize biological products, air, other gases, ophthalmic solutions, and heat-labile injections before they are supplied to aseptic locations. It might also be required in manufacturing settings, where they are a part of ventilation systems on freeze-dryers, centrifuges, and autoclaves.

4.3.1.3 IRRADIATION

The method of subjecting surfaces or items to different forms of radiation in order to sterilize them is known as radiation. Sterilization mostly involves electromagnetic radiation. It is believed that microbial DNA is the main target of these radiations, which can be damaged by excitation (UV light) or ionization, leading to the generation of free radicals (gamma rays and electrons). There are two varieties of it.

4.3.1.3.1 Nonionizing Radiation

The object is exposed to ultraviolet rays, which the microbes' nucleic acids absorb. The resulting thymine and cytosine in DNA produce the replicative mistake, ultimately resulting in the microbe's death. Nonionizing waves only kill bacteria that are on the surface since they have a low penetration power. When these waves are exposed to different chemicals, including nucleic acids, they are absorbed by them. Consequently, the waves produce thymine and cytosine dimers, which cause mistakes in the replication of DNA and, in the end, cause microorganisms to die through mutation. Because typical packaging materials are not as permeable to UV radiation, it is not a viable method for sterilizing pharmaceutical dosage forms. Nonetheless, it is used for water treatment for manufacturing, surface sterilization of aseptic workspaces, and air sterilization.

4.3.1.3.2 Ionizing Radiation

Oxidative distress, including superoxide ions and hydrogen peroxide, is created when exposed to ionizing radiations like gamma rays and X-rays. These species oxidize the microbe's biological components, causing it to perish. The most often utilized ionizing radiation for sterilization is gamma and X-ray radiation. These are high-energy radiations that ionize water and other substances. When water is ionized, various hazardous O_2 metabolites are created, such as H_2O_2, superoxide ions, and hydroxyl radicals. These metabolites are strong oxidizers that oxidize several bacterial cell components, killing the bacteria. In the presence of moisture or dissolved oxygen, microbial resistance to ionizing radiation decreases at high temperatures (owing to increased formation of free radicals). Surgical equipment, sutures, prosthesis, unit-dose ointments, plastic syringes, and dry pharmaceutical products are among the items that are frequently sterilized by radiation.

4.3.2 CHEMICAL STERILIZATION

Plastic equipment and biological material in microbiology are sterilized by the chemical method of sterilization. Several substances function as bactericidal agents in this manner. They come in two varieties: liquid and gaseous.

4.3.2.1 GASEOUS STERILIZATION

Gas sterilization is the process of exposing an object to gas in a sealed, heated, and pressurized chamber. Gaseous chemical agents which are used in sterilization are formaldehyde, nitrogen dioxide, ozone, and ethylene oxide. The filters used for this are often made of aluminum or Kraft paper corrugated sheets used in laminar air flow cabinets, wall or ceiling panels, or ducts. The pleated glass microfiber sheets are separated and supported by these sheets. These high-efficiency particulate air (HEPA) filters function as depth filters since they can remove up to 99.997% of particles larger than 0.3 mm in diameter. Since most bacteria are linked to dust particles, their microbe eradication effectiveness is considerably higher in practice. Filters can also be used to clean and sterilize medical gases, decontaminate air in mechanical ventilators, treat exhausting air from microbiological safety cabinets (HEPA filters), and sterilize displacement or venting air in culture medium (hydrophobic membrane filters and carbon filters).

4.3.2.2 LIQUID STERILIZATION

Liquid sterilization is the process of immersing an object in a liquid to destroy all living microorganisms and their spores. Hypochlorite solution, hydrogen peroxide, and glutaraldehyde are common liquid chemical agents used for sterilization. This method is less effective than gaseous sterilization to remove small levels of contamination. Membrane filters are disc-shaped and can be mounted in a vacuum filtration unit for liquid filtration or placed in pressure-operated filters for syringe mounting and in-line use. The ideal method is pressure-fed filtration because it enables high-flow loading directly into final containers without the risk of foaming, solvent evaporation, or air leaks. In order to improve membrane filters' capacity to handle dirt, a coarse-grade fiberglass depth prefilter is commonly used in tandem with them.

4.4 VALIDATION OF STERILIZATION METHODS AND EQUIPMENT

According to Tavalsky et al. (2013), creating recorded evidence that a certain process will reliably produce a product that satisfies its predetermined criteria and quality features is known as validation. Food and Drug Administration (FDA) published guidelines for validation, and according to the FDA, the three guiding concepts for the validation process are as follows:

1. To include sterility in an item
2. To show the highest degree of confidence that the sterilization processes have created sterility for every batch of units, and
3. To increase the assurance regarding the finished product's sterility test results.

Tests that gather information about the sterilization process and statistically demonstrate that it can reliably sterilize goods or medical equipment in "worst-case scenario" circumstances are known as validations of the sterilization process.

4.4.1 OBJECTIVES OF VALIDATION

- To reduce dependence on final product testing
- To incorporate sterility into a product
- Raise the sterility assurance limit (SAL) to every unit, and
- To increase the support and guarantee of sterility testing for final products.

4.4.2 MOIST HEAT STERILIZATION

The material to be sterilized by moist heat sterilization is sanitized using steam as a source. Steam is used as an arbitrator to convey the heat energy to the substance because of its higher enthalpy of 438 KJ/mol, which makes it a more effective heat carrier than dry air (Mendes et al., 2007). The fact that steam sterilization can soften even the protective layers of bacteria is another factor in the argument for steam sterilization's superiority. As a result, sterility is imparted because the protein structures necessary for bacteria to proliferate are disrupted (Van Doornmalen and Kopinga, 2008).

The standard steam sterilization conditions are 121°C for 15–30 min at 115 pounds (1.2 bars) of pressure. However, depending on the sterilization technique, parameters often change. Two possible approaches are the overkill approach and the bioburden approach. Since the kill strategy is typically applied to heat-stable materials, under the worst-case scenario with a Decimal reduction time (D-value) of 121°C, we can anticipate a minimum 12-log reduction in microbes. When a substance is heat sensitive, the bioburden technique is employed, necessitating the calculation of both the D-value and bioburden data. As a result, log to the base 10 of 134, or 2.14, may be the predicted cycle time and must be computed to decrease the bioburden from 134 colony-forming units to 1 (Sultana, 2007).

The cycle consists of three phases: heating, where steam replaces air; sterilizing, where steam is exposed to the product; and finally, heating. Subsequently, the product undergoes a cooling phase during which air circulation is resumed to achieve atmospheric pressure. Generally, wrapped materials and utensils need to be sterilized for 15 min at 121°C and 30 min at 132°C, while unwrapped items need to be sterilized for 1 minute at 121°C and 3 min at 132°C (Dion and Parker, 2013).

4.4.3 DRY HEAT STERILIZATION

In contrast to moist sterilization, this method involves eliminating or killing germs at a somewhat higher temperature. This process takes a prolonged exposure period of 1.5–3 h. This process sterilizes items that could be spoiled if moist sterilization is used, like granules, hydrocarbon compounds, or some harsh objects, using a dry heat sterilizer, or burners (Karlsson et al., 2002). Heat is absorbed on the outside of the object and then transferred, layer by layer, to the center during the conduction process. The drawback of this method is the destruction it causes to the oxygen molecules, which can destroy biological components and result in the organism's death. Jacobs and Wills (1988) state that the temperature required for the same is 170°C for 30 min, 160°C for 60 min, and 150°C for 150 min or more, depending on the volume. Forced air and static air are the types of dry-heat sterilizers available. Static air sterilizers work like oven sterilizers, with the warming coil located at the bottom of the device, causing heated air inside the chamber to ascend. As a result, this method is considerably slower and takes longer to reach sterilization. However, the process is less consistent than the second kind, called forced static, which uses a motor-driven blower to circulate hot air quickly, allowing for a quick energy transfer (Hemphill et al., 2015). Regarding the benefits of this system, this kind of sterilization is very economical because it can easily permeate the material and is not harmful to the environment or the metals. However, the procedure takes a long time and calls for a higher temperature, which is inappropriate for some materials (Masuishi et al., 2013).

The dry-heat sterilizers cannot be validated using any particular technique. However, its physical variables, such as temperature, belt speed, and air particle matter, could be validated (Schmidt et al., 2015). Validation of the depyrogenation cycle must also be performing, and the Limulus Amebocyte Lysate test must be run to determine whether the endotoxin has been rendered inactive by a reduction of about 1000 times or a three-log reduction. Less than 2 h are spent doing the cycles at 170°C (the entire range is 180–300°C). While a greater temperature is appropriate for depyrogenation, a lower one will result in sterilization. The D value of toughest microbial spore at 170°C is 6–10 min, while this D value is only a few seconds at the temperature of depyrogenation. Z values for endotoxins are 54°C, and microbiological resistance is 20°C. As the Z value rises, endotoxin becomes more resistant to the dry-heat sterilization technique. The bioburden and resistance investigations may not be necessary if the overkill strategy is employed alone. The ideal bioburden reduction is thought to be 12 logs (Purohit and Gupta, 2017).

4.4.4 STERILIZATION BY FILTRATION AND ITS VALIDATION

It describes eliminating germs from a fluid stream without negatively impacting the end product. For example, it is frequently used to sterilize vitamins and medicines. Its foundation uses membranes with pores that prevent bacteria from passing through. It is beneficial for liquid and gas samples. Because of the water's viscosity, viruses can typically be eliminated with this kind of sterilization, which typically has a prolonged flow rate (Shinde et al., 2013). In this process, three different types of filters are typically utilized. The first type is called a depth filter, consisting of layers upon layers of fibrous sheets made of glass, asbestos, or paper. As a result, it forges a winding route that aids in capturing the particles inside to keep the materials from getting blocked during the actual filtration process. These can be used as a prefilter. The membrane filter is an extra filter that is frequently used in microbiology. It is composed of polymers with high tensile strength. It resembles a dense web of linked strands with distinct gaps between the polymers. Thus, we may efficiently manage the pore size of a membrane of variable sizes by varying the polymerization process (Ariffin et al., 2014). Another is a nucleopore polycarbonate membrane, which is made by first subjecting to nuclear radiation and then using an etching solution to produce weak spots so the membrane eventually has pores. In particular, it is employed to arrest bacteria on the membrane for microscopic examination. Since the aerobic process uses a lot of air, air sterilization is the primary application for this kind of filtration. As a result, the filters are changed regularly when they become unclean (Li et al., 2013). This process's main benefits are its low cost, applicability to heat-sensitive materials, and capacity to eliminate different-sized particles. However, the drawbacks include the nominal pore size of each filter, the inability to separate microorganisms of similar sizes, and the need for great differential pressure throughout the whole process (Kumar et al., 2015).

4.4.5 GASEOUS STERILIZATION

By exposing the material to gas, germs are killed during the gaseous sterilization. According to Bhatarah and Greenwood (2013), formaldehyde and ethylene oxide (EtO) have a broad spectrum of biocidal activity. The gases primarily used to sterilize pharmaceutical powders, surgical tools, and equipment are formaldehyde and EtO. Specifically, EtO is preferred over formaldehyde because it treats bacterial spores more effectively (Galante et al., 2017). Because EtO is highly explosive, it must be mixed with 10% CO_2 for sterilization. EtO concentration and relative humidity have standard operating limits of 500–1000 mg/L and 30%–60%, respectively. The alkylation reaction serves as the foundation for the sterilization procedure.

The sterilizers typically used for this purpose are explosion- and leak-proof, with a volume and capacity of 100–300 L. Through evaporation, humidification, and steam passage at subatmospheric pressure, the technique extracts air from the chamber. It is encased in a hot water jacket. Injecting additional gas at the start of the process or when the pressure drops improves the absorption of EtO by the load, and forced gas circulation is provided to reduce changes in atmospheric conditions. Afterwards, the exhaust system is used to remove the gases. Therefore, the EtO must be removed safely to lessen the operator's exposure to harmful dangers. The teratogenous nature of the gas, its carcinogenic and odorous qualities, and its nasal mucosa, conjunctiva, and skin toxicity are some of the disadvantages of the method. At 55°C, the operation takes 2–5 h (Carbone et al., 2014). Another gas that might be utilized is formaldehyde, which is produced by heating formalin to an extremely high temperature. The sterilization procedure is the same for this gas as well. Preconditioning is used to keep the compartment at the optimum pressure and relative humidity. The fluctuation is reduced by heating the jacket and forcing steam or water through it. After that, gas is injected into the compartment with steam at a precise humidity level to start the sterilization process. Maintaining the gas's concentration is necessary since it may be adsorbed onto specific materials, causing variations in the concentration level. Finally, the load is subjected to a temperature range of 30–50°C during the degassing process by flowing air filtered by HEPA over it. The same must be done for 48 h because any remaining gas can damage healthy body tissues, necessitating extensive aeration. Thus, infrastructure and a close-fitting ventilation arrangement are required (Fichet et al., 2007).

When verifying the sterility of gaseous sterilization, the first validation is crucial. The gas concentration, temperature, pressure, and humidity all affect the thermochemical death time in this situation. Therefore, it is necessary to establish the functions of various environmental factors in aeration and sterilization. The overkill approach is generally employed for this process, wherein the spore population and D value are determined using a biological indicator (BI). The sites of the worst cases must be identified to pinpoint the point at which the BI is not inactivated throughout the sterilization cycle (Van Doornmalen and Kopinga, 2008). It is also possible to determine the half cycle, the lowest point at which the BI inactivates, and the significant value for the same, which is the point at which the BI reduces by six logs. It is necessary to ascertain the bioburden in a minimum of three batches and the survival of BI.

Along with a specific gas concentration and relative humidity, microbiological evaluation should be carried out (Acosta-Gnass and Stempluk, 2010). *Bacillus atrophaeus* is the BI that the pharmacopoeia recommends, and the United States Pharmacopeia states that its concentration is 13,106 spores (vegetative bacterial and fungal spores display partial resistance to the sterilizing agent). Spore persistence suggests that additional sterilization sessions are needed. For compartments with up to 5000 L of usable space, the number of BI utilized is usually 20 (or more), which increases with larger chambers. To find the sublethal dose, experiments are typically conducted in triplicate. The sublethal cycle timing should be selected to get positive testing so that 30–80% of the BI should survive. Three cycles should be the bare minimum that can be allowed at each time point. Requalification and measurement of the gas concentration have to be carried out on a regular basis. This revalidation includes half-cycle, one sublethal cycle, bioburden testing, and EtO residual testing. A comprehensive revalidation is necessary whenever any significant changes are made to the product, packaging, or manufacturing procedure (Vaughn et al., 2014).

4.5 FACTORS AFFECTING STERILIZATION

4.5.1 NUMBER AND SPATIAL ARRANGEMENTS OF MICROBES

Keeping other factors entirely equal, the primary factor influencing sterilization is the population of microorganisms; the amount of time needed for the sterilization process to destroy is directly correlated with the amount of microorganisms (Dagsuyu et al., 2016). Furthermore, it can be more difficult to eradicate clustered or group microorganisms than dispersed ones; sometimes the sterilization capacity is not enough to destroy every microbe; sometimes an inadequate sterilization plan indicate the formation of condensed masses of microbial cells and biofilms or extracellular components; and lastly, the steps that reduce the quantity of microorganisms and improve the margin of protection during the sterilization process are disinfection and cleaning (Wong and Smith, 2014).

4.5.2 RESISTANCE WITHIN MICROBES

Depending on the sterilization techniques employed, microbes can have fluctuating levels of resistance to various antibiotic classes. Microbial spores are more resistant to the sterilizing procedure than actual germs. The bacterial spore's coat and cortex, which serve as a barrier, are the cause of this (Ben Belgacem et al., 2017). The type of material that needs to be disposed of may affect the sterilization process. Different viruses have different levels of resistance to different germicides; for example, bacterial spores are more resistant than vegetative bacteria, mycobacteria, fungus, and viruses. Even bacterial spores are used as a biological contaminant and are essential in a number of experiments that assess the efficacy of sterilizations techniques.

4.5.3 PHYSICOCHEMICAL FACTORS

Temperature and relative humidity are the two primary physical and chemical factors that influence sterilization. For instance, when the temperature rises, sterilization effectiveness rises as well. On the other hand, a temperature increase that is too great could also compromise the integrity of the product and change its intended quality. Relative humidity and temperature can significantly affect how active gaseous sterilants like formaldehyde, chlorine dioxide, and EtO increase the rate of microbial inactivation. The sterilizing procedure may be harmed by an increase in humidity because most bacteria grow best in humid environments (Gerba, 2015).

4.5.4 STORAGE REQUIREMENT

Royalty et al. (2014) examined the impact of varying storage conditions (freezing, −15°C, refrigeration temperature 5°C, and room temperature 22°C) on the EtO D-value resistance of spore bands. All three of the tested batches that were kept in freezers displayed a decrease in D value when compared to spore bands kept at 22°C. Two of the three batches had a minor increase in resistance, or D-value, during the nine months while they were refrigerated. This experiment clearly shows that the resistance to the sterilizing process was enhanced by the length of the storage period.

4.6 STERILITY TESTING METHODS

A sterility investigation is typically necessary for the sterile element to be certified. The terminal sterilization procedure is required for the sterilization of consumables. This involves measuring the product's bioburden before sterilization and comparing it to the microorganisms' authentication cycles (Niazi, 2016). Most sterility tests included in pharmacopoeias rely on traditional bacterial growth. Despite the quick sterility test, various regulatory organization guidelines and specific national legislation require a growth-based microbiological method to examine sterility (Daniell et al., 2016). The sterility of pharmaceuticals can be parametrically analyzed using a sample of articles examined from a cluster and a physical data review. The parametric release is unacceptable for aseptically filled items and can only be achieved by the sterility test.

4.6.1 KINETICS OF MICROBIAL DESTRUCTION

Radiation sterilization, chemical reactions, and temperature increases are examples of microbial destruction techniques. A logarithmic relationship can be seen between the number of live bacteria and the radiation dose or exposure time, depending on the sterilization method used. One log of surviving cells can be reduced in time and dose by using the relationship, which can be either linear or nonlinear. The computation uses the following parameters (Holdsworth and Simpson, 2016).

4.6.2 METHODS FOR TESTING STERILITY

The three significant pharmacopoeias (European, American, and Japanese) provide the most widely used sterility testing method. The US FDA has permitted alternative rapid microbiological techniques since 2012. The modification of the sterility test is frequently employed in the case of medical equipment, as opposed to the direct inoculation method, which maintains the device in a culture for a while after post-sterilization (Sandle, 2013).

4.6.3 MEMBRANE SEPARATION

The membrane filtering technique is valuable due to its large-scale applicability and capacity to sterilize larger batches. The procedure requires the development of tiny holes in the product and then passage through the membrane. Half the filled amount of a significant volume product must be subjected to a membrane filter. In addition, a few milliliters of a liquid substance are transferred into the test media during the direct inoculation procedure (Hayashi et al., 2014). The best method for aqueous, alcoholic, greasy, and solvent compounds is membrane filtration. The standard filter is made of similar plastics, such as cellulose esters. Since the filter membrane separates the material from microorganisms, in the product, any microbes may become lodged inside the filter milieu as the material passes through the filter (Ghugare et al., 2017). To remove any remaining substance, use a rinse solution such as Ringer's, phosphate-buffered, or saline. The filter is divided into binary sections, or in certain situations, an additional filter is used for that persistence (the polycarbonate membrane is a famous example). Microorganisms may adhere to the filter membrane; hence, a culture medium must be provided for each filtration cycle (Warkiani et al., 2015). The most fashionable culture media are those that pharmacopoeias suggest. These include soyabean casein digest media (tryptone soy broth (TSB); incubated at 20–25°C to separate fungi and aerobic bacteria) and fluid thioglycollate medium (FTM), which is incubated at 30–35°C to separate aerobic and anaerobic bacteria (Zitron et al., 2016).

For developing aerobic and anaerobic bacteria, resazurin, a redox indicator included in FTM, forms a chemical coating that is observed by a pink color. However, some products, such as protein-based goods that can clog the filter holes, would not filter out immediately because the direct inoculation method is necessary due to their inherent antibacterial properties (Chen et al., 2018).

4.6.4 DIRECT INOCULATION

Sometimes, the membrane filtration approach must be validated, in which case the direct inoculation method is preferred. Based on the membrane filtering approach, the straightforward inoculation technique involves adding two distinct culture media, like FTM and TSB, to which a varied amount of the product is added. A concentrated culture medium is incorporated with substances produced in large quantities. The neutralizer or product dilution is added to achieve this (Zitron et al., 2016).

4.6.5 INCUBATION AND ANALYSIS OF STERILITY TESTS

FTM is incubated at 30–35°C, and TSB is incubated at 20–25°C. Except for the subculture containers, test and control containers must be incubated without microbial contamination for at least 14 days to be detected. During the incubation period, turbidity, precipitation, or other signs of microbial development are seen. Using colonies of each microbe and gram stain, the growth is then quantified microscopically (Thornsberry and Swenson, 1980). It is difficult to see flocculation, turbidity, and the presence of microbial growth in suspensions. It needs a subculture stage as a result. To perform subculturing, a suitable portion of the culture medium is transferred to the same medium in an appropriate vessel and incubated for an additional duration. On the incubated substance, the product description, the culture medium, the incubation temperature, and the testing time are fundamentally labelled. When examining the tested materials, it might be cautious to prevent unnecessary agitation, especially when dealing with FTM. If anaerobic conditions are not maintained, the resazurin indicator must show it. The material must be gently spun during the last incubation period to check for any apparent turbidity under the light source (Goulet et al., 2013).

4.6.6 VALIDATION OF STERILITY ASSESSMENT METHOD

A sterile finished material has many distinguishing characteristics, such as being free of microorganisms, pyrogens, and particles and meeting strict purity and quality requirements. Validation procedures for the sterilization processes must be intricate and comprehensive. The official sterility test determines the choice of sterility (Wood, 2015). Data gathering and evaluation from the start of the project to the end of production provide the evaluation proof. Among the standards used in the assessment of the sterilization process are probability of maximum level, formulation sterility, assurance improvement, specification and performance distinctive establishment, specific technique, method, and manufacturing apparatus. An evaluation with a great degree of confidence results in a consistent output that satisfies predefined requirements and offers quality assurance. To demonstrate that the culture medium has no antibacterial activity, each product type needs to be confirmed (Peris-Vicente et al., 2015).

4.7 NEW PERSPECTIVES ON THE TECHNICAL DEVELOPMENT OF STERILIZATION

4.7.1 FINAL STERILIZATION

Final sterilization is characteristically used to fill and seal dose vessels under specified circumstances, aiding in the following sterilization procedure (Maquille et al., 2008). Final sterilization is not the same as aseptic treatment, which involves sterilizing each material, item of dose or medicines, vessel, and closure separately before being collected. Consequently, the vessel was packed in the desired configuration without the need for any further sterilization. This also increases the likelihood of microbial infection and its unpredictable nature. In addition, a number of sterilization methods were considered for the aseptic procedure, such as sterile filtration, wet heat sterilization, and dry heat sterilization for rubber closures, liquid dosage forms, and glass containers, correspondingly (Izumi et al., 2016).

4.7.2 STERILIZATION BY RADIATION

Radiation such as high-energy electron and γ radiation are used in this sterilization test as effective sterilization agents for a variety of heat-labile medicinal items, as well as those that cannot be sterilized with ETO. Radiation sterilization has various effects (depending on the type of radiation and the interaction between radiation and material) because of the physicochemical features of the material (Nguyen et al., 2013). For example, the most important use of sterilization by radiation was that it would damage the material's physicochemical and medicinal characteristics. Additionally, there are two types of radiation: particle-type, such as accelerated electrons, and natural/artificial, electromagnetic, such as UV light and γ radiation (Amery and Myntti, 2014). A microbe's DNA is directly impacted by radiation sterilization, which also causes microorganisms to perish. A 25-kGy dosage of γ radiation was suggested as an appropriate method for sterilizing specific surgical materials and equipment in the British Pharmacopoeia. According to standards published by the International Atomic Energy Agency, medical materials and devices can be radiation-sterilized with an actual dosage of radiation of up to 25 kGy (Freeman et al., 2015; Marsit et al., 2014). The temperature, concentration of active substances, dose rate, and absorbed dose are some variables that could impact sterilization. Because of the unique effects of radiation on people and the environment, both the environment and the workforce involved in the sterilization process require extreme caution. In addition, improper disposal of radioactive waste contributes significantly to the process' high cost. Primarily in medical items and polymer-related medical devices, which are susceptible to radiation-induced chemical deterioration. Thus, a technique that would both lessen radiation damage and improve cost-effectiveness in the future was needed. Radiation sterilization is an easy way to sanitize objects that contain radioactive chemicals and drugs. These days, drug delivery methods include liposomal systems, microspheres, nanospheres, and microemulsions, delivered to the target tissue or organ using e-beam sterilization techniques and gamma (γ) and beta (β) radiation. Due to these delivery systems' advantages over traditional systems, they are receiving a lot of attention these days (Tekade et al., 2017; Lalu et al., 2017; Darwis et al., 2015; Maheshwari et al., 2012).

A method of sterilizing biological materials using ionizing radiation that combines c irradiation and e-beam was recently devised. It is hypothesized that radiation causes the generation of free radicals in microbial organization due to peptide backbone scission, hydrogen bond disruption, and cross-link creation. A biological scaffold was created by Dearth et al. as a medicinal device for pig dermal remodeling. Türker et al. (2014) evaluated the effects of various radiation, for example, ethylene oxide, γ-radiation, and e-radiation, on the characteristics of the biological material and the *in vivo* remodeling effect.

Furthermore, the final sterilization of an extracellular matrix scaffold is related to a number of variables. For example, the effects of temperature (frozen vs room temperature) and hydration grade (lyophilized vs hydrated) during the sterilization process were noted on the biological scaffold material. The biological materials displayed were exposed to ethylene oxide, γ-radiation, and e-radiation (Dearth et al., 2016).

4.8 CONCLUSION

Providing goods that are effective, safe, and efficient is the primary goal of the pharmaceutical sector. One of the most important steps in ensuring the safety of pharmaceutical formulations is sterilization, which keeps the formulation microorganism-free. These microorganisms are hazardous to the public and impact the products' effectiveness. The sterility of medical equipment and pharmaceuticals is covered in this chapter. This chapter emphasized the value, application, and use of sterility.

Additionally, the salient features of endotoxins and bacterial by products and their impact on sterility are discussed. The many approaches to achieving sterility are highlighted; these approaches use various harmful agents and eliminate, incapacitate, or kill the microorganisms, which are also covered in this chapter. There is a description of the techniques and how they are divided into physical, chemical, and physiochemical categories. These techniques' guiding concepts and how they are used are described. BI, physical indicator, and chemical indicator are only a few indicators used to validate and assess sterilization techniques. These signs aid in determining the completion of the processes and provide reassurance regarding the success of sterilization. The broad categories used to achieve sterilization through aseptic filling or terminal sterilization are listed. There is a risk of contamination with aseptic filling because the final container is sterilized during terminal sterilization. EtO gas, electron beam radiation, or irradiation are used to fix the terminal. The most used technique among the others is heat sterilization. The chapter makes explicit the distinctions between the two forms of heat sterilization: steam sterilization and dry heat sterilization.

Furthermore, steam sterilization kills microorganisms more effectively than heat sterilization, which is limited to materials that can tolerate moisture and heat. The effectiveness of the procedures depends on a variety of factors. For heat sterilization, for example, temperature and duration are essential considerations. This chapter discusses the relationship between temperature and time, showing that it is inversely proportional. As the temperature rises, it takes less time to destroy a live organism. The population of microorganisms is generally the standard variable across all sterilization techniques; nevertheless, this variable has a dramatic relationship with temperature, implying that more critical populaces require higher dosages and temperatures to accomplish sanitization. The type of microorganisms should also be taken into account; the more resistant the germs, the longer it will take to eradicate them. The resistant microorganisms are employed as BI to support technique validation and bioburden assessment. Understanding the type and quantity of microorganisms is essential to prevent these issues. Other aspects must also be considered, such as the surrounding conditions, the type of soil, the materials utilized, and any organic matter on the substance. Preventing contamination from the environment and items used is crucial. Also discussed is the sterility test, as specified in pharmacopoeias. This aids in evaluating the sterility's efficacy. Since sterility can be quantified precisely as an absolute, SAL is usually cited as a likelihood in this context. At long last, it is vital to note that sanitization is a complex but essential need. Depending on the number of microorganisms present, kinetic parameters of microbial death like Z-value and D-value assist in determining the extent of dose and time. Sterilization can be accomplished and helps to reduce the risk of contamination and injury to people if procedures are created with enough validation parameters. A continuous process watch is sustained along with perfect compliance with Good Manufacturing Practices.

KEYWORDS

- **sterilization**
- **validation**
- **microorganism**
- **sterility test**
- **kinetics of microbial destruction**
- **biological indicator**

REFERENCES

Abuhanoglu, G., Ozer, A. Y. (2014). Radiation sterilization of new drug delivery systems. *Interventional Medicine and Applied Science*, *6*(2), 51–60.

Acosta-Gnass, S. I., Stempliuk, V. D. A. (2010). *Sterilization Manual for Health Centers*. Pan American Health Organization.

Amery, D. P., Myntti, M. F. (2014). U.S. Patent No. 8,653,319. U.S. Patent and Trademark Office: Washington, DC.

Ariffin, A. A., Ghazali, H. M., Kavousi, P. (2014). Validation of a HPLC method for determination of hydroxymethylfurfural in crude palm oil. *Food Chemistry*, *154*, 102–107.

Basu, D., Bhattacharya, S., Mahajan, A., Ramanan, V. R., Chandy, M. (2014). The importance of the central sterile supply department in infection prevention and control. *Infection Control and Hospital Epidemiology*, *35*(10), 1312–1314.

Ben Belgacem, Z., Carré, G., Charpentier, E., Le-Bras, F., Maho, T., Robert, E., Pouvesle, J. M., Polidor, F., Gangloff, S. C., Boudifa, M., Gelle, M. P. (2017). Innovative non-thermal plasma disinfection process inside sealed bags: Assessment of bactericidal and sporicidal effectiveness in regard to current sterilization norms. *PLoS One*, *12*(6), 1–18.

Bhatarah, P., Greenwood, K. A. (2013). U.S. Patent No. 8,541,399. U.S. Patent and Trademark Office: Washington, DC.

Carbone, P., Benedek, K., Ruffo, M. O., Luongo, W. (2014). U.S. Patent No. 8,721,984. U.S. Patent and Trademark Office: Washington, DC.

Chen, J. L., Steele, T. W., Stuckey, D. C. (2018). Metabolic reduction of resazurin; location within the cell for cytotoxicity assays. *Biotechnology and Bioengineering*, *115*(2), 351–358.

Cooper, P. D., Barclay, T. G., Ginic-Markovic, M., Petrovsky, N. (2014). Gamma ray sterilization of delta inulin adjuvant particles (Advax™) makes minor, partly reversible structural changes without affecting adjuvant activity. *Vaccine*, *32*(5), 552–557.

Dagsuyu, C., Gocmen, E., Narli, M., Kokangul, A. (2016). Classical and fuzzy FMEA risk analysis in a sterilization unit. *Computers and Industrial Engineering*, *101*, 286–294.

Daniell, E., Bryans, T., Darnell, K., Hansen, J., Hitchins, V. M., Saavedra, M. (2016). Product sterility testing to test or not to test? that is the question. *Biomedical Instrumentation and Technology*, *50*(S3), 35–43.

Darwis, D., Erizal, Abbas, B., Nurlidar, F., Putra, D. P. (2015). Radiation processing of polymers for medical and pharmaceutical applications. *Macromolecular Symposia*, *353*(1), 15–23.

Dearth, C. L., Keane, T. J., Carruthers, C. A., Reing, J. E., Huleihel, L., Ranallo, C. A., Kollar, E. W., Badylak, S. F. (2016). The effect of terminal sterilization on the material properties and *in vivo* remodeling of a porcine dermal biologic scaffold. *Acta Biomaterialia*, *33*, 78–87.

Dion, M., Parker, W. (2013). Steam sterilization principles. *Pharmaceutical Engineering*, *33*(6), 1–8.

Fichet, G., Antloga, K., Comoy, E., Deslys, J. P., McDonnell, G. (2007). Prion inactivation using a new gaseous hydrogen peroxide sterilisation process. *Journal of Hospital Infection*, *67*(3), 278–286.

Freeman, A., Riggs, B., Harrison, R., Simmons, G. S. (2015). U.S. Patent No. 9,155,806. U.S. Patent and Trademark Office: Washington, DC.

Galante, R., Ghisleni, D., Paradiso, P., Alves, V. D., Pinto, T. J., Colaco, R., Serro, A. P. (2017). Sterilization of silicone-based hydrogels for biomedical application using ozone gas: Comparison with conventional techniques. *Materials Science and Engineering: C*, *78*, 389–397.

Gerba, C. P. (2015). Disinfection. In: Pepper, I. L., Gentry, T. J., Gerba, C. P. (Eds.), *Environmental Microbiology* (pp. 645–662). Academic Press: San Diego.

Ghugare, G. S., Nair, A., Nimkande, V., Sarode, P., Rangari, P., Khairnar, K. (2017). Membrane filtration immobilization technique—a simple and novel method for primary isolation and enrichment of bacteriophages. *Journal of Applied Microbiology*, *122*(2), 531–539.

Goulet, V., King, L. A., Vaillant, V., de Valk, H. (2013). What is the incubation period for listeriosis. *BMC Infectious Diseases*, *13*, 1–7.

Hasanain, F., Guenther, K., Mullett, W. M., Craven, E. (2014). Gamma sterilization of pharmaceuticals—a review of the irradiation of excipients, active pharmaceutical ingredients, and final drug product formulations. *PDA Journal of Pharmaceutical Science and Technology*, *68*(2), 113–137.

Hayashi, K., Douhara, K., Kashino, G. (2014). Evaluation of the bubble point test of a 0.22-μm membrane filter used for the sterilizing filtration of PET radiopharmaceuticals. *Annals of Nuclear Medicine*, *28*, 586–592.

Hemphill, W. K., Eason, M. P., Olson, M. E., Sims, J. P. (2015). U.S. Patent No. 9,011,786. U.S. Patent and Trademark Office: Washington, DC.

Holdsworth, S. D., Simpson, R., Holdsworth, S. D., Simpson, R. (2016). Kinetics of microbial death and factors for quality attributes. In: *Thermal Processing of Packaged Foods* (pp. 89–24).

Izumi, M., Fujifuru, M., Okada, A., Takai, K., Takahashi, K., Udagawa, T., Miyake, M., Naruyama, S., Tokuda, H., Nishioka, G., Yoden, M., Aoki, M. (2016). Evaluation of *Bacillus oleronius* as a biological indicator for terminal sterilization of large-volume parenterals. *PDA Journal of Pharmaceutical Science and Technology*, *70*(1), 30–38.

Jacobs, G. P., Wills, P. A. (1988). Recent developments in the radiation sterilization of pharmaceuticals. *International Journal of Radiation Applications and Instrumentation. Part C. Radiation Physics and Chemistry*, *31*(4–6), 685–691.

Karlsson, A. K., Larrivee-Elkins, C., Molin, O. (2002). U.S. Patent No. 6,392,036. U.S. Patent and Trademark Office: Washington, DC.

Kumar, A., Martin, J., Kuriyel, R. (2015). Scale-up of sterilizing-grade membrane filters from discs to pleated cartridges: Effects of operating parameters and solution properties. *PDA Journal of Pharmaceutical Science and Technology*, *69*(1), 74–87.

Lalu, L., Tambe, V., Pradhan, D., Nayak, K., Bagchi, S., Maheshwari, R., Kalia, K., Tekade, R. K. (2017). Novel nanosystems for the treatment of ocular inflammation: Current paradigms and future research directions. *Journal of Controlled Release*, *268*, 19–39.

Li, L., Mak, K. Y., Shi, J., Leung, C. H., Wong, C. M., Leung, C. W., Mak, C. S. K., Chan, K. Y., Chan, N. M. M., Wu, E. X. and Pong, P. W. T. (2013). Sterilization on dextran-coated iron oxide nanoparticles: Effects of autoclaving, filtration, UV irradiation, and ethanol treatment. *Microelectronic Engineering*, *111*, 310–313.

Maheshwari, R. G., Tekade, R. K., Sharma, P. A., Darwhekar, G., Tyagi, A., Patel, R. P., Jain, D. K. (2012). Ethosomes and ultradeformable liposomes for transdermal delivery of clotrimazole: A comparative assessment. *Saudi Pharmaceutical Journal*, *20*(2), 161–170.

Maquille, A., Jiwan, J. L. H., Tilquin, B. (2008). Radiosterilization of drugs in aqueous solutions may be achieved by the use of radioprotective excipients. *International Journal of Pharmaceutics*, *349*(1–2), 74–82.

Marsit, N., Dwejen, S., Saad, I., Abdalla, S., Shaab, A., Salem, S., Khanfas, E., Hasan, A., Mansur, M., Abdul Sammad, M. (2014). Substantiation of 25 kGy radiation sterilization dose for banked air-dried amniotic membrane and evaluation of personnel skill in influencing finished product bioburden. *Cell and Tissue Banking*, *15*, 603–611.

Masuishi, R., Fukuda, H., Murase, H. (2013). Optimal arrangement of the dry-heat sterilizer in a plant factory. *IFAC Proceedings*, *46*(4), 293–296.

McCrudden, M. T., Alkilani, A. Z., Courtenay, A. J., McCrudden, C. M., McCloskey, B., Walker, C., Alshraiedeh, N., Lutton, R. E., Gilmore, B. F., Woolfson, A. D., Donnelly, R. F. (2015). Considerations in the sterile manufacture of polymeric microneedle arrays. *Drug Delivery and Translational Research*, *5*, 3–14.

Mehmood, Y. (2014). Sterility assurance level and aseptic manufacturing process in pharmaceuticals. *International Journal of Pharmaceutical Research and Allied Sciences*, *3*(4), 10–15.

Mendes, G. C., Brandao, T. R., Silva, C. L. (2007). Ethylene oxide sterilization of medical devices: A review. *American Journal of Infection Control*, *35*(9), 574–581.

Moondra, S., Raval, N., Kuche, K., Maheshwari, R., Tekade, M., Tekade, R. K. (2018). Sterilization of pharmaceuticals: Technology, equipment, and validation. In: *Dosage form Design Parameters* (pp. 467–519). Academic Press.

Nguyen, H., Cassady, A. I., Bennett, M. B., Gineyts, E., Wu, A., Morgan, D. A., Forwood, M. R. (2013). Reducing the radiation sterilization dose improves mechanical and biological quality while retaining sterility assurance levels of bone allografts. *Bone*, *57*(1), 194–200.

Niazi, S. K. (2016). Formulations of semisolid drugs. In: *Handbook of Pharmaceutical Manufacturing Formulations Semisolid Products* (pp. 151–56). CRC Press.

Peris-Vicente, J., Esteve-Romero, J., Carda-Broch, S. (2015). Validation of analytical methods based on chromatographic techniques: An overview. *Analytical Separation Science*, *5*, 1757–1808.

Purohit, I. K., Gupta, N. V. (2017). Temperature mapping of hot air oven (Dry heat sterilizer). *Journal of Pharmacy Research*, *11*(2), 120–123.

Royalty, W., Ware, M., Nyberg, R. (2014). *Effect of Storage Conditions Upon the Resistance (D-value) of Spore Strip Biological Indicators (BIs) used in EtO Sterilization Monitoring* (pp. 1–8). Raven Biological Laboratories: Omaha, Nebraska.

Rutala, W. A., Weber, D. J. (2013). Disinfection and sterilization: An overview. *American Journal of Infection Control*, *41*(5), S2–S5.

Rutala, W. A., Weber, D. J. (2016). Disinfection, sterilization, and antisepsis: An overview. *American Journal of Infection Control*, *44*(5), e1–e6.

Sandle, T. (2013). *Sterility, Sterilisation and Sterility Assurance for Pharmaceuticals: Technology, Validation and Current Regulations* (p. 370). Woodhead Publishing Ltd.: Oxford, UK.

Schmidt, M., Gail, L., Hemel, H. (2015). Air filtration challenges and answers for dry heat sterilisation tunnels. https://ispe.org/pharmaceutical-engineering/ispeak/air-filtration-challenges-answers-dry-heat-sterilization-tunnels.

Shinde, S. J., Jain, P. S., Kale, N. K. (2013). Critical review on qualification of sterilization equipment in aseptic processing. *Journal of Pharmaceutical and BioSciences*, *1*, 24–35

Sultana, Y. (2007). *Pharmaceutical Microbiology and Biotechnology*. Jamia Hamdard: New Delhi.

Tavalsky, D. (2013). Sterilization validation, qualification requirements. ISPE—Boston Chapter Framingham MA. https://www.ispeboston.org->2013-09-19-CIP-SIP-Sterilization-DTavalsky.pdf

Tekade, R. K., Maheshwari, R., Soni, N., Tekade, M., Chougule, M. B. (2017). Nanotechnology for the development of nanomedicine. In *Nanotechnology-based Approaches for Targeting and Delivery of Drugs and Genes* (pp. 3–61). Academic Press.

Thornsberry, C., Swenson, J. M. (1980). Antimicrobial susceptibility tests for *Streptococcus pneumoniae*. *Laboratory Medicine*, *11*(2), 83–86.

Türker, N. S., Özer, A. Y., Kutlu, B., Nohutcu, R., Sungur, A., Bilgili, H., Ekizoglu, M., Özalp, M. (2014). The effect of gamma radiation sterilization on dental biomaterials. *Tissue Engineering and Regenerative Medicine*, *11*, 341–349.

Van Doornmalen, J., Kopinga, K. (2008). Review of surface steam sterilization for validation purposes. *American Journal of Infection Control*, *36*(2), 86–92.

Vaughn, E., Doletski, B. G., Dunn, T. M., Raulli, R. E. (2014). U.S. Patent No. 8,703,066. Washington, DC: U.S. Patent and Trademark Office.

Warkiani, M. E., Tay, A. K. P., Guan, G., Han, J. (2015). Membrane-less microfiltration using inertial microfluidics. *Scientific Reports*, *5*(1), 1–10.

Wong, G. M., Smith, D. J. (2014). Microorganisms in the Stratosphere (MIST), In-Flight Sterilization with UVC LEDs (No. KSC-E-DAA-TN16983).

Wood, T. (2015). Validation and implementation of alternate sterility test for cell therapy products. *Cytotherapy*, *17*(6), S28–S29.

Zitron, R., Wajsfeld, T., Klautau, G. B., da Silva, C. B., Nigro, S., Mercadante, M. T., Polesello, G. C., Cury, R. P, L., Salles, M. J. C. (2016). Concentration of sonication fluid through centrifugation is superior to membrane filtration for microbial diagnosis of orthopedic implant-associated infection. *Journal of Clinical Microbiology*, *54*(3), 788–790.

CHAPTER 5

Microbial Biofilms and Their Applications in Pharmaceuticals

SONIA SETHI

Dr. B. Lal Institute of Biotechnology, Malviya Nagar, Jaipur, Rajasthan, India

ABSTRACT

The development of biofilms is a major concern in various areas and presents significant hazards to business, healthcare, and the public at large. Bacterial biofilm formation is a significant ongoing problem because it raises morbidity and mortality, which puts tremendous financial strain on the healthcare industry. Additionally, bacterial biofilms make biofouling worse, which has an impact on offshore industry and shipping operations in their natural habitat. Additionally, they play significant roles in the corroding industrial pipelines. Bacterial pathogens are substantially more resistant to external attack at the biofilm state, including antibiotics, chemicals, and disinfectants. They lack empathy toward medication and host immunological reactions inside of cells. For bacterial infections to propagate and stay in the host, complete biofilm formation is essential. Additionally, bacteria create biofilms on every likely substrate, and human, animal, and plant illnesses have all been linked to them. There has been concern for the creation of fresh techniques for new methods for treating and preventing the formation of biofilms. A workable method that may target adhesion characteristics without impairing bacterial viability is required to stop the emergence of resistant mutants. The field of research that has been sparked to find workable controls to stop the production of biofilms is expanding quickly.

Advances in Pharmaceutical Microbiology: From Bench to Bedside. Harpreet Singh, Arun Kumar Mishra, Jeyabalan Sangeetha, and Devarajan Thangadurai (Eds.)

DOI: 10.1201/9781779640918-7

5.1 INTRODUCTION: UNVEILING THE WORLD OF MICROBIAL BIOFILMS

In the intricate tapestry of microbial life, a remarkable phenomenon has captivated the scientific community is the existence of microbial biofilms. Unlike the solitary existence of planktonic microorganisms, biofilms embody a collective and cooperative lifestyle, where microbial communities join forces to form intricate structures bonded by an EPS that is created by the cell itself. This concealed world, hidden within the crevices of medical devices, natural surfaces, and even the human body, presents a realm of challenges and opportunities that have far-reaching implications across various disciplines. Microbial biofilms have emerged as a subject of intense scrutiny, reshaping our understanding of microbiology, ecology, and medicine. From their initial attachment to surfaces to the establishment of resilient communities, the life cycle of biofilms weaves a complex narrative of adaptation, communication, and survival strategies. Beyond their mere existence, these microbial enclaves possess an innate resilience against traditional treatment methods, paving the way for a new era in pharmaceutical research. The dangerously high death and morbidity rates are significantly correlated with the sharp increase in the prevalence of infectious diseases (Leventhal et al., 2015). The dynamics of disease and the numerous elements that could support and promote disease transmission (both acute and chronic) have captured the interest of many medical professionals. Microbes cause acute infections when they are in their planktonic condition, but they can eventually adapt to their harsh habitats and evolve survival strategies. As a result, a "biofilm" is a term used to describe a type of cellular community capable of intercellular communication.

The term "extracellular polymeric substances (EPS)" describes a matrix that enables microbes to cling to both biological and nonbiological surfaces permanently, such as those present in microbial biofilms, which can represent a wide range of species (such as an interspecies relationship between bacteria and fungi). Microbial biofilms and other sites contain EPS (Burmølle et al., 2014).

Biofilms have an effect on every aspect of human existence, including public health, industrial problems, the economy, energy use, equipment deterioration, contaminated goods, and infections. Modern tools including scanning and confocal microscopy have assisted researchers in comprehending the incredibly complex structure of biofilms. These innovative methodologies have revealed that biofilms are intricate communities of cells encased in an EPS framework with permeable water channels, homogeneous cell deposition, and accumulated slime. Many human diseases and the colonization of medical equipment are linked to microorganisms that form biofilms and exhibit significant resistance to antimicrobial therapies. Biofilm formation initiates the disease process through a number of mechanisms, such as the separation of individual bacterial cells or groups of bacterial cell aggregates, the production of endotoxins, increased evasion of host immune system surveillance, and the creation of a protective barrier that is favorable to the emergence of immune-resistant organisms (Sharma et al., 2023).

Neutral or harmful biofilms are possible (Rose, 2023). In contrast to biofilms that develop on exposed wounds after infection, those that are a part of a natural ecosystem are neutral. In the case of an oil spill, biofilms might help reduce ground contamination. Biofilms have a key role in human healthcare-associated infections, which account for 70% of all microorganism-induced diseases. The microbe that is a component of the biofilm exhibits distinctive traits such group cooperation, source capture, and improved resistance to antimicrobial treatment. Biofilms are in charge of persistent chronic infections due to their improved ability to survive and avoid detection by the host immune system.

5.2 FORMATION AND CHARACTERISTICS OF MICROBIAL BIOFILMS

5.2.1 THE BIOFILM LIFE CYCLE: FROM ATTACHMENT TO MATURATION

Bacterial biofilms are collections of microorganisms whereby cells are covered in an EPS that the bacteria have self-assembled (Maier, 2021). In contrast to planktonic bacteria, which move around freely in a bulk solution, this state is very different. Cells in a multilayered biofilm interact with one another, either directly in the biofilms themselves that are in contact with the solid surface, or in flocs of mobile biofilms that are created on surfaces. A complex microbiological process, known as biofilm production involves various developmental stages, some of which are unique to the types of bacteria involved (Garrett et al., 2008).

A insulating layer of organic and inorganic molecules that are either released by the bacteria reaching the surface or settled from the bulk solution helps planktonic bacteria stick to a surface in the first place (i.e., early adhesion). Early bacterial adhesion occurs when planktonic cells stick to the surface due to interactions between the bacteria, elements of the conditioning layer, and the bacterial appendages (cilia, flagelli, and curli). The first stage of the biofilm is formed when the bacteria begin to multiply, cluster, and release EPS after the adhesion is irreversible and finally lose their ability to move. Once the biofilm reaches its maximal volume that reflects the maturation period (stage 2), bacteria continue to multiply to produce more of it. In order to colonize new surfaces, the biofilm begins to discharge planktonic bacteria when it reaches a sufficient thickness (stage 3).

Five steps are involved in the formation and growth of biofilms: (1) initial attachment of single bacteria (reversible and irreversible), (2) gathering of microbes, (3) formation of microcolonies, (4) maturity, and (5) dispersion or separation (Juhlin et al., 2017). The first phase is characterized by the production of bacterial adhesins, which promote adherence to surfaces. Free-floating planktonic bacteria perform the initial colonization of any surface. These loose floating creatures stick to the surface, develop, become sessile, absorb characteristics from their environment, and stick to the surface covalently.

5.2.1.1 INITIAL ADHERENCE

When the planktonic bacteria are free to drift in contact with any surface, attachment starts. They adhere to the surface via either physical force or bacterial appendages like flagella and/or pili. Hydrophobic, steric, electrostatic, van der Waals, and protein adhesion are some of the forces that might affect the strength of attachment. The combined action of these forces enables the bacteria to continue adhering reach the surface and defeat the opposing troops in order to form a monolayer that is permanently adhered to the surface (Buttner et al., 2015).

5.2.1.2 BACTERIAL ADHESION AND AGGREGATION

The anchoring or latching phase, also known as the second stage of adhesion, is characterized by a molecularly coordinated interaction between certain adhesins and the outermost layer. The EPS produced at this step interacts with surface components and/or receptor-specific ligands found on pili, fimbriae, and fibrillae, or both, to consolidate the loosely linked organisms through the adhesion process. By doing this, the organisms' attachment to the surface is strengthened. Planktonic bacteria are capable of sticking to different types of surface-bound organisms as well as to one another during this stage in the adhesion process, leading to the creation of an aggregation on the substrate. Different adhesins are produced by each bacterium, and the transcriptional level regulates a portion of these adhesins (D'Acunto et al., 2015).

5.2.1.3 MICROCOLONY FORMATION

Following bacterial adhesion, bacteria multiply and divide their cells to form microcolonies. In the EPS and microcommunities, unique chemical communication is what initiates this process. The interchange of substrates, the movement of important byproducts of metabolism, and the removal of metabolic waste all depend on this cooperation (D'Acunto et al., 2015).

5.2.1.4 MATURATION

The linked cells mature and continue to develop during the fourth stage of biofilm formation, called maturation. The connected bacterial cells' production of signaling molecules, which causes the expression of genes specific to biofilms, facilitates maturation. To improve bacterial virulence, signaling factors change gene regulation. EPS, which stabilizes the biofilm structure and protects it against antimicrobial agents, is released from the cells at the start of the process. In general, maturation happens in two phases: In stage I, there is direct contact between cells and the generation of autoinducer signal molecules, such as N-acylated homoserine lactone (AHL). In stage II, however, the microcolony must grow to a size and thickness of around 100 m, which is the standard for an established microcolony.

5.2.1.5 DISPERSION

A critical step in the formation of biofilms is dispersion, which is the process by which bacteria spread disease from one part of an infected person's body to another. A biofilm normally consists of two distinct layers. The surface layer serves as a dispersal zone where the bacteria disperse into their surroundings, allowing their spread and persistent presence. The fundamental layer is one component where the bacteria primarily live. This stage results in chronic infection and other severe disorders such embolic issues, which call for urgent medical care. After being freed, the bacteria either form new biofilms in various body organs or float on the surface by inducing the synthesis of proteins that helps in movement.

5.2.1.6 QUORUM SENSING (QS)

QS, a technique of cell–cell communication, synchronizes gene expression in response to the density of the population's cells. QS and the development of biofilms are interrelated processes. The QS gene directs the biofilm's formation, development, and disintegration when it is turned on. Only when there are very few bacteria in a given volume is the phenomena of QS possible. The number of bacteria in each volume of a microcolony can be calculated using the amount of autoinducer signaling molecules released by the bacteria (He et al., 2015).

5.3 UNDERSTANDING BIOFILM RESISTANCE AND ADAPTATION

5.3.1 ANTIBIOTIC TOLERANCE: DEFYING TRADITIONAL TREATMENT

A biofilm is a complex assemblage of proteins, polysaccharides, and DNA in an extracellular polymeric matrix that is made up of bacteria. Biofilms have been found on a range of surfaces, including living tissues, medical devices, and naturally occurring aquatic or drinking water systems. Numerous studies have been done on how bacteria escape phagocytosis, antibiotics, and other disinfecting agents by forming biofilms. In the natural world, biofilm communities such as macro- and micro-colonies exhibit distinctive architectural characteristics due to interstitial voids. The voids allowed nutrients, gases, and antimicrobial agents to diffuse through the biofilms; however, the architecture of the biofilms is modulated in response to these alterations in the internal and external processes. Cells exchange quorum-sensing molecules, additional chromosomal plasmids, and displayed varied characteristics in each biofilm community as a result of their close proximity.

A number of factors, such as the antibiotics' slow or ineffective penetration into the biofilm, the biofilm's changed chemical microenvironment, and a subpopulation of microbes displaying "a type of cell differentiation similar to spore formation" can lead to antibiotic resistance in biofilm communities. The multicellular nature of biofilms leads to antibiotic resistance of biofilm communities and treatment strategy failure. These processes are the outcome of this, coupled with the well-known conventional resistance mechanisms. The true source of the resistance mechanisms outlined above is the multicellular form of biofilms, which plays a significant role in the antibiotic resistance of the biofilm communities.

Use of antibiotics, sanitizers, and germicidal chemicals can be done for biofilms and related infections control. Bacteria living in biofilms show a 10–1000-fold increase in drug resistance, especially antibiotic resistance, as compared to their planktonic state (Dan et al., 2023). For instance, it has been noted that all *Staphylococcus epidermidis* biofilm isolates were vancomycin sensitive when tested planktonically. However, nearly 75% of the bacteria that were isolated from a biofilm showed resistance to antibiotics. The same findings were made about *Klebsiella pneumoniae*. When tested from a biofilm, this strain is highly resistant to particular antibiotics but is vulnerable when separated from an aqueous solution.

Antimicrobial resistance is brought on by various functional changes, varying growth rates of the microbial species that make up biofilms, and inadequate or delayed diffusion of anti-microbial drugs through biofilms. It is well recognized that bacteria in the planktonic form can evolve resistance to medications by using either enzymes, efflux pumps, or mutations. A high rate of mutation and the existence of selective pressure against microorganisms, persistence of persisters (Li et al., 2014), localized competition between mutants in the compartmentalized structure of the biofilms, and the preservation of a large population of microorganisms resistant to antibiotics are additional factors that promote the emergence of antibiotic resistance in biofilms. Prior research has identified antibiotic resistance in *Pseudomonas aeruginosa*, which was recovered from a biofilm that had been repeatedly exposed to ceftazidime (Liu et al., 2022).

5.3.2 MECHANISMS OF RESISTANCE: GENETIC AND PHENOTYPIC CHANGES

The ability of some germs to persist despite exposure to substances deemed fatal is known as antimicrobial resistance. It can be divided into three categories: (1) intrinsic, (2) acquired, and (3) adaptive since it is made possible by various methods. All inhibitory mechanisms that are built into the microbe are included in intrinsic resistance (I). This kind of resistance allows strains to persist even if they have never come into touch with the antibiotic. The process of acquired resistance (II) involves the inclusion of genetic material or mutations. Given the close proximity of the cells in this environment, this kind is extremely prevalent in biofilms (Mahamuni-Badiger et al., 2020). Adaptive resistance (III) is the capacity of a microorganism to endure due to modifications in gene or protein expression brought on by encounter to physiological distress (Blair et al., 2015). The expression of intrinsic defense systems can be altered by genetic mutations and changes brought on by environmental pressures, which can promote resistance to antimicrobials. This latter phenomenon, however, can represent a link between intrinsic and acquired resistance.

The two processes that are most frequently seen in biofilms and may be implicated in all three types of resistance are QS and horizontal gene transfer (HGT). However, other tactics to boost resistance to biocides can also be used, particularly by multidrug resistance (MDR) microorganisms. These include altering the antimicrobial target, inactivating the antimicrobial, and reducing intracellular accumulation by controlling efflux pumps and decreasing membrane permeability. In actuality, QS or HGT coordinates these strategies.

5.3.2.1 QS

A mechanism of cell-to-cell communication called QS uses chemical cues to facilitate cooperative gene expression. These genes affect a wide range of biological procedures, such as the development of biofilms, spore production, conjugation, flexibility, regulation of bacterial luminescence, and the synthesis of virulence factors such adhesins, proteases, and toxins. QS is dependent on population density and is based on communication via autoinducers, signaling substances that are identified by cell surface receptors or in the cytoplasm. As these molecules are produced, they accumulate in the biofilm environment. After the receptor is identified, transcription of genes encoding surface proteins, virulence factors, transcription factors, and proteins involved in the formation of biofilms occurs. Autoinducing peptides are the autoinducers utilized by Gram-positive bacteria, while acylated homoserin is the autoinducer used by Gram-negative bacteria (Ghasemi et al., 2018).

Recalcitrance (tolerance and antimicrobial resistance [AMR]) is favorably influenced by QS. The majority of authors do, however, suggest a clear connection and a great impact on AMR. Additionally, while QS is an inherent resistance mechanism, it also appears to have an impact on adaptive resistance. This process enables brief adaptive changes in the expression of biofilm genes; however, this event can only happen when such genes were present in the past. Some investigations discovered the genes icaA, icaB, icaD, and icaC in MDR *Staphylococcus aureus*, MDR *Salmonella*, and MDR *Listeria*, as well as the genes adrA, bapA, csgB, csgD, fimA, and fimH, and observed high biofilm generation (Bissong and Ateba, 2020).

In response to stressors, QS boosts the creation of microcolonies, favors the formation of biofilms, and increases sanitizer resistance. It also controls how proteins that are involved in the permeability of the outer membrane are produced. Since their structure is impacted by this process, mutants with QS deficiency appear to create less organized biofilms and are thus more sensitive to antimicrobials. Additionally, QS is closely related to two crucial AMR strategies: the alteration of antimicrobial targets and the management of drug efflux pumps. These tactics have previously been linked to higher antibiotic and sanitizer resistance. In a recent research investigation, investigators examined the relationship between MDR infections and QS, and they hypothesized that MDR bacteria's capacity to form biofilms enhanced antibiotic resistance (Ghasemi et al., 2018).

5.3.2.2 TRANSMISSION OF GENES HORIZONTALLY (HGT)

Another widely recognized process of adaptation in bacteria that contributes to the spread of MDR biofilms' resistance to antimicrobial agents is HGT, which happens in acquired resistance through the incorporation of genetic material and the uptake of resistance genes or mutations (Rizzo et al., 2013).

The first of the three primary pathways that make up the HGT mechanism—transduction, transformation, and plasmid-mediated conjugation—is most commonly seen in biofilms. Circular sequences of extra-chromosomal DNA are called plasmids. Antibiotic resistance is assumed to spread mostly through a process called plasmid-mediated conjugation (A). Moreover, HGT can assist MDR bacteria in acquiring pathogenicity factors and situation adaptation (Stanley et al., 2022).

In biofilms, gene transfer rates are higher due to denser and more stable populations. ARGs are absorbed partly as a result of mobile genomic element accumulation and increasing cell density. Plasmids have the ability to swiftly transfer ARGs between phyla and taxa. The T6SS secretion system is another HGT mechanism that requires cell-to-cell contact. It transfers virulence factors and effector proteins from one bacterial cell to another in a single step. This highlights the important significance that biofilms' high cell density and close proximity play in bacterial resistance (Dell'Annunziata et al., 2021).

System type VIII (T8SS), in addition to the T6SS secretion, has been linked to biofilms. T8SS is made up of three protein parts that help curli fibers assemble in the extracellular environment and are employed by Enterobacteriaceae to secrete amyloid fibers, one of the major components of biofilms. Numerous antimicrobials are resistant to this mechanism (Li et al., 2022).

Biofilms facilitate the exchange and recycling of nucleic acids because of the close proximity and prolonged retention time of cells within the EPS matrix. Various environmental factors affect the Bacteria's genetic makeup. The early stages of variation in genetics of bacteria may take place through mutations resulting in modification. Both vertical transmission and HGT can transfer genetic material. This method has the ability to transform benign bacteria into frequent human diseases. HGT includes the following methods of transferring DNA: conjugation, which involves direct contact between donor and recipient cells; transformation, which involves competent cells assimilating extracellular naked DNA; and bacteriophages, which assist DNA transfer (transduction).

A fourth process describes the exchange of genetic material that occurs during cell fusion and is mediated by outer membrane vesicles (OMVs). It is covered in the literature less extensively than other HGT mechanisms. OMVs are produced by Gram-negative bacteria, whereas membrane vesicles (MVs) are produced by Gram-positive bacteria. OMVs can act as gene-transfer vectors. Among other genetic components, they could have plasmid DNA, chromosomal DNA, phage DNA, or RNA. The contributions of OMVs to HGT have recently been examined. Numerous biofilm-forming organisms, including *Escherichia coli*, *Acinetobacter baylyi*, *P.*

aeruginosa, *Acinetobacter baumannii*, and *Porphyromonoas gingivalis*, have been demonstrated to transmit via OMV (Li et al., 2022).

In a recent study, it was shown that OMVs released by *K. pneumoniae* serve as cargo for ARGs (Dell'Annunziata et al., 2021). OMVs exposed phylogenetically diverse bacteria, including *E. coli*, *Salmonella enterica*, *P. aeruginosa*, and *Bacillus cerevisiae*, to two unique-lactam resistance plasmids. Furthermore, plasmids containing the blaCTX-M-55 and blaOXA-24 genes, respectively, can be released by *E. coli* and *A. baumannii* OMV. The mechanisms behind MV-mediated HGT in Gram-positive bacteria are poorly understood.

In *Aeromonas* spp., *P. aeruginosa*, *Pseudomonas putida*, *Helicobacter pylori*, and *Vibrio cholerae*, OMVs have been demonstrated to encourage the development of biofilms. OMVs and MVs, on the other hand, have been shown in numerous studies to be effective antibiofilm agents, such as *Burkholderia thailandensis* MVs for *Streptococcus mutans* biofilms (Wang et al., 2021). In a dual-species biofilm, *P. aeruginosa* OMVs were found to be important in suppressing *S. aureus* growth. OMVs protect DNA from exonuclease degradation, freezing-induced inactivation, and thermodegradation.

Another HGT process that was discovered in *B. subtilis* involves nanotubes as a mediator. These lengthy, membrane extracellular structures enable cell communication between adjacent cells. This makes contact-dependent chemical exchange between cells easier. It is yet unclear how they affect and change the physiological significance of genetic diversity in biofilms. The primary drivers of HGT are mobile genetic elements (MGEs), such as integrons, transposons, ICEs, and plasmids. Since most bacteria in nature live in biofilms rather than between planktonic cells, it makes likely that HGT happens more frequently there (Dubey et al., 2016).

5.4 APPLICATION OF MICROBIAL BIOFILMS IN PHARMACEUTICALS

5.4.1 DRUG DISCOVERY AND TESTING: MIMICKING IN VIVO CONDITIONS

Biofilm-based drug screening provides a more realistic model for testing antimicrobial compounds compared to traditional planktonic cultures.

Researchers can evaluate drug efficacy under conditions that closely resemble *in vivo* environments, where bacteria often exist in biofilm form. This approach enhances the likelihood of identifying compounds that effectively target biofilm-related infections, overcoming the limitations of conventional drug testing methodologies. Living organisms create biofilms, which have been linked to the development of antibiotic resistance as well as tissue and implant infections. For the successful development of antibiofilm medicines and therapies, it is crucial to comprehend biofilm production and be able to imitate such processes. The groundwork for creating *in vitro* and *in vivo* biofilm models has been developed over many decades of research. However, there is currently no such thing as "all fit" *in vitro* or *in vivo* biofilm model.

According to the National Institutes of Health, biofilms have a role in the etiology of over 80% of microbial illnesses (NIH, 2002). Biofilm microbiological infections can generally be divided into: associated with in dwelling medical devices and intrinsic to host tissues (Sun et al., 2013). For the most part, the earlier types are persistent opportunistic infections that affect various tissues and organs, such as cystic fibrosis (CF), osteomyelitis, conjunctivitis, vaginitis, urethritis, nonhealing wounds, native valve infectious endocarditis, some pediatric respiratory infections like otitis media and rhinosinusitis, as well as a variety of oral diseases such as caries, periodontitis, halitosis, and gingivitis (Filardo et al., 2019).

The protracted occurrence of biofilm-related illnesses and their high level of antibiotic and antimicrobial resistance place a financial strain on healthcare systems around the globe. Microbial biofilms are the source of many chronic infections, such as those caused by prosthetic joints, pneumonia in CF, urinary and central venous catheters, periodontitis, and persistent cutaneous wounds. Localized, slow-moving, resistant to antimicrobial treatment, and recurrent infections are typical characteristics of these conditions. They place a heavy financial strain on society as well as a heavy toll on patients, doctors, and healthcare workers. Can new medications assist to solve this issue? Because their activities and routes differ from those that are crucial for free-floating microbial cells, bacteria in biofilms present a variety of potential therapeutic targets, which is one reason to say "yes" to this question (Kostakioti et al., 2013).

It is frequently discovered that microorganisms in biofilms are particularly resistant to traditional antibiotic therapy. The majority of currently used antibiotics target a macromolecular biosynthetic process, like the creation of cell walls, DNA replication, or translation. It is widely acknowledged that biofilms exhibit physiological variability; next to dynamically growing cells that have switched to a nongrowing or latent state can also be found in them (persistant). Finding medicines that more potently target nongrowing or persistent cells is one tactic for overcoming a biofilm infection. A novel antimicrobial agent, for instance, was described by Podos et al. (2012) and is more effective than traditional antibiotics at killing staphylococci in stationary phase. According to reports, acyldepsipeptide derivatives destroy the cells that remain by triggering an endogenous protease, which causes persisters to self-digest (Conlon et al., 2013). A third instance is the anticancer medication mitomycin C, which irreversibly crosslinks DNA without requiring the cell to be actively growing (Kwan et al., 2015). Finally, by giving the right metabolic stimuli to "wake-up" persister cells, it should be feasible to enhance the effectiveness of a traditional antibiotic (Allison et al., 2011).

The adherence of a cell to an epithelial or biomaterial surface is the first stage in the fabrication of a biofilm. An efficient way to stop biofilm infection might be to stop this first stage. In the area of urinary tract infections brought on by enteric bacteria, a sophisticated pharmaceutical version of this strategy is evolving. For adhesion, these microbes rely on proteinaceous appendages like pili and curli. It is now possible to find inhibitors of the pilus and curli biosynthesis, export, and assembly processes thanks to the elucidation of their intricate molecular pathways. These substances, also known as pilicides or curlicides, have shown promise in animal models and specifically target the bacterium and the biofilm (Guiton et al., 2012).

Disrupting intercellular communication has been among a number of well-known nontraditional treatment approaches to fight biofilms. Since then, both the popular and technical press have been consistently enthusiastic about the potential of QS inhibitors. Homoserine lactones (Hense and Schuster, 2015), cis-2-unsaturated fatty acids (Ryan et al., 2015), and a furanosyl borate diester are a few examples of signaling compounds for which the interaction with biofilms has been investigated. Both agonists and antagonists of the native signal molecule have the potential to impair the regular operation of these systems.

A viable alternative method is to target the biofilm matrix since microorganisms in a biofilm might be so resistant to being killed by antimicrobial agents. Dissolving the biofilm can make the liberated cells more vulnerable to the host's defenses or common antibiotics and antiseptics, as well as to the biofilm's remaining cells. It is believed that extracellular proteins, nucleic acids, and polysaccharides make up the bulk of the biofilm matrix. It is possible to directly target these EPS or to obstruct the cellular mechanisms necessary for their formation.

Using enzymes to break down the polymers that make up the biofilm matrix is a very simple method of spreading a biofilm. The host's defenses or conventional antibiotics may be able to control bacteria that have been freed from a biofilm since they are usually more vulnerable to antimicrobial attack. Two examples of enzymes that have been shown to break down EPS in particular biofilms are polysaccharide lyases and DNAses (Nijland et al., 2010).

5.4.2 MODEL SYSTEMS FOR RESEARCH: STUDYING CHRONIC INFECTIONS

Biofilms play a pivotal role in chronic infections, such as those associated with medical implants or CF. By creating *in vitro* biofilm models, scientists can better understand the mechanisms underlying these persistent infections and explore strategies to disrupt or prevent biofilm formation. This insight can lead to the development of targeted therapies and interventions.

Following the identification of confined bacteria and the comprehension of their role in chronic illnesses in humans, *in vitro* models of bacterial infection and biofilm formation were created. Since then, numerous *in vitro* models have been developed, the majority of which are intended to replicate the production of biofilms employing certain bacteria under regulated settings. *In vitro* models, despite being frequently criticized for being overly basic, are nevertheless widely employed they are still relevant today and are essential to our mechanistic comprehension of the biology of bacterial infections and biofilms. Due to a number of benefits they provide, including low cost, simple setup, and suitability for high-throughput designs and automation in addition to their responsibilities in clarifying the underlying biology, they are highly depended upon in the current drug development paradigm as screening methods to examine libraries of antimicrobial drugs.

But there is growing recognition that these simplistic *in vitro* models sometimes leave out crucial environmental factors like a host immune system and other mammalian cells, which may mean they have poor predictive potential. In reality, a paucity of *in vitro* models that can accurately predict a drug's long-term antimicrobial effectiveness *in vivo* contributes to many promising antimicrobial medications failing to reach the bedside. To rule out false positive or false negative conditions in this regard, complementary assays must be employed, and results from these models *in vitro* must be taken extremely cautiously. Here, the general setup, benefits, and drawbacks of frequently employed *in vitro* model systems are given, with the aim that they would be helpful guidelines for both the choice of models and the interpretation of findings.

5.4.3 IN VITRO BIOFILM MODEL SYSTEMS

In vitro models serve as valuable tools for researchers to study infections and biofilms in a controlled environment that mimics certain aspects of host–pathogen interactions. These models offer a bridge between simplified laboratory experiments and complex *in vivo* conditions, allowing scientists to investigate the mechanisms of infection, biofilm formation, and potential therapeutic interventions.

5.4.4 MICROTITRE PLATE ASSAY

In these systems, biofilms grow on the surface of a coupon inserted into the wells of the microtiter plate (MTP; most frequently a 6-, 12-, or 24-well plate) or on the bottom and wall (Moreira et al., 2013) of the MTP wells (most frequently a 96-well plate). These simple and user-friendly systems have a lot of benefits, which accounts for why they are so widely used. Additionally, a number of accepted assays are accessible for figuring out various aspects of the biofilm in MTPs. They can be divided into three groups: matrix quantitation assays (via specific labeling of matrix components), viability assays (determination of viable cells), and biofilm biomass assays (matrix and live/dead cell quantification). In clinical research, MTPs are frequently used for biofilm inhibition, biofilm development, and antimicrobial compound screening. The most widely used methodology for tracking biofilm production in MTPs is crystal violet (CV) staining. This technique was modified from the original Christensen et al. (1985) method, which only quantified biofilm biomass at the bottom of the well. The fundamental dye CV stains both living and dead cells by binding to negatively charged surface molecules and polysaccharides in the EPS of biofilms.

Subsequently, the CV assay was modified to increase precision and allow for the use of dye solubilization to quantify biofilm biomass throughout the whole well. Therefore, this technique can be regarded as a bulk technique that reveals information about the total number of biofilms formed without disclosing any details on biofilm localization. Dynamic circumstances, such as shaking the MTP in an orbital motion, have been demonstrated to cause the biofilm distribution in the wall of a 96-well MTP to be less uniform. For example, using ordinary optical microscopy, confocal laser scanning microscopy (CLSM), or scanning electron microscopy, this biofilm heterogeneity can be examined under a microscope.

The "Biofilm Ring Test," an adapted MTP-based technique, was developed based on the ability of bacteria to impede magnetized beads during the biofilm-forming process. The objective of this technique is to investigate the kinetics of the early stages of biofilm formation, specifically the initial adhesion of bacteria during this phase. The kinetics of biofilm formation can be tracked by employing a plate reader to measure magnetic bead mobility.

5.4.5 SUSPENDED SUBSTRATUM REACTORS (SSRS)

A planktonic batch culture of any material of interest, such as glass beads, dental enamel, bits of biomaterial, or glass wool, can be supplemented with substrata to create the simplest biofilm model in this class. But because continuous growth has so many useful benefits, "chemostats" have frequently been preferred for use in biofilm investigations. The creation of stable states with regard to bacterial biomass and homogeneity is essential for the validity of research conducted in chemostats. Wall growth, or the establishment of a biofilm on the glass surface of the fermentation tank, was an issue that needed to be avoided since it would force the abandonment of experimental runs and lower the quality of the data that was produced. SSRs leverage the inclination of planktonic bacteria to generate biofilms at solid–liquid interfaces by incorporating detachable and colonizable materials into reactor vessels such as "chemostats" (Ahmed et al., 2007).

5.4.6 SSRS AND GENE EXPRESSION

SSRs have emerged as a valuable tool for studying gene expression within biofilms, offering insights into the intricate mechanisms governing microbial communities. By creating controlled environments where biofilms develop on suspended substrates, researchers can investigate how different factors impact gene expression patterns. For instance, in environmental microbiology, SSRs can be employed to explore how biofilm gene expression responds to varying nutrient levels, temperature shifts, or the presence of specific contaminants. The ability to sample and analyze gene expression from biofilms growing on suspended substrates provides a more accurate representation of *in situ* conditions than traditional laboratory-grown biofilms. This approach has the potential to uncover new avenues for understanding microbial behavior, developing biotechnological applications, and enhancing our knowledge of complex microbial ecosystems in diverse settings, ranging from industrial processes to natural environments.

For instance, Whiteley et al. (2001) investigated the differences between *P. aeruginosa* cells growing in biofilms formed on glass beads inside a "chemostat" vessel and those growing freely using DNA microarrays. Remarkably few genes (about 1% of all genes) displayed expression differences between the two growth phases. The study's authors sought to elucidate the mechanisms of tobramycin resistance specific to biofilms. Merely 20 genes exhibited altered expression upon exposure of biofilms to the antibiotic. Pysz et al. (2004) supported the anaerobic, thermophilic bacterium *Thermotoga maritima* biofilms in a chemostat vessel using a variety of suspended substrata.

5.4.7 THE CENTERS FOR DISEASE CONTROL AND PREVENTION (CDC) BIOFILM REACTOR

The CDC biofilm reactor is a standardized laboratory apparatus designed for the controlled cultivation and study of microbial biofilms. It is a widely recognized tool in microbiology and environmental engineering, particularly in investigating the formation, growth, and behavior of biofilms. The CDC biofilm reactor consists of multiple cylindrical glass or plastic coupons that serve as substrates for biofilm development. These coupons can be immersed in a liquid medium to simulate various environments, such as water distribution systems or medical devices, where biofilms often form. By controlling factors like flow rate, temperature, nutrient concentration, and shear forces, researchers can replicate conditions relevant to real-world scenarios.

This reactor allows scientists to explore biofilm-related phenomena, including bacterial adhesion, colonization, detachment, and resistance to antimicrobial agents. It is also used to evaluate the efficacy of different materials, coatings, or treatments in preventing or controlling biofilm growth. The CDC biofilm reactor's versatility and reproducibility make it an essential tool for advancing our understanding of biofilm-related issues and developing strategies to manage biofilms in industries like healthcare, water treatment, and more (Goeres et al., 2005).

5.4.8 ROTATING REACTORS FOR CONTROL OF SHEAR STRESS

The composition and recalcitrance of biofilms that grow at solid-liquid interfaces can be significantly impacted by the fluid dynamic forces they are exposed to (Dunsmore et al., 2002; Crabbe et al., 2008). Therefore, attempts to achieve maximum realism in biofilm models or studies aimed at studying fluid flow as a crucial variable have looked for models that enable its control. Submerged substratum reactors with integrated rotating cylinders have been developed and validated for a range of applications aimed at better understanding the effects of fluid dynamic forces upon nascent and mature biofilms, although this can also be accomplished by adjusting the flow rate and bore width in flow cells and within Robbins devices.

5.4.9 THE ROBBINS DEVICE AND FLOW CELLS

The Robbins Device and flow cells are both experimental setups used in microbiology and biotechnology to study microbial biofilms and their behavior. They provide controlled environments for observing the formation, growth, and interactions of biofilms in real time.

The Robbins Device, also known as the Robbins Device Biofilm Reactor, is a specialized apparatus used for studying biofilms under controlled hydrodynamic conditions. It consists of a rotating disk made of a material suitable for biofilm growth, such as glass or metal. This disk is partially submerged in a liquid medium, allowing microorganisms to colonize and form a biofilm on its surface. The rotation of the disk generates hydrodynamic shear forces, mimicking the dynamic conditions often found in natural environments. Researchers can adjust the rotation speed to simulate different flow rates and shear stresses, enabling the study of how biofilms respond to mechanical forces and facilitating investigations into biofilm detachment, growth patterns, and resistance to shear-induced stress (Rogers et al., 2001).

Flow cells are transparent chambers that allow for the cultivation of biofilms on surfaces while maintaining a continuous flow of liquid medium. They consist of one or more channels through which the liquid flows over a substrate, providing a consistent supply of nutrients and oxygen to the biofilm. Flow cells are often used in conjunction with microscopy techniques, such as CLSM, to observe and analyze the biofilm structure and dynamics in situ. Researchers can introduce different treatments, environmental factors, or genetic modifications to the biofilm and observe their effects in real time. Flow cells are valuable tools for gaining insights into biofilm architecture, microbial interactions, and the impact of various factors on biofilm development (Araujo et al., 2004).

5.4.10 CONTROLLED DRUG DELIVERY: UTILIZING BIOFILM MATRIX

ECM accumulation and turnover are a defining feature of tissue damage, remodeling, and repair in human disorders. Collagen, microcellular protein, elastin, proteoglycans, and fibronectin are just a few of the ECM components that have been shown to influence drug absorption, distribution, and effectiveness. Furthermore, it has been discovered that integrin, a few proteases, and other ECM biomaterials work well to support the targeted administration of medications for the treatment of a number of illnesses, including cancer (Schaefer and Reinhardt, 2016). In addition to loading drugs with integrin, it has also been reported that using interin-loaded nanoparticles (NPs) improves the drug's biodistribution and uptake into malignant cells (Arosio and Casagrande, 2016).

A substantial adaptive role in tissue repair, disease management, and treatment of tissue injury is played by hyaluronan, a key component of the ECM. Interactions, position, size, and binding partners all affect how the function works. The genes of distinct cell types control the fragmented production of hyaluronan, which controls inflammation and tissue healing.

The pathogenesis of the disease is influenced by its interactions with binding proteins, and these interactions may hold fresh promise for the development of novel therapies for inflammatory and fibrosis diseases (Liang et al., 2016). Collagen interacts with certain enzymes such as metalloproteinases and cell surface receptors to regulate a variety of cellular processes. High-resolution structures of triple-helical peptide connections formed by collagen interactions with its natural partner have been studied and tested for the goal of liposomal delivery to melanoma Elastin-like recombinant materials, Elastin-like recombinamers-based delivery methods, or recombinant technology-prepared formulations have also been evaluated for drug delivery, demonstrating the intricacy of the interplay to enable the trapping medication at the site of action (Rodríguez-Cabello et al., 2016).

5.5 BIOFILM DISRUPTION STRATEGIES: ENHANCING ANTIBIOTIC EFFICACY

Agents that prevent and eliminate the growth of biofilms are known as antibiofilm agents. While numerous chelating agents and synthetic compounds have been discovered to demonstrate some anti-biofilm action, the established anti-biofilm substances are primarily derived from natural sources. According to Plakunov et al. (2019) recent assessment, the agents should be divided into four groups depending on how they behave at different stages of biofilm formation (Table 5.1).

TABLE 5.1 Classification of Antibiofilm Agents with Functions

Antibiofilm Agents	Functions
Class I	Infiltrate the membrane of biofilm EPS and inhibit cell growth
Class II	Disrupt the bacterial adhesion and biofilm phenotypic creation
Class III	Regulates the production of EPS and the growth of bacteria with the biofilm phenotype
Class IV	Spread the developed biofilms

5.6 RECENT THERAPEUTIC APPROACHES TO INHIBIT BIOFILM GROWTH

Apart from traditional antibiotics, a few intriguing underlying methods supported by the widely used biofilm inhibitors stop biofilm formation and decrease the pathogenicity of microorganisms. 80% of human infections and disease are brought on by the majority of the bacteria that create biofilms. They are immune-resistant to the human immune system because of the EPS matrix of the biofilm. Defensins and other biofilm inhibitors have a significant role in how antimicrobial peptides work on the matrix.

5.6.1 APPROACH FOR QS BLOCKAGE

Since microorganisms' unique behavior is what causes biofilm to form, a number of studies have helped to clarify that inhibiting the QS system is a crucial strategy for stopping biofilm. Furthermore, the QS signals can be triggered by bacterial pathogens within the host to generate virulence factors and form biofilms. Therefore, the human immune system and antibiotic responses can more successfully fight the bacterial illnesses by preventing this bacterial communication with QS inhibitors (Li et al., 2020). This makes QS a more accessible therapeutic target in the fight against bacterial illnesses caused by biofilms (Li et al., 2020). As a result, it makes QS an easier therapeutic target for preventing biofilm-mediated bacterial infections. Quorum quenching is the term used to describe the phenomena of the QS system being downregulated or silenced. Three key methods can generally be used to disrupt the QS system of Gram-negative bacterial pathogens: AHL inactivation or breakdown, blocking the production of the AHL molecule, and interfering with the signal receptor are the three main effects.

5.6.2 INTERFERING WITH THE BIOSYNTHESIS OF AHL SIGNAL MOLECULES

The catalysis of the AHL molecule's synthesis in sequentially ordered processes has previously been tested *in vitro*. As the amino donor, S-adenosyl methionine forms the homoserine lactone ring moiety. An appropriately charged acyl carrier protein serves as the building block for the acyl side chain of the AHL signal (Li et al., 2016). According to research by Zano et al. (2013), AdoMet may also serve as a precursor for the synthesis of two distinct QS signal molecules. As a result, blocking AdoMet can prevent the growth of biofilm in a variety of Gram-negative bacterial pathogens. Consequently, QS inhibitors that target the production of the AHL molecule can be developed by comprehending signal generation.

5.6.3 BIODEGRADATION OR MODIFICATION OF AHL SIGNAL MOLECULE

Enzymatic degradation of AHL molecules by various enzyme classes keeps AHL from building up in the body. The homoserine lactone ring can be opened by the AHL lactonases by breaking the connection to the left of the double-bonded oxygen. The same property is also possessed by the enzyme decarboxylases, which break the double-bonded oxygen link to the right of the AHL molecule without changing the remainder of its structure. A recent study by Shastry et al. (2019) found that *Aeromonas hydrophila* biofilm formation is successfully inhibited by the lactonase enzyme AHL.

5.6.4 ANALOG COMPOUNDS' INTERFERENCE WITH RECEPTOR PROTEINS

By attaching the antagonistic molecules, the membrane receptors can be stopped from interacting with AHL signaling molecules. The physiological behavior of the bacterial population changes if there is no signal recognition, especially in terms of decreased biofilm activity, decreased pathogenicity, and decreased antibacterial tolerance. *S. epidermidis*' ability to produce biofilms has been successfully inhibited by a powerful QS inhibitor known as furanone (Hume et al., 2004). Additionally, studies conducted by Lonn-Stensrud et al. (2009) on furanone, which was isolated from the marine alga *Delisea pulchra*, have demonstrated the antagonistic activity of furanone together with a significant halt in QS signaling. Apart from the aforementioned three principal techniques, a number of antimicrobial peptides possess the capability to obstruct the QS system by disrupting the translocation of signal molecules within or outside the cell, thereby impeding the signal transduction cascade and biofilm formation (Sharma et al., 2019).

5.6.5 AN ELECTROCHEMICAL METHOD FOR THE DEGRADATION OF BIOFILMS

The electrochemical strategy is one of the most fascinating and prospective way to dramatically retard the growth of bacterial biofilms. Applying a mild electric field with a lower dose of antibiotics to remove the forming or mature biofilm is known as the "Bioelectric effect," or electrochemical approach. Numerous studies have shown that the electric potential kills biofilm organisms and lowers the amount of antibiotics required to deactivate the biofilm.

The biofilm matrix is usually difficult for antibiotics to penetrate. The shift in biofilm permeability is associated with the release of biocide ions brought on by the antimicrobial agents when exposed to an electrical field. The biofilm is thereby rendered inactive when these biocide ions penetrate the biofilm matrix. It electrophoresizes and electro-osmoses the bacterial cells to death, even at low concentrations. Wolfmeier et al. (2018) claim that the increased generation of oxygen molecules is expressed by the hydrolysis of water and pH shift in electrical impulses, which raises the minimal inhibitory concentration and makes drug-resistant bacteria and biofilm more susceptible to antibiotics.

5.6.6 MODIFYING SURFACE OF BACTERIAL ADHESION

Biofilm formation is the cause of many issues in the food, pharmaceutical, aquatic, and commercial industries. Lately, antifouling has become increasingly important, especially in the maritime environment. Due to the significant harm that biofouling caused to the marine ecosystem, marine enterprises faced many challenges. The disruption of the nutrition source in the surrounding ecosystem by biodeposition causes the biological niche in the benthic zone to become disordered. Numerous investigations have been conducted in an effort to find fresh and creative antifouling component technologies. Barnacles and other deposits, such as microbial biofilms on the surface of the ocean, are prevented or countered by antifouling substances.

Bacteriocins have the ability to suppress biofilms, making them a useful tool for managing biofilms. Furthermore, bacteriocin derived from *Lactobacillus sakei* has been shown to be effective in inhibiting the growth of *Listeria monocytogenes* biofilms on stainless steel. Several bacteriocin variations affect bacterial adherence and biofilm formation even at sub-inhibitory concentrations. By altering the hydrophobicity of the microbial cell and the substrate at the sub-inhibitory concentration, the bacteriocins bovicin HC5 and nisin targeted the microbial cellular adhesion (de Jesus Pimentel-Filho et al., 2014). This study found that bacteriocin suppresses the expression of *S. aureus* genes that regulate biofilm formation, such as icaD, fnbA, clfB, and rnaIII. Surfaces of ingestible medical equipment covered with a bactericidal substance like aryl rhodanines have prevented the biofilm development (Chung and Toh, 2014).

5.6.7 ANTIMICROBIAL LIPIDS (AML) AS INHIBITORS OF BIOFILM FORMATION

Fatty acids and monoglycerides are examples of AML, also referred to as single-chain lipid amphiphiles. Monoglycerides and fatty acids have been repeatedly shown to have antibacterial activity against a variety of infections (Wang et al., 2020). It is well known that AML work via a variety of pathways, including persistent membrane holes, preventing the activity of bacterial enzymes, destruction of cells, targeting of the bacterial surface communication system, and disruption of the electron transport chain (Verderosa et al., 2019).

Glycerol monolaurate (GML), a fatty acid made of glycerol and lauric acid, possesses antibacterial or immunomodulatory properties. The U.S. Food and Drug Administration has approved GML as a cosmetic and nutritional ingredient and has given it the general recognition as safe designation. Additionally, Schlievert and Peterson (2012) confirmed GML's ability to prevent the growth of biofilms from *Haemophilus influenzae* and *S. aureus*. They support GML's bactericidal effects on the development of mature biofilms from both bacterial pathogens. Atomic force microscopy has recently been used by Lopes et al. (2019) to support the biofilm inhibitory capacity of GML nanocapsules against *P. aeruginosa* biofilm.

In a study by Harvey et al. (2019), fluorescent microscopy with Alexa Fluor® 647 and SYTO® 9-labeled dextran conjugate was used to determine the biofilm limiting efficiency of antibacterial lipids on the cariogenic bacterium *Streptococcus mutans*. Additionally, several unsaturated fatty acids like oleic acid, linoleic acid, and palmitoleic acid have been shown to successfully prevent the biofilm growth of Gram-positive bacterial pathogens such *S. epidermidis*, *S. aureus*, and *S. mutans*. Recently, Sun et al. (2016) investigated the inhibitory efficiency of the two fatty acids docosahexaenoic acid and eicosapentaenoic acid against the biofilms of *P. gingivalis* and *Fusobacterium nucleatum*.

5.6.8 BREAKDOWN OF THE BIOFILM'S EPS MATRIX

One strategy for suppressing biofilms is to target the EPS, which is mostly composed of polysaccharides, proteins, and nucleic acids (e-DNA). The biofilm disintegration is enabled by the malfunctioning of the EPS matrix components. Lipopolysaccharide, alginate, Psl (Polysaccharide synthesis locus), and Pel (Pellicle) are the primary EPS of the *P. aeruginosa* biofilm (Rabin et al., 2015). Alginate lyase, DNase, and hydrolase-based methods are additional significant processes associated with the effect on the biofilm's EPS matrix breakdown.

5.6.9 REPRESSION OF THE ALARMONE STRATEGIES

Under stress conditions like nutrient depletion, bacteria are thought to take an essential phase in their production of some substances in the alarmone system, such as guanidine 3′diphosphate 5′triphosphate (pppGpp) and guanidine 3′5′bis-diphosphate (ppGpp), which are collectively communicated as (p)ppGpp by the cassette of RelA and SpoT. With the assistance of the bifunctional enzyme Rel/Spo for both the hydrolysis and synthesis, the signal molecule (p)ppGpp, which is produced by RelA and hydrolyzed by SpoT, controls the stringent response in Eubacteria, particularly in Gram-negative bacteria and in Gram-positive bacteria. The stringent response mediation that regulates the growth of biofilms in *S. mutans* and *E. coli* is brought about by these molecules. AMP 1,018 acts as a biofilm inhibitor, eliminating the alarmone ((p)ppGpp) signal. In a previous work (De La Fuente-Nunez et al., 2014), the biofilm inhibitory effectiveness of the peptides 1018 was revealed.

5.6.10 ENZYME-MEDIATED BIOFILM CONTROL

The dissolution of different bacterial species' biofilms is mediated by specific enzymes. However, certain endogenous matrix-degrading enzymes produced by the bacteria themselves, such as glycosidases, proteases, and DNase, may promote the dispersal of the biofilm. Gram-positive and Gram-negative bacteria are both sensitive to the biofilm-inhibitory effects of DNase. As e-DNA is necessary for the EPS's primary adherence and agglomeration onto the substrate, which will keep the biofilm robust for an extended period of time. DNase also plays a role in breaking down the phosphodiester linkage in the backbone of e-DNA molecules in the produced biofilm. Additionally, according to Chagnot et al. (2013), e-DNA is one of the elements required for the development, maintenance, and control of biofilms.

5.6.11 PHOTODYNAMIC APPROACH

The most cutting-edge technique recently developed for the dissolution of biofilms is the photodynamic approach. The fundamental idea behind this strategy is the use of photosensitizing compounds, which attach to the target biological components including lipid, protein, and nucleic acid and absorb light intensity of a particular wavelength. It causes reactive oxygen radicals to form, which then lead to toxic/lethal effects on the target in the form of hydrogen peroxide, hydroxyl radicals, and superoxide anion. The most recent efforts to demonstrate biofilm inhibition in this area can be found in Gholibegloo et al. (2018). The photosensitive agent and the source of light utilized are crucial for this kind of automated clearance of biofilms through photodynamic intervention. The photosensitive substances that are frequently employed are methylene blue, toluidine blue, and toluidine blue O.

According to Sadekuzzaman et al. (2015), further photosensitizers include 23H-porphine, tetrakis (1-methyl-pyridino)-21H, tetrakis (phenylthio)-29H, 31H-phthalocyanine, and tetra-p-tosylate salt. Methylene blue has an absorption spectrum at 664 nm, while toluidine blue has an absorption spectrum at 638 nm and is in the 600–1000 nm area of the UV-visible spectrum. The ability of methylene blue photosensitizer to kill Gram-positive bacteria outweighs its effectiveness against other bacterial diseases. It is because the presence of teichoic acid makes it more successful at transmitting the negative charge to the target cell with a negative charge cell wall (de Oliveira et al., 2019).

5.7 OTHER THERAPEUTIC APPROACHES

5.7.1 PHAGE THERAPY AND CRISPR–CAS 9

Treatment of wound biofilm infections and device-related infections has demonstrated a remarkable impact, according to recent experimental and clinical research. Large populations of bacteria in the biofilms allow the bacteriophages to infect their host and multiply thereafter. This process happens swiftly and efficiently. Numerous characteristics of bacteriophages may make biofilms susceptible to them. Enzymes that break down the ECM are known to be produced by or induced by them. Additionally, they can infect persister cells. According to Tkhilaishvili et al. (2018), bacteriophages like Sb-1 improved antibiotic action against biofilm.

A unique method for editing the genome in some prokaryotes and eukaryotes is the CRISPR-Cas9 system, which combines clustered regularly interspaced short palindromic repeats and CRISPR–associated protein 9 (Gou et al., 2019). For managing biofilm-associated infections, Zuberi et al. (2017) most recently used CRISPRi technology to suppress the luxS gene and the fimbriae-associated gene (fimH). CRISPRi appears to be another viable tool for managing biofilms as a result.

5.7.2 VACCINES

Antibiotic-resistant organisms develop the ability to colonize and circumvent host defenses. Because vaccinations are unique to a certain microbe and exhibit significant heterogeneity when vaccine-targeted peptides are expressed, utilizing vaccines to target biofilms presents various challenges. However, a number of conjugative vaccines have recently been developed that focus on generally preserved EPS components. Staphvax is a conjugative vaccine that targets the CP5 and CP5 capsular polysaccharide serotypes of *S. aureus* (Parastan et al., 2020). The integration host factor, a member of the DNABII family of DNA-binding proteins, gives eDNA in biofilms structural stability.

5.7.3 BIOMATERIALS AND NPS

Global healthcare is at great risk as a result of pathogenic biofilms that have developed on human tissues or implantable medical devices (IMDs). Functionalized biomaterials might represent a fresh way to fight and get rid of pre-existing biofilms. IMD-associated infections begin with bacterial adhesion, which allows germs to colonize the implants. Biofilms could be prevented by enveloping the implants in biomaterials possessing antifouling and antibacterial properties. Drugs with NP coatings could be used to disperse biofilms in order to eradicate them (Huang et al., 2020).

NPs are viewed as an alternative to antibiotics for treating infections that are biofilm-associated and multidrug-resistant. The interaction between the biofilm and NP occurs in three steps: NP transit across the biofilm, NP adsorption to the biofilm EPS, and NP piercing and migration via dissemination inside the biofilm are all possible outcomes of NP transport. These processes can be impacted by the biofilm's pore sizes, charges, hydrophobicity, and chemical gradient (Ikuma et al., 2015). Antibiotic therapy has several drawbacks, like decreased penetration into the biofilm, but these might be easily remedied by using their nano-formulations, which can pass the biological barrier.

5.8 CASE STUDIES: BIOFILM-RELATED PHARMACEUTICAL INNOVATIONS

5.8.1 ANTIBIOTIC-ELUTING WOUND DRESSINGS

A pharmaceutical company developed wound dressings embedded with antibiotics that are released slowly over time to treat infected wounds. The biofilm formed on chronic wounds often hinders healing and leads to treatment-resistant infections. These dressings not only provide a physical barrier to protect the wound but also deliver antibiotics directly to the biofilm, targeting the bacteria responsible for the infection. This approach improves wound healing outcomes and reduces the risk of antibiotic resistance.

5.8.2 CF TREATMENT

Patients with CF often suffer from chronic lung infections caused by bacterial biofilms. Researchers have developed inhaled antibiotics that specifically target the biofilm-forming bacteria in CF patients' lungs. These antibiotics disrupt the biofilm structure and enhance the effectiveness of treatment, leading to improved lung function and reduced exacerbations in CF patients.

5.8.3 BIOFILM-TARGETING NPS

NPs have been engineered to target and disrupt bacterial biofilms. These NPs are designed to carry antimicrobial agents and can penetrate the biofilm matrix. Once inside, they release the antimicrobial agents, effectively killing bacteria within the biofilm. This approach has potential applications in medical implants and catheters, where biofilm-related infections are a significant concern.

5.8.4 ORAL HEALTH PRODUCTS

Dental plaque is a type of biofilm that forms on teeth, leading to cavities and gum disease. Some toothpaste and mouthwash formulations now contain biofilm-disrupting agents that prevent the adhesion of bacteria to teeth surfaces and interfere with the biofilm formation process. This innovation contributes to improved oral hygiene and reduces the risk of dental diseases.

5.8.5 IMPLANT COATINGS

Biofilm formation on medical implants, such as joint replacements, can lead to device-related infections. Researchers have developed implant coatings that release antimicrobial agents, preventing biofilm formation and reducing the risk of infection. These coatings improve the longevity of implants and minimize the need for revision surgeries.

These case studies showcase the diverse applications of biofilm-related pharmaceutical innovations across various medical and healthcare fields. By targeting biofilms, these innovations address challenges related to antibiotic resistance, chronic infections, and medical device-related complications, ultimately improving patient outcomes and quality of life.

5.9 FUTURE PROSPECTS AND CHALLENGES

Advances in understanding the diversity of biofilm compositions and behaviors could lead to personalized treatment strategies tailored to specific biofilm types and environments. Targeting pressing issues in health, materials, energy, and the environment, synthetic biology (SB) is a promising interdisciplinary research field. It has the potential to design and build newer manufactured devices, artificial metabolic pathways, and organisms, as well as reform existing natural and biological systems. Utilizing SB, researchers might engineer biofilms for beneficial purposes, such as bioremediation, bioproduction, and drug delivery. Harnessing biofilms for innovative technologies, such as bioenergy production, biosensors, and bioreactors, holds potential for sustainable applications.

Developing combination therapies that target multiple aspects of biofilm formation, such as both QS and matrix disruption, could enhance treatment efficacy. Continued development of nanomaterials and nanotechnologies could offer precise ways to disrupt and control biofilms on various surfaces.

5.10 CHALLENGES IN BIOFILM RESEARCH

Biofilm communities are highly heterogeneous, posing challenges in terms of treatment effectiveness, as different parts of the biofilm may respond differently to interventions. Developing rapid and accurate methods for diagnosing biofilm-related infections remains a challenge, as biofilms are often hard to detect using standard techniques. Biofilms inherently exhibit increased resistance to antibiotics and immune responses, necessitating the exploration of alternative treatment strategies. Understanding the complex interactions between different microorganisms within biofilms and their adaptations to changing environments is crucial. Incorporating biofilm-related innovations into medical practices might require navigating regulatory pathways due to the unique challenges biofilms present. Even after successful treatment, dormant bacteria within biofilms can re-emerge, leading to relapses in infections. Lack of standardized protocols for studying and characterizing biofilms makes comparisons across studies challenging. The manipulation of biofilms for various purposes raises ethical questions, particularly in environmental and medical contexts.

5.11 CONCLUSION: PAVING THE WAY FOR BIOFILM-BASED PHARMACEUTICALS

In the realm of pharmaceutical innovation, biofilm research is illuminating new paths to address complex challenges that have long posed significant hurdles. Biofilms, intricate communities of microorganisms embedded within self-produced matrices, have shown remarkable resilience and adaptability. While once primarily associated with persistent infections and industrial fouling, biofilms are now being harnessed as a source of inspiration for ground breaking pharmaceutical solutions. The journey of exploring biofilm-based pharmaceuticals has led to remarkable strides in several directions. By deciphering the intricate communication systems within biofilms, researchers are designing QS inhibitors and other molecules that disrupt bacterial coordination, potentially curbing biofilm formation and enhancing treatment outcomes. The development of biofilm-targeting NPs and controlled drug delivery systems capitalizes on the unique matrix architecture of biofilms, enabling precise and sustained therapeutic interventions.

In the realm of wound care, biofilm-based pharmaceuticals are reshaping chronic wound management through antibiotic-eluting dressings that tackle biofilm-related infections head-on. Moreover, the utilization of biofilm engineering to cultivate therapeutic biofilms for environmental cleanup, bioproduction, and personalized drug delivery highlights the transformative potential of this field. However, challenges remain. The intricate nature of biofilms demands a comprehensive understanding of their biology and behavior. The journey toward regulatory approval for novel biofilm-based pharmaceuticals requires careful navigation, as does the ethical consideration of manipulating biofilms for human and environmental benefit.

As we stand on the precipice of an era characterized by precision medicine, personalized therapies, and sustainable solutions, biofilm-based pharmaceuticals hold the promise of a paradigm shift. By leveraging the very structures that once confounded us, we are crafting innovative tools to combat infections, enhance medical treatments, and contribute to a more harmonious coexistence with our microbial counterparts. The journey has just begun, and as we navigate the complexities, one thing remains clear: biofilm-based pharmaceuticals are illuminating a promising path toward a healthier and more resilient future.

KEYWORDS

- **biofilm**
- **microbial community**
- **adhesion**
- **aggregation**
- **bioreactors**
- **genetic changes**
- **phenotypic changes**

REFERENCES

Ahmed, S., Macfarlane, G. T., Fite, A., McBain, A. J., Gilbert, P., Macfarlane, S. (2007). Mucosa-associated bacterial diversity in relation to human terminal ileum and colonic biopsy samples. *Applied and Environmental Microbiology, 73*, 7435–7442.

Allison, K. R., Brynildsen, M. P., Collins, J. J. (2011). Metabolite-enabled eradication of bacterial persisters by aminoglycosides. *Nature, 473*, 216–220. https://doi.org/10.1038/nature10069.

Araujo, J. C., Mortara, R., Campos, J. R., Vazoller, R. F. (2004). Development and analysis of anaerobic biofilms onto hydrophobic and hydrophilic surfaces. *Environmental Technology, 25*, 809–817.

Arosio, D., Casagrande, C. (2016). Advancement in integrin facilitated drug delivery. *Advanced Drug Delivery Reviews, 97*, 111–143.

Bissong, M. E. A., Ateba, C. N. (2020). Genotypic and phenotypic evaluation of biofilm production and antimicrobial resistance in *Staphylococcus aureus* isolated from milk, North West Province, South Africa. *Antibiotics, 9*, 156.

Blair, J., Webber, M. A., Baylay, A. J.,Ogbolu, D. O., Piddock, L. J. (2015). Molecular mechanisms of antibiotic resistance. *Nature Reviews Microbiology, 13*, 42–51.

Burmølle, M., Ren, D., Bjarnsholt, T., Sørensen, S. J. (2014). Interactions in multispecies biofilms: Do they actually matter? *Trends in Microbiology, 22*, 84–91. https://doi.org/10.1016/j.tim.2013.12.004

Buttner, H., Mack, D., Rohde, H. (2015). Structural basis of *Staphylococcus epidermidis* biofilm formation: Mechanisms and molecular interactions. *Frontiers in Cellular and Infection Microbiology, 5*, 14.

Chagnot, C., Zorgani, M. A., Astruc, T., Desvaux, M. (2013). Proteinaceous determinants of surface colonization in bacteria: Bacterial adhesion and biofilm formation from a protein secretion perspective. *Frontiers in Microbiology, 4*, 303.

Christensen,G. D., Simpson, W. A., Younger, J. J. (1985). Adherence of coagulase-negative staphylococci to plastic tissue cultureplates: A quantitative model for the adherence of staphylococci to medical devices. *Journal of Clinical Microbiology, 22*(6), 996–1006.

Chung, P. Y., Toh, Y. S. (2014). Anti-biofilm agents: Recent breakthrough against multi-drug resistant *Staphylococcus aureus*. *Pathogens and Disease, 70*, 231–239. https://doi.org/10.1111/2049-632x.12141

Conlon, B. P., Nakayasu, E. S., Fleck, L. E., LaFleur, M. D., Isabella, V. M., Coleman, K., Leonard, S. N., Smith, R. D., Adkins, J. N., Lewis, K. (2013). Activated ClpP kills persisters and eradicates a chronic biofilm infection. *Nature, 503*, 365–370. https://doi.org/10.1038/nature12790.

Crabbe, A., De Boever, P., Van Houdt, R., Moors, H., Mergeay, M., Cornelis, P. (2008). Use of the rotating wall vessel technology to study the effect of shear stress on growth behaviour of *Pseudomonas aeruginosa* PA01. *Environmental Microbiology, 10*, 2098–2110

D'Acunto, B., Frunzo, L., Klapper, I., Mattei, M. R. (2015). Modeling multispecies biofilms including new bacterial species invasion. *Mathematical Biosciences, 259*, 20–26. https://doi.org/10.1016/j.mbs.2014.10.009

Dan, B., Dai, H., Zhou, D., Tong, H., Zhu, M. (2023) Relationship between drug resistance characteristics and biofilm formation in *Klebsiella pneumoniae* strains. *Infection and Drug Resistance, 16*, 985–998.

De La Fuente-Nunez, C., Korolik, V., Bains, M., Nguyen, U., Breidenstein, E. B., Horsman, S.(2012). Inhibition of bacterial biofilm formation and swarming motility by a small synthetic cationic peptide. *Antimicrobial Agents and Chemotherapy, 56*, 2696–2704. https://doi.org/10.1128/aac.00064-12

de Oliveira, A. B., Ferrisse, T. M., Marques, R. S., De Annunzio, S. R., Brighenti, F. L., Fontana, C. R. (2019). Effect of photodynamic therapy on microorganisms responsible for dental caries: A systematic review and meta-analysis. *International Journal of Molecular Sciences, 20*, 3585. https://doi.org/10.3390/ijms20143585

Dell'Annunziata, F., Folliero, V., Giugliano, R., de Filippis, A., Santarcangelo, C., Izzo, V., Daglia, M., Galdiero, M., Arciola, C. R., Franci, G. (2021). Gene transfer potential of outer membrane vesicles of gram-negative bacteria. *International Journal of Molecular Sciences*, *22*, 5985.

Dubey, G. P., Malli Mohan, G. B., Dubrovsky, A.,Amen, T.,Tsipshtein, S.,Rouvinski, A., Rosenberg, A., Kaganovich, D., Sherman, E., Medalia, O., (2016). Architecture and characteristics of bacterial nanotubes. *Developmental Cell, 36*, 453–461

Dunsmore, B. C., Jacobsen, A., Hall-Stoodley, L., Bass, C. J., Lappin-Scott, H. M., Stoodley, P. (2002). The influence of fluid shear on the structure and material properties of sulphate-reducing bacterial biofilms. *Journal of Industrial Microbiology and Biotechnology,* 29, 347–353.

Filardo, S., Di Pietro, M., Tranquilli, G., Sessa, R. (2019). Biofilm in genital ecosystem: A potential risk factor for *Chlamydia trachomatis* infection. *Canadian Journal of Infectious Diseases and Medical Microbiology* 1672109.

Garrett, T.R., Bhakoo, M., Zhang, Z.B. (2008). Bacterial adhesion and biofilms on surfaces. *Progress in Natural Science: Materials International, 18*, 1049–1056, https://doi.org/10.1016/j.pnsc.2008.04.001.

Ghasemi, M., Hense, B. A., Eberl, H. J., Kuttler, C. (2018). Simulation-based exploration of quorum sensing triggered resistance of biofilms to antibiotics. *Bulletin of Mathematical Biology, 80*, 1736–1775

Gholibegloo, E., Karbasi, A., Pourhajibagher, M., Chiniforush, N., Ramazani, A., Akbari, T. (2018). Carnosine-graphene oxide conjugates decorated with hydroxyapatite as promising nanocarrier for ICG loading with enhanced antibacterial effects in photodynamic therapy against *Streptococcus mutans*. *Journal of Photochemistry and Photobiology B: Biology, 181*, 14–22. https://doi.org/10.1016/j.jphotobiol.2018.02.004

Goeres, D. M., Loetterle, L. R., Hamilton, M. A., Murga, R., Kirby, D. W., Donlan, R. M. (2005). Statistical assessment of a laboratory method for growing biofilms. *Microbiology, 151*, 757–762.

Gou, Y., Liu, W., Wang, J. J., Tan, L., Hong, B., Guo, L., Liu, H., Pan, Y., Zhao, Y. (2019). CRISPR-Cas9 knockout of *qseB* induced asynchrony between motility and biofilm formation in *Escherichia coli*. *Canadian Journal of Microbiology*, *65*(9), 691–702. https://doi.org/10.1139/cjm-2019-0100

Guiton, P. S., Cusumano, C. K., Kline, K. A., Dodson, K. W., Han, Z., Janetka, J. W., Henderson, J. P., Caparon, M. G., Hultgren, S. J. (2012). Combinatorial small-molecule therapy prevents uropathogenic *Escherichia coli* catheter-associated urinary tract infections in mice. *Antimicrobial Agents and Chemotherapy, 56*, 4738–4745. https://doi.org/10.1128/AAC.00447-12.

Harvey, V., Brady, D., Kealey, C. (2019). Effect of antibacterial lipids on biofilm formation by *Streptococcus mutans. Access. Microbiol. 1*, 871.

He, Z., Liang, J., Tang, Z., Ma, R., Peng, H., Huang, Z. (2015). Role of the luxS gene in initial biofilm formation by *Streptococcus mutans. Journal of Microbiology and Biotechnology,25*, 60–68.

Hense, B. A., Schuster, M. (2015). Core principles of bacterial autoinducer systems. *Microbiology and Molecular Biology Reviews, 79*, 153–169. https://doi.org/10.1128/MMBR.00024-14.

Huang, D., Wang, J., Ren, K., Ji, J. (2020). Functionalized biomaterials to combat biofilms. *Biomaterials Science, 8*, 4126–4140. https://doi.org/10.1039/D0BM00526F.

Hume, E., Baveja, J., Muir, B., Schubert, T., Kumar, N., Kjelleberg, S. (2004). Thecontrol of *Staphylococcus epidermidis* biofilm formation and in vivo infection rates bycovalently bound furanones. *Biomaterials, 25*, 5023–5030. https://doi.org/10.1016/j.biomaterials.2004.01.048

Ikuma, K., Decho, A. W., Lau, B. L. T. (2015). When nanoparticles meet biofilms—interactions guiding the environmental fate and accumulation of nanoparticles. *Frontiers in Microbiology, 6*, 591. https://doi.org/10.3389/fmicb.2015.00591.

Juhlin, A., Svensson, S.,Thomsen, P., Trobos, M. (2017). Staphylococcal biofilm gene expression on biomaterials—a methodological study. *Journal of Biomedical Materials Research Part A, 105*, 3400–3412.

Kostakioti, M., Hadjifrangiskou, M., Hultgren, S. J. (2013). Bacterial biofilms: Development, dispersal, and therapeutic strategies in the dawn of the postantibiotic era. *Cold Spring Harbor Perspectives in Medicine, 3*, a010306. https://doi.org/10.1101/cshperspect.a010306.

Kwan, B. W., Chowdhury, N., Wood, T. K. (2015). Combatting bacterial infections by killing persister cells with mitomycin C. *Environmental Microbiology* https://doi.org/10.1111/1462-2920.12873.

Leventhal, G. E., Hill, A. L., Nowak, M. A., Bonhoeffer, S. (2015). Evolution and emergence of infectious diseases in theoretical and real-world networks. *Nature Communications, 6*, 6101. https://doi.org/10.1038/ncomms7101.

Li, L., Mendis, N., Trigui, H., Oliver, J. D., Faucher, S. P. (2014). The importance of the viable but non-culturable state in human bacterial pathogens. *Frontiers in Microbiology, 5*, 258.

Li, D., Ramanathan, S., Wang, G., Wu, Y., Tang, Q., Li, G. (2020). Acetylation of lysine 7 of AhyI affects the biological function in *Aeromonas hydrophila. Microbial Pathogenesis, 140*, 103952. https://doi.org/10.1016/j.micpath.2019.103952

Li, C., Wen, R., Mu, R., Chen, X., Ma, P., Gu, K., Huang, Z., Ju, Z., Lei, C., Tang, Y. (2022) Outer membrane vesicles of avian pathogenic *Escherichia coli* mediate the horizontal transmission of *bla*CTX-M-55. *Pathogens, 11*, 481.

Li, W., Yao, Z., Sun, L., Hu, W., Cao, J., Lin, W. (2016). Proteomics analysis reveals a potential antibiotic cocktail therapy strategy for *Aeromonas hydrophila* infection in biofilm. *Journal of Proteome Research, 15*, 1810–1820. https://doi.org/10.1021/acs.jproteome.5b01127

Liang, J., Jiang, D., Noble, P. W. (2016). Hyaluronan as a therapeutic target in human diseases. *Advanced Drug Delivery Reviews, 97*, 186–193.

Liu, Q.,Yin, L., Zhang, X., Zhu, G., Liu, H., Bai, F., Cheng, Z.,Wu, W., Jin, Y. (2022). Reversion of ceftazidime resistance in *Pseudomonas aeruginosa* under clinical setting. *Microorganisms, 10*, 2395.

Lonn-Stensrud, J., Landin, M. A., Benneche, T., Petersen, F. C., Scheie, A. A. (2009). Furanones, potential agents for preventing *Staphylococcus epidermidis* biofilm infections? *Journal of Antimicrobial Chemotherapy, 63*, 309–316. https://doi.org/10.1093/jac/dkn501

Lopes, L. Q. S., De Almeida Vaucher, R., Giongo, J. L., Gündel, A., Santos, R. C. V. (2019). Characterisation and anti-biofilm activity of glycerol monolaurate nanocapsules against *Pseudomonas aeruginosa. Journal of Antimicrobial Chemotherapy, 130*, 178–185. https://doi.org/10.1016/j.micpath.2019.03.007

Mahamuni-Badiger, P. P., Patil, P. M., Badiger, M. V., Patel, P. R., Thorat-Gadgil, B. S., Pandit, A., Bohara, R. A. (2020). Biofilm formation to inhibition: Role of zinc oxide-based nanoparticles. *Materials Science and Engineering C, 108*, 110319

Maier, B. (2021). How physical interactions shape bacterial biofilms. *Annual Review of Biophysics, 50*, 401–417, https://doi.org/10.1146/annurev-biophys-062920-063646.

Moreira, J. M. R., Gomes, L. C., Araujo, J. D. P. (2013). The effect of glucose concentration and shaking conditions on *Escherichia coli* biofilm formation in microtiter plates. *Chemical Engineering Science, 94*, 192–199.

NIH. (2002). Available at: https://grants.nih.gov/grants/guide/pa-files/PA-03-047.html

Nijland, R., Hall, M. J., Burgess, J. G. (2010). Dispersal of biofilms by secreted, matrix degrading, bacterial DNase. *PLoS One, 14*, e15668. https://doi.org/10.1371/journal.pone.0015668.

Parastan, R., Kargar, M., Solhjoo, K., Kafilzadeh, F. (2020). *Staphylococcus aureus* biofilms: Structures, antibiotic resistance, inhibition, and vaccines. *Gene Reports, 20*, 100739. https://doi.org/10.1016/j.genrep.2020.100739.

Plakunov, V. K., Zhurina, M. V., Gannesen, A. V., Mart'yanov, S. V., Nikolaev, Y. A. (2019). Antibiofilm agents: Therminological ambiguity and strategy for search. *Microbiology, 88*, 747–750. https://doi.org/10.1134/S0026261719060146

Podos, S. D., Thanassi, J. A., Leggio, M., Pucci, M. J. (2012). Bactericidal activity of ACH-702 against nondividing and biofilm Staphylococci. *Antimicrobial Agents and Chemotherapy, 56*, 3812–3818. https://doi.org/10.1128/AAC.00092-12.

Pysz, M. A., Conners, S. B., Montero, C. I., Shockley, K. R., Johnson, M. R., Ward, D. E., Kelly, R. M. (2004). Transcriptional analysis of biofilm formation processes in the anaerobic, hyperthermophilic bacterium *Thermotoga maritima. Applied and Environmental Microbiology, 70*, 6098–6112

Rabin, N., Zheng, Y., Opoku-Temeng, C., Du, Y., Bonsu, E., Sintim, H. O. (2015). Biofilm formation mechanisms and targets for developing antibiofilm agents. *Future Medicinal Chemistry, 7*, 493–512. https://doi.org/10.4155/fmc.15.6

Rizzo, L., Manaia, C., Merlin, C., Schwartz, T., Dagot, C., Ploy, M. C., Michael, I., Fatta-Kassinos, D. (2013). Urban wastewater treatment plants as hotspots for antibiotic resistant bacteria and genes spread into the environment: A review. *Science of the Total Environment, 447*, 345–360.

Rodríguez-Cabello, J. C., Arias, F. J., Rodrigo, M. A., Girotti, A. (2016). Elastin-like polypeptides in drug delivery. *Advanced Drug Delivery Reviews, 97*, 85–100.

Rogers, J. D., Palmer, R. J., Jr., Kolenbrander, P. E., Scannapieco, F. A. (2001). Role of *Streptococcus gordonii* amylase-binding protein A in adhesion to hydroxyapatite, starch metabolism, and biofilm formation. *Infection and Immunity, 69*, 7046–7056.

Rose, J. B. (2023). Biofilms: The good and the bad. Available at: https://waterandhealth.org/safe-drinking-water/drinking-water/biofilms-good-bad-2/. Access 5 May, 2023.

Ryan, R. P., An, S. Q., Allan, J. H., McCarthy, Y., Dow, J. M. (2015). The DSF family of cell-cell signals: An expanding class of bacterial virulence regulators. *PLoS Pathogens, 11*, e1004986. https://doi.org/10.1371/journal.ppat.1004986.

Sadekuzzaman, M., Yang, S., Mizan, M., Ha, S. (2015). Current and recent advanced strategies for combating biofilms. *Comprehensive Reviews in Food Science and Food Safety, 14*, 491–509. https://doi.org/10.1111/1541-4337.12144

Schaefer, L., Reinhardt, D. P. (2016). Extracellular matrix: Therapeutic tools and targets in cancer treatment. *Advanced Drug Delivery Reviews, 97*(1–3), 116.

Schlievert, P. M., Peterson, M. L. (2012). Glycerol monolaurate antibacterial activity in broth and biofilm cultures. *PLoS One, 7*, e40350. https://doi.org/10.1371/journal.pone.0040350

Sharma, D., Misba, L., Khan, A. U. (2019). Antibiotics versus biofilm: An emerging battleground in microbial communities. *Antimicrobial Resistance & Infection Control, 8*, 1–10.

Sharma, S., Mohler, J., Mahajan, S. D., Schwartz, S. A., Bruggemann, L., Aalinkeel, R. (2023), Microbial biofilm: a review on formation, infection, antibiotic resistance, control measures, and innovative treatment. *Microorganisms, 11*, 1614. https://doi.org/10.3390/microorganisms11061614.

Shastry, R. P., Rekha, P., Rai, V. R. (2019). Biofilm inhibitory activity of metallo-protein AHL-lactonase from cell-free lysate of endophytic *Enterobacter* species isolated from *Coscinium fenestratum* Gaertn. *Biocatalysis and Agricultural Biotechnology, 18*, 101009. https://doi.org/10.1016/j.bcab.2019.01.047

Stanley, D., Batacan, R., Bajagai, Y. S. (2022). Rapid growth of antimicrobial resistance: The role of agriculture in the problem and the solutions. *Applied Microbiology and Biotechnology, 106*, 6953–6962.

Sun, F., Qu, F., Ling, Y., Mao, P., Xia, P., Chen, H., Zhou, D. (2013). Biofilm-associated infections: Antibiotic resistance and novel therapeutic strategies. *Future Microbiology, 8*, 877–886.

Sun, M., Zhou, Z., Dong, J., Zhang, J., Xia, Y., Shu, R. (2016). Antibacterial and antibiofilm activities of docosahexaenoic acid (DHA) and eicosapentaenoic acid (EPA) against periodontopathic bacteria. *Microbial Pathogenesis, 99*, 196–203. https://doi.org/10.1016/j.micpath.2016.08.025

Tkhilaishvili, T., Lombardi, L., Klatt, A. B., Trampuz, A., Di Luca, M. (2018). Bacteriophage Sb-1 enhances antibiotic activity against biofilm, degrades exopolysaccharide matrix and targets persisters of *Staphylococcus aureus*. *International Journal of Antimicrobial Agents, 52*, 842–853. https://doi.org/10.1016/j.ijantimicag.2018.09.006.

Verderosa, A. D., Totsika, M., Fairfull-Smith, K. E. (2019). Bacterial biofilm eradication agents: A current review. *Frontiers in Chemistry, 7*, 824.

Wang, Y., Hoffmann, J. P., Baker, S. M., Bentrup, K. H., Wimley, W. C., Fuselier, J. A., Bitoun, J. P., Morici, L. A. (2021). Inhibition of *Streptococcus mutans* biofilms with bacterial-derived outer membrane vesicles. *BMC Microbiology*, *21*, 234.

Wang, W., Wang, R., Zhang, G., Chen, F., Xu, B. (2020). In vitro antibacterial activities and mechanisms of action of fatty acid monoglycerides against four foodborne bacteria. *Journal of Food Protection, 83*, 331–337. https://doi.org/10.4315/0362-028x.jfp-19-259.

Whiteley, M., Bangera, M. G., Bumgarner, R. E., Parsek, M. R., Teitzel, G. M., Lory, S., Greenberg, E. P. (2001). Gene expression in *Pseudomonas aeruginosa* biofilms. *Nature*, *413*, 860–864.

Wolfmeier, H., Pletzer, D., Mansour, S. C., Hancock, R. E. (2018). New perspectives in biofilm eradication. *ACS Infectious Diseases, 4*, 93–106.

Zano, S. P., Bhansali, P., Luniwal, A., Viola, R. E. (2013). Alternative substrates selective for S-adenosylmethionine synthetases from pathogenic bacteria. *Archives of Biochemistry and Biophysics, 536*, 64–71.

Zuberi, A., Misba, L., Khan, A. U. (2017). CRISPR interference (CRISPRi) inhibition of luxS gene expression in *E. coli*: An approach to inhibit biofilm. *Frontiers in Cellular and Infection Microbiology, 7*, 214. https://doi.org/10.3389/fcimb.2017.00214.

CHAPTER 6

Microbiome and Drug Response

RASHMI PATHAK[1*] and HIMANSHU SHARMA[2]

[1]*Department of Pharmacy, Invertis University, Bareilly, Uttar Pradesh, India*

[2]*Department of Pharmacology, Nims Institute of Pharmacy, Nims University Rajasthan, Jaipur, Rajasthan, India*

*Corresponding author

ABSTRACT

The human microbiome, consisting of diverse bacterial communities inside and outside the body, plays a crucial role in influencing health and drug responses. Growing evidence shows that the microbiome affects drug toxicity, safety, pharmacokinetics, and therapeutic outcomes. Its enzymes and metabolic activities are involved in bioactivation, biotransformation, and detoxification of medicines, directly shaping how drugs work. Moreover, the microbiome interacts bidirectionally with pharmaceuticals: while it modifies drug metabolism, drugs particularly antibiotics can alter the microbiome's composition and function, potentially disrupting treatment effectiveness. Variations in microbiota among individuals add further complexity, as they may explain differences in therapeutic and adverse drug effects. These insights hold promise for advancing treatments for conditions like cancer, autoimmune disorders, psychological illnesses, and metabolic diseases. However, challenges remain in standardizing approaches and translating findings into clinical practice. To harness the microbiome effectively in precision medicine, interdisciplinary collaboration among clinicians, microbiologists, pharmacologists, and bioinformaticians is essential. Such integration could minimize side effects, enhance

Advances in Pharmaceutical Microbiology: From Bench to Bedside. Harpreet Singh, Arun Kumar Mishra, Jeyabalan Sangeetha, and Devarajan Thangadurai (Eds.)

DOI: 10.1201/9781779640918-8

drug efficacy, and improve patient care. Ultimately, deeper investigation into microbiome–drug interactions is vital to developing personalized therapeutic strategies that align with individual microbial profiles, paving the way for more effective and safer precision medicine.

6.1 INTRODUCTION

6.1.1 BACKGROUND ON THE HUMAN MICROBIOME

The term "human microbiome" denotes the massive and varied community of microbes on the body's mucosal membranes, including the stomach, skin, and mouth. This composite ecology of microbes poses a serious danger to human health. Advances in DNA sequencing technology and a growing understanding of microorganisms' role in physiological functioning have led to studying human microbiota, a diverse composition influenced by genetics, nutrition, environment, and upbringing (Ursell et al., 2012). The human microbiome is crucial in various physiological processes, including digestion, biotransformation, and immune system regulation. It aids in breaking down complex meals, providing vitamins, and preventing diseases from colonizing. The microbiome is linked to various health issues, including obesity, mental health, autoimmune illnesses, and cancer. Understanding this relationship could lead to personalized therapies (Bull and Plummer, 2014).

6.1.2 SIGNIFICANCE OF MICROBIOME IN HEALTH AND DISEASE

The human microbiome is crucial in physiological activities like digestion, immune system regulation, and biotransformation. It produces essential vitamins, aids in mineral decomposition, and prevents pollutants. The microbiome has been linked to health issues like obesity, autoimmune disorders, mental health, and cancer. Maintaining a diverse bacterial population is essential for overall health (Ipci et al., 2017; Ogunrinola et al., 2020). The microbiome is crucial in personalized medicine, influencing therapeutic therapies. Understanding interactions between medications and the microbiome can lead to more effective treatments. Fecal microbiota transplantation and microbial community modification can deliver novel treatments while maintaining homeostasis. A holistic medical strategy recognizes the microbiome's connection to human biology, enabling innovative diagnostic, therapeutic, and preventative approaches (Kashyap et al., 2017; Behrouzi et al., 2019).

6.1.3 EMERGING ROLE OF MICROBIOME IN DRUG RESPONSE

The growing significance of microbiota in pharmacologic responses influences medical therapy and customization. The microbiome, comprising billions of bacteria, is crucial for evaluating prescription drugs for safety and effectiveness, challenging traditional thinking (Kashyap et al., 2017). The gut microbiota plays a crucial role in drug biotransformation and absorption, with different configurations potentially causing adverse effects and affecting pharmacokinetics and therapeutic components, thus requiring a comprehensive understanding (Tsunoda et al., 2021). Recent studies indicate a link between gut microbiota and the immune system, suggesting gut bacterial populations may influence body reactions to immunotherapies and suppressed immune systems. Additionally, the relationship between edema and the microbiota may affect the efficiency of medication, absorption, and distribution. As they investigate these intricate relationships, scientists are becoming increasingly motivated to alter the microbiome to bring the most significant possible benefits and the least possible negative ones (Gopalakrishnan et al., 2018a).

Precision medicine may be able to adapt treatment tactics for particular patients based on the data collected from the microbiome. If doctors can identify microbiological indicators linked to drug reactions, they may be able to predict pharmaceutical effects more precisely and facilitate treatment. Utilizing this information might lead to the development of novel treatment plans, such as manufacturing medications that consider and harmoniously interact with each patient's unique biological profile. In conclusion, a paradigm change in medicine has increased our awareness of the role the microbiota plays in pharmaceutical reactions. There is potential to increase treatment efficacy, reduce side effects, and achieve more efficient and individualized healthcare *via* microbiome data in pharmaceutical research and clinical practice. Future developments in this study area will undoubtedly impact pharmacological treatment and increase the precision of drug age (Zmora et al., 2016; Lamb et al., 2022).

6.2 OVERVIEWS OF THE HUMAN MICROBIOME

A collection of microorganisms that live in and interact with the human body is known as the human microbiota. Three types of interactions are possible: harmful, communalistic, and mutualistic. The term "human microbiome" refers to the genetic composition of microorganisms (microbiota) living in a specific human body region. Numerous anatomical locations inside the body, including the skin, mucosa, gastrointestinal system, respiratory tract, urogenital tract, and mammary gland, are colonized by microorganisms. Together, they create a unique and complex ecosystem that adapts to the environmental needs of each niche (Whiteside et al., 2015; Ogunrinola et al., 2020). A constant relationship (symbiosis) between the human body and its indigenous microbiota is established at delivery. These relationships have a significant impact on maintaining general health and well-being. The organisms that comprise the microbiota have coevolved to inhabit specific niches inside the human body and actively adapt to their particular habitats (Whiteside et al., 2015). These organisms' biological activity, which results in various alterations from conception to death, makes them regarded as parts of the human body. The microbiomes of humans are ever-changing in reaction to their hosts. Several variables, including inherited genes, age, nutrition, lifestyle, hormonal swings, and underlying disorders, influence the microbiome at any time. Nonetheless, alterations in the makeup of the human microbiota might lead to fatal illnesses (dysbiosis). It has been shown that a healthy microbiome is essential for sustaining good health. The human microbiota is most concentrated in the stomach. The primary agents responsible for preserving human health are these organisms. According to prior studies on the human microbiome project, a dysbiotic gut flora may be directly connected to changes in the immune environment. Necessary medical conditions such as intestinal inflammation, cancer, cardiovascular disease, and bacterial contaminations that are difficult to treat and resistant to antimicrobial agents have all been connected to dysbiosis (Morgan and Huttenhower, 2012; Pascal et al., 2018).

6.2.1 THE CONSTITUTION AND VARIATION OF MICROBIAL COMMUNITIES

The term "human microbiome" denotes the complex and diverse population of microorganisms within the body. Microorganisms reside in the mouth, skin, stomach, and reproductive organs, forming active infective communities influenced by environmental contact, lifestyle, nutrition, and genetics (Dekaboruah et al., 2020). The gut microbiome, a diverse ecosystem of billions of microorganisms in the human gut, plays a crucial role in digestion, immune system regulation, and nutrient absorption. Its diverse composition, including hundreds of distinct microorganisms, enhances its ability to break down complex carbohydrates and synthesize essential vitamins (Thursby and Juge, 2017). Human microbial ecosystems are linked to various health and disease aspects, with diseases like overweightness, autoimmune disorders, and inflammatory bowel disease (IBD) linked to dysbiosis. Understanding these interrelations helps develop innovative studies and therapeutic methods aimed at changing the microbiome to improve well-being and prevent illness (DeGruttola et al., 2016). Researchers are investigating the human microbiome to an unprecedented level due to progressions in DNA sequencing technologies. The direct examination of the DNA of microorganisms from samples made possible by metagenomic study discloses the vast genetic range seen in these groups. Consequently, new microbes have been recognized, and our understanding of the microbiome's function in human well-being and disease has grown. (Handelsman, 2004). In summary, the multifaceted connections between microbes and the human body depend on the wealth and makeup of human microbial groups. These communities significantly impact human well-being and are vital to many physical functions. Future studies in this area might provide fresh viewpoints on the intricate connections between the state of the human microbiome and general well-being, opening the door to more specific disease prevention and treatment methods (Aggarwal et al., 2023).

6.2.2 MICROBIOME VARIABILITY ACROSS INDIVIDUALS

The range of bacteria on and inside the human body is called the ""micro-biome," and it varies widely across people. Numerous variables, such as nutrition, geography, environmental exposure, manner of life, and heredity, influence this diversity. Humans have a separate microbiota, similar to a modified microbial fingerprint that syndicates intrinsic and extrinsic mechanisms. An individual's sensitivity to specific bacterial interactions and colonization, as well as the arrangement of their baseline microbiota, are determined by genomic variables (Ahn and Hayes, 2021). The microbial community in the human body is significantly affected by diet. Deviations in the kinds of carbohydrates, fats, and other nutrients consumed may affect the diversity and quantity of certain microbiological species. Compared to a high-fiber diet, a low-fiber diet may encourage the growth of bacteria that are accomplished of breaking down complex carbohydrates, resulting in a unique microbial outline (Singh et al., 2017).

Antibiotic use, physical activity routines, and hygiene standards are a few lifestyle choices impacting microbiome diversity. Antibiotics may disturb the delicate balance of microbial communities, which may lead to long-term alterations in the microbiome, even while they are required for treating bacterial infections. Exercise is linked to a more diverse and robust microbiome, influencing lifestyle and environmental factors like urbanization and exposure to ambient microbes. The microbial profiles of rural dwellers may differ from those of urban dwellers, indicating the impact of environmental factors on microbial colonization. Understanding the heterogeneity of microbiomes is crucial for developing customized medications and interventions. The complex interactions between the microbiome and human health are still being explored, highlighting the need for an all-encompassing plan considering each person's unique potential. The variety of microbiomes offers new opportunities for improving and treating health, highlighting the flexibility and complexity of these microorganism communities (Ejtahed et al., 2017).

6.2.3 FACTORS INFLUENCING MICROBIOME COMPOSITION

Even though the gut microorganisms grow early in infancy, several aspects may later affect their growth and variability, as shown in Figure 6.1.

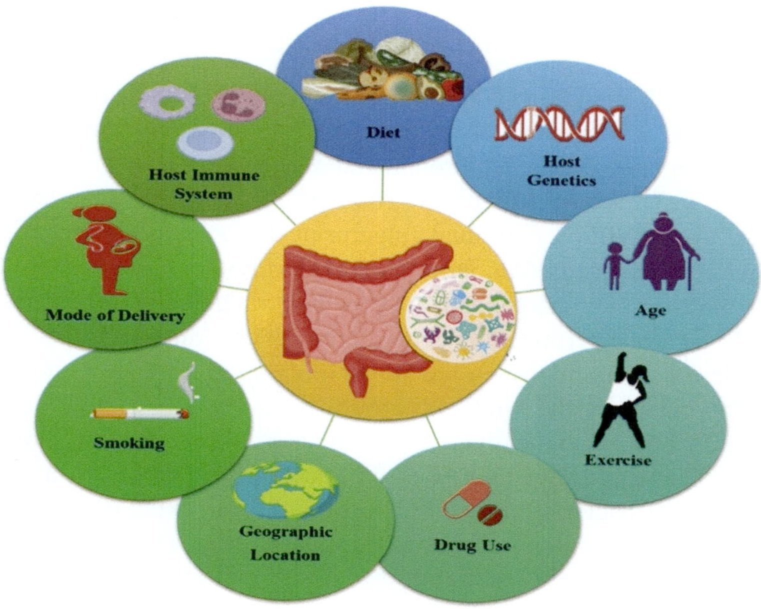

FIGURE 6.1 Factors influencing microbiome composition.

6.2.3.1 AGE AND DELIVERY PATTERN

When microbiota colonizes the placenta and amniotic fluid during pregnancy, microbial intestinal colonization begins. Research has shown that bacteria and their metabolites, including DNA, are present in meconium, amniotic fluid, and the placenta. Maternal germs may transfer to the placenta and amniotic fluid. Research on pregnant mice found that oral delivery of tagged *Enterococcus faecium* isolated the bacterium from the babies' stool samples. The postnatal delivery mode affects the early development of the gut flora. The babies delivered by cesarean section obtain their gut microbiota from the skin are influenced by *Corynebacterium*, *Streptococcus*, and *Propionibacterium* sp., whereas infants delivered vaginally have a foremost gut microbiota influenced by *Prevotella* and *Lactobacillus*, which are generated from the mother's vaginal microbiota. Over time, these significant microbiome changes have become more stable and diversified. At about three years old, they resemble an adult's gut flora (Collado et al., 2016; Nagpal et al., 2017; Wampach et al., 2017).

6.2.3.2 DIET

After birth, the baby's diet first affects the gut flora (breast or formula milk). The milk's composition shaped the early gut microbiome. The oligosaccharides in mother's milk are quickly broken down by these species, increasing the amount of short-chain fatty acids (SCFAs) and stimulating the immune system to release more immunoglobulin G. The two main species in breastfed babies' gut microbiota are *Bifidobacterium* and *Lactobacillus*. Conversely, the most prevalent species in infants given formula are *Bacteroides*, *Enterobacteria*, *Enterococcus*, *Streptococcus*, and *Clostridia*. Since the central microbiota that newborns acquire throughout infancy may contribute significantly to their initial immunity as they develop, it is vital to understand the composition of the primary microbiota during this period to protect infants from illnesses associated with compromised immune systems. Breastfeeding produced a more consistent population of gut microbiota and a better mucosal immunological response than formula feeding, according to several studies comparing these two parameters (Guaraldi and Salvatori, 2012; Groer et al., 2014; Sherman et al., 2015). Beyond infancy, the ecosystem's composition, variety, and organization are still greatly influenced by nutrition, and the gut microbiota continually changes.

While nonvegetarian diets (Western diets) have been linked to an increase in *Bacteroides* and a decrease in *Firmicutes*, vegetarian diets have been linked to a healthy, broad gut microbiota defined by the supremacy of species that can metabolize insoluble carbohydrates, such as *Eubacterium*, *Roseburia*, and *Ruminococcus*. Diet may cause significant changes, even in short-term outcomes. After consuming Western cuisine, the gut bacteria ferment amino acids to produce SCFAs for energy and hazardous compounds. A vegetarian diet prevents this since it encourages the microbiota's primary function, which is the fermentation of carbohydrates (Table 6.1) (Walker et al., 2011; Windey et al., 2012; David et al., 2014).

TABLE 6.1 Summary of Diet–Microbiota Interactions in Health and Disease

Healthy Microbiota	Gut Dysbiosis	Other Consequence	References
High dietary fiber intake	Junk food; low core diversity	High in choline/fat/ added sugar	Haiser et al. (2013); Sonnenburg and Backhed (2016)
Vegetables and fruits; prebiotic consisting of foods	Low fiber consumption	Beer, sugar, bread	Trompette et al. (2014); Valdes et al. (2018); Halmos and Gibson (2019)
Anti-inflammatory omega-3	High-omega-6 fatty acid diet	Pro-inflammatory	Hills and Erpenbeck (2018); Watson et al. (2018)
Lipid and glucose homeostasis	Insulin resistance and the invasion of bacteria	Heart disease	Chassaing et al. (2017); Grosso et al. (2017); Chambers et al. (2018)
Gut and brain relations	Emotional distress or internal discomfort	Leaky gut, emulsifiers, psychological stress, plasma endotoxin	Foster and McVey Neufeld (2013); Skonieczna-Żydecka et al. (2018); Miclotte and van de Wiele (2020)
Intermittent fasting	Excess sugar intake	Overgrowth of *Candida*; intolerance to gluten	Zhernakova et al. (2016); Li et al. (2017); Skodje et al. (2018);
Beneficial bacteria/ probiotics: *Bifidobacterium*, *Lactobacillus*	Oxidative stress; *E. coli*	Prescription dysbiosis and broad-spectrum antibiotics	Blaser (2016); Kadooka et al. (2013)

6.2.3.3 ANTIBIOTICS

Antibiotics have two drawbacks: they indiscriminately destroy both beneficial and harmful bacteria, resulting in the loss of the gut microbiota, dysbiosis, and the growth of pathogenic germs. Antibiotic usage affects the colon's secondary bile acid and serotonin metabolism, which results in a decline in microbiota and a delay in intestinal motility, according to studies done on lab mice. Antibiotics interfere with the fundamental mechanism by which harmful bacteria are eliminated by microbiota, the competitive exclusion machinery. Other diseases like *Clostridium difficile* thrive more readily due to this disturbance. Studies have shown the long-lasting effects of ciprofloxacin, metronidazole, clarithromycin, and clindamycin on the structure of the microbiota (Klingensmith and Coopersmith, 2016; Ge et al., 2017). Clindamycin modifies the microbiota over two years, and the diversity of *Bacteroides* does not reappear. Comparatively, when *Helicobacter pylori* are treated with clarithromycin, *Actinobacteria* populations drop, and when ciprofloxacin is administered, *Ruminococcus* populations have been shown to decrease. Vancomycin is the best antibiotic for curing *C. difficile* infection (CDI). Still, like other antibiotics, it alters the gut microbiota, which might promote the development of dangerous strains of *Escherichia coli* or cause recurrent CDI. Vancomycin treatment is associated with decreases in *Faecalibacterium*, *Ruminococcus*, and *Bacteroidetes* and increases in *Proteobacteria* species while depleting much of the gut microbiota, including *Bacteroidetes*. Individual differences impact the duration of recovery and the particular impacts of antibiotic medication on the microbiota, such as the impact of pretreatment modifications on the gut microbiota (Lewis et al., 2015; Vrieze et al., 2014; Isaac et al., 2017; Lee et al., 2017).

6.3 MICROBIOME-DRUG INTERACTIONS

Over the last 10 years, many noteworthy findings have been produced that relate a variety of prevalent illnesses and characteristics to the makeup and activities of the human gut microbiome. Studies linking alterations in the diversity of gut microbiota to disorders of other organs and systems, including autoimmune diseases, mental disorders, metabolic and cardiovascular diseases, and gastrointestinal phenotypes like IBD, colorectal cancer, and irritable bowel syndrome, have been conducted (Lloyd-Price et al., 2019; Thomas et al., 2019; Zhou et al., 2019). In addition to association analysis, animal studies and intervention trials have shown the causal link and correlation between many diseases and the gut microbiota. Moreover, we are becoming increasingly aware of the effects of extrinsic and intrinsic factors on the microbiome's composition. Metformin and proton pump inhibitors (PPIs) are two common nonantibiotic drugs that modify the microbiome's composition and activity. This is an important new finding regarding PPIs, and these changes might affect patient outcomes or reduce the efficacy of the medicine (in the case of metformin). However, further information indicates that the gut microbiota may adjust a drug's toxicity, bioavailability, or bioactivity *via* enzymatic changes, directly impacting an individual's reaction to that therapy. These days, this phenomenon is known as pharmacomicrobiomics (Figure 6.2). Finally, by influencing the host's overall immunological condition, the gut microbiome may indirectly influence a person's reaction to immunotherapy in the treatment of cancer (Zitvogel et al., 2017; Vila et al., 2018; Petersen et al., 2020).

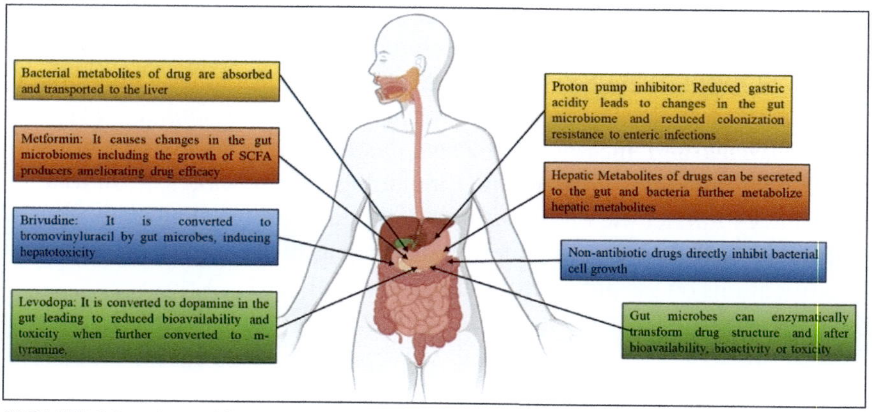

FIGURE 6.2 A graphical representation of the interactions between typical nonantibiotic medications and the gut microbiota (short-chain fatty acids (SCFAs)).

6.3.1 BASICS OF MICROBIOME-DRUG METABOLISM

The intricate and ever-changing process of drug metabolism and human microbiota interaction substantially impacts the effectiveness and safety of medicinal therapies. The billions of bacteria that reside in the gut, known as the microbiome, perform a variety of roles in drug metabolism. One essential component is the enzymatic activity of microorganisms, which may alter medications before or during systemic circulation (Belkaid and Hand, 2014). The relationship between drug biotransformation and the microbiome is complicated by variations in microbial populations, leading to unique medicine biotransformation processes and individual variations in drug reactions. Understanding the role of the microbiota in medicine breakdown offers predictions for enhancing pharmacological treatment, mitigating side effects, and generating more active and customized treatment schedules. A rising corpus of investigation in this range designates that the microbiota largely determines the destiny of pharmacological substances inside the individual. Understanding the purpose of microbiota in medical biotransformation would allow us to treat individuals more surely and successfully by customizing their treatment schedules (Zhang et al., 2023).

6.3.2 IMPACT ON DRUG ABSORPTION AND BIOAVAILABILITY

It is a prevalent choice because of its affordability, comfort of use, high oral administration, and safety compliance. Regrettably, the poor intestinal absorption of many oral medicines limits their efficacy. The symbiotic microbiota has a vital but recurrently overlooked function in drug biotransformation, the drug transport system, and the alteration of specific gut properties, all of which may affect how bioavailable oral medications are (Zhang et al., 2021).

6.3.3 MICROBIAL MODULATION OF DRUG METABOLISM

The pharmacokinetics of many medicines exhibit an intriguing interaction with the microbiome *via* bacterial modification of drug biotransformation. Research has depicted that the gastrointestinal microbiome, a heterogeneous group of microorganisms, significantly affects drug biotransformation *via* many mechanisms. One vital method is the enzymatic action of microorganisms, which may directly destroy medicines in the GIT before they are absorbed into the systemic circulation. This method could affect a medicine's effectiveness and safety, perhaps altering the way it acts therapeutically (Swanson, 2015; Jourova et al., 2016). Numerous enzymes found in gastrointestinal bacteria can damage a broad spectrum of medications. Two medicine inactivations, which result in decreased efficiency, and medication alteration into active forms, which upsurge therapeutic aids, are effects of this microbial biotransformation. Interestingly, this bacterial influence is significant for longer first-pass metabolizing medications. Understanding the specific enzymes and metabolic pathways involved in bacterial drug metabolism is vital to estimate and enhance treatment reactions (Jandhyala et al., 2015; Vemuri et al., 2018).

6.4 COMMONLY USED TREATMENT FOR THE GASTROINTESTINAL SYSTEM

6.4.1 PROTON PUMP INHIBITORS

PPIs are among the drugs administered most often worldwide. They are used to prevent bleeding and gastroduodenopathy caused by nonsteroidal anti-inflammatory drugs, as well as to treat acid-related diseases such as dyspepsia, stomach ulcers, and gastro-esophageal reflux. Because of PPI's superior effectiveness and favorable safety profile, its use has augmented dramatically over the last 20 years (Forgacs and Loganayagam, 2008; Othman et al., 2016). Metagenomic sequencing data were used in recent research to examine the impact of 41 regularly used medications on the gut flora. This allowed for the investigation of anticipated routes and high-resolution classification. Once again, it was shown that PPIs were responsible for the most significant number of connections (Vila et al., 2020). When the effects of concurrent drug use were taken into account, PPIs were shown to be significantly correlated with 133 pathways and 24 taxa. The expected functional changes were increased lipid and fatty acid biosynthesis, purine deoxyribonucleoside breakdown, and L-arginine production. These differences in pathways may have an explanation related to the detected fluctuations in the abundance of certain species. For example, the microbiomes of PPI users produced more L-arginine. Statistical analysis showed that the only changes linked to PPI consumption were connected to *Streptococcus mutans*, despite the expectation that other bacterial taxa, including *Ruminococcus* and *Bifidobacterium* sp., may contribute to these paths (Vila et al., 2020). Because a decrease in PPI-induced stomach acidity creates space for oral bacteria to colonize the gut microbiome and alter taxonomic homeostasis, this reduction will likely be the origin of the observed microbial alterations (Figure 6.2). This is maintained by discovering that the gut microbiomes of PPI users had experienced "oralization" (Floris et al., 2016). However, studies conducted *in vitro* to evaluate the direct impact of routinely used medications, such as PPIs, on gut commensals discovered significant variations in the rates of bacterial proliferation. This raises the likelihood that PPI binding to bacterial H^+/K^+ ATPases will mediate a direct impact (Maier et al., 2018).

PPIs have significantly favorable efficacy and safety profiles when recommended for evidence-based reasons. Still, the medical community has to start thinking again about these drugs' over-the-counter availability and chronic, widespread use. The long-term effects of PPI-induced changes in the microbiome in up to 15% of the population in Western culture now need serious consideration. In the history of humanity, there has been a prominent and relatively recent transition. We must pay close attention to how early modifications to the gut microbiota impact health and illness in later life (Bajaj et al., 2018).

6.4.2 METFORMIN

Metformin, an oral drug that lowers blood glucose, treats type 2 diabetes. Metformin does lower hepatic gluconeogenesis, albeit it has a complex and poorly understood exact mechanism of action. Additionally, some research is starting to point to the possibility that the gut flora mediates some of the sound effects of the medicine (Shin et al., 2014; L. Sun et al., 2018). PPIs are used for several purposes, but metformin is almost exclusively used in the treatment of diabetes. This makes it more challenging to discern changes in the gut microbiota linked to the underlying disease from the effects of the medicine on the microbiome. However, this was made possible by a groundbreaking study that showed that the underlying type 2 diabetes was the reason for the previously experiential gut flora changes linked to metformin therapy (Forslund et al., 2015). In a different intervention experiment with healthy adults, metformin use changed over 80 species when equated to a control group that received a placebo. Surprisingly, metformin therapy results in an increase in *E. coli* and a reduction in *Intestinibacter*. These findings align with cross-sectional cohorts that looked at the differences between type 2 diabetes patients receiving metformin treatment and those who did not (Wu et al., 2017). After that, the scientists gave germ-free mice fecal samples from donors who received either a placebo or metformin treatment. They found that when the mice were given fecal samples from people who were on metformin, their blood glucose levels decreased, suggesting that the gut microbiota directly affects blood glucose levels. It is believed that the frequency of *Akkermansia muciniphila* and the impact of metformin on bacteria that make butyrate, or SCFAs, mediate this effect. Metalloproteins may be encoded by biological mechanisms and genes often spotted in bacteria linked with metformin. Also, clinical investigations specify that GIT side effects such as vomiting, bloating, and diarrhea may affect up to one-third of metformin consumers. These detrimental effects, generally brought on by an upsurge in *E. coli* species, have been linked to variations in the biotransformation of gas and virulence factors (Wu et al., 2017). The complicated connection between gut microbiota and metformin demonstrates how a generally used treatment may change gut microbiota, and clarifies both the therapeutic and adverse effects of the drug. It also highlights how vital it is to prudently control for factors like the usage of drugs in microbiome studies that concentrate on precise conditions (Imhann et al., 2017).

6.4.3 MORE WIDELY USED NONANTIBIOTIC MEDICATIONS

Many population-based microbiome research studies have used cross-sectional information from the UK, Netherlands, and Belgium cohorts to assess various variables involving drug usage. In addition to metformin and PPIs, usually consumed drugs such as opioids, statins, laxatives, and antidepressants may account for some of the heterogeneity in the gut microbiome's structure, according to related research (Falony et al., 2016; Imhann et al., 2017; Jackson et al., 2018). When analyzing microbial modifications brought on by laxative administration, it is vital to bear in mind that intestinal transit time, bacterial numbers, and stool consistency (such as microbial load per sample) all impact microbiome natures (Vandeputte et al., 2016, 2017). For example, the quantity of *Bacteroides* species was more significant in feces samples with poor consistency and in individuals who were taking laxatives. Nevertheless, the second research that used mice treated with polyethylene glycol (PEG) revealed a comparable rise in *Bacteroides*. In this study, the administration of PEG injections to induce moderate osmotic diarrhea led to changes in the gut flora over time, a transient disturbance of the mucus layer, and consequent adaptive and innate immunological reactions (Tropini et al., 2018). The S24-7 Family, a subsection of the *Bacteroidales* order, disappeared after receiving PEG treatment and was entirely replaced by *Bacteroidaceae* outgrowth. This effect would not go away if the S24-7 Family were not altered. Some taxa, including *Verrucomicrobia* and *Gammaproteobacteria*, experienced short-lived changes before returning to their former forms. Despite the absence of comprehensive research, small human data in individuals receiving bowel preparations have also demonstrated transitory, temporary alterations in microbiome diversity indices. However, given the outcomes in mice, it is plausible that the use of laxatives influences the gut microbiome's composition both temporarily and permanently in ways unrelated to the number of bacteria in each sample and the consistency of the feces (Nagata et al., 2019).

6.5 THE DRUGS INFLUENCED BY GUT MICROBIOME

6.5.1 THE GENESIS OF PHARMACOMICROBIOMICS

In the last several decades, the discipline of pharmacogenomics, which examines how differences in the human genome impact the distribution and action of drugs, has grown significantly. With the rising recognition of the gut microbiome as the second biological genome, pharmacomicrobiomics has developed as a logical evolution of pharmacogenomics. The concept that the gut microbiome might affect therapeutic effectiveness is not new; it was first recognized in 1937 when it was discovered that gut microorganisms could activate the antibacterial antibiotic prontosil (Fuller, 1937; Doestzada et al., 2018). Drugs taken orally go from the upper gastrointestinal tract into the intestinal system, where they come into contact with the myriad of species that live in our digestive tracts (Figure 6.2). This results in two-way exchanges. As was already noted, drugs may change the microenvironments of the intestines and affect the development, makeup, and activity of bacteria. On the other hand, *via* enzymatic drug structure transformation, the gut microbiota may directly affect an individual's reaction to a particular medicine, changing its toxicity, bioactivity, or bioavailability. Since the gut microbiota may be altered, unlike human heredity, it is a desirable therapeutic target for optimizing treatment (Koppel et al., 2017).

6.5.2 THE RECIPROCAL RELATIONSHIP BETWEEN MEDICATIONS AND MICROORGANISMS IN BOTH IN VITRO AND ANIMAL RESEARCH

Many animal investigations have uncovered the action mechanisms of drug–microbe interactions and their possible effects on medication effectiveness and safety, coinciding with human gut–microbe relationships.

6.5.2.1 HYPOTHESIZED METHODS BY WHICH DRUGS AFFECT THE GUT MICROBIOTA

The makeup of the gut microbiota may be affected by medication use in two different ways. First, taking some drugs may force the microbiota from other body areas to migrate to the stomach. As was already established, PPIs may reduce the acidity barrier in the stomach, which makes it possible for oral bacteria to pass through and reach the gut, leading to microbial dysbiosis. The capacity of drugs to alter intestinal microenvironments and directly affect bacterial growth is one potential mechanism of action. For instance, research indicates that metformin promotes the growth of bacteria in the stomach that produce SCFAs. These bacteria eventually assist metformin in achieving its therapeutic effects, which include improving glucose homeostasis and decreasing insulin resistance. In this second phase, there is potential for bidirectional activity. Moreover, drugs may inhibit the growth of certain bacteria rather than promote it, for example, by functioning as antibiotics with antimicrobial qualities. This was shown by an unprecedented high-throughput study that assessed the antibacterial qualities of over a thousand drugs, including 835 drugs aimed explicitly at humans and working on human cells. Surprisingly, the antibacterial activity of 24% of these drugs affected the growth rate of at least one of the 40 bacterial strains that were analyzed. At least half of the strains' growth rate was impacted by eight of them, which seemed to be detrimental to the bacteria. These included four anticancer drugs (floxuridine, streptozotocin, daunorubicin, and 5-fluorouracil), one anti-gout drug (benzbromarone), two anti-inflammatory and antirheumatic drugs (diacerein and auranofin), and one treatment for peptic ulcer disease (oxethazaine). Because cancer treatments are often cytotoxic, this study emphasizes the negative consequences of cancer treatment on the gut flora (Maier et al., 2018).

6.6 THE ANTITUMOUR AND GUT MICROBIOME RESPONSE IN CANCER TREATMENT

We have discussed how commonly used nonantibiotic pharmaceuticals may affect the makeup of the gut microbiota and how this may affect the effectiveness and accessibility of medications. Moreover, growing evidence shows that a patient's gut microbiome affects how they react clinically to cancer therapy. This only occurs while undergoing immunotherapy with monoclonal antibodies that specifically target the receptor for cytotoxic T lymphocyte antigen 4 (CTLA-4) and programmed cell death protein one ligand (PD-L1), programmed cell death protein 1 (PD-1). Here, the role of the gut microbiome in controlling the host's overall immunological state is assumed to be responsible for the immune system's antitumor activation on checkpoint inhibition (Figure 6.3) (Momtaz and Postow, 2014; Gopalakrishnan et al., 2018b).

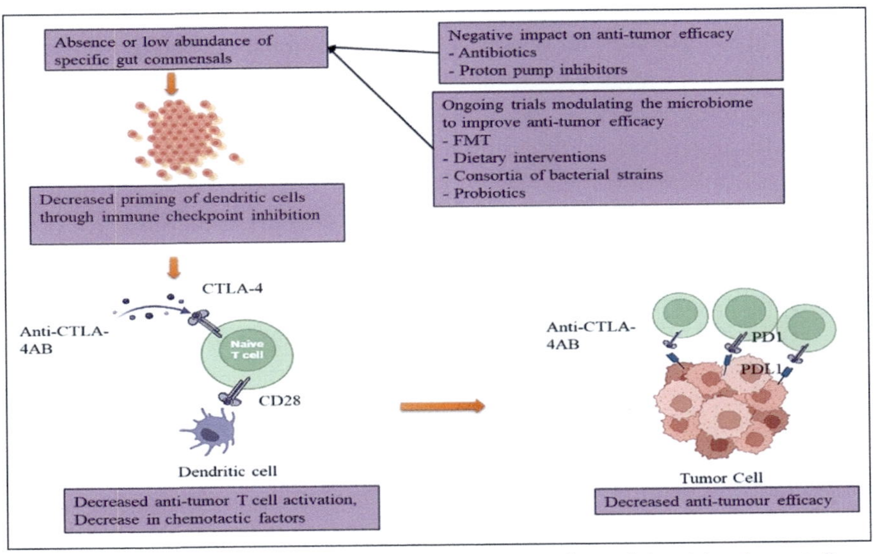

FIGURE 6.3 The clinical outcome to cancer therapy is modulated by the gut flora. CTLA-4, cytotoxic T lymphocyte antigen 4; PD-1, programmed cell death protein 1; FMT, fecal microbiome transplantation; PD-L1, programmed cell death protein one ligand.

The first groundbreaking study to demonstrate how the gut microbiota influences the body's response to tumors was conducted on mice; later, human clinical and microbiome data confirmed these findings. Anti-CTLA-4 treatment was less effective in pathogen-free animals. After that, *Bacteroides fragilis* and either *Burkholderia cepacia* or *Bacteroides thetaiotaomicron* were administered orally to the mice, which induced the growth of intratumorous dendritic cells and a Th1-mediated immune response. This led to an improved antitumor response to anti-CTLA-4 treatment. In a later phase, the mice were given the excrement of individuals with higher levels of *B. fragilis*, and this did improve the antitumor response to anti-CTLA-4 treatment (Vetizou et al., 2015). How the gut microbiota affects the immune response to immunotherapy is still unclear. General peripheral immunological homeostasis is assumed to be primarily mediated by the microbiome, and increased T-cell reactivity induced by microbial antigens may facilitate tumor-specific responses. Both adaptive and innate immune cells exposed to certain gut bacteria have been shown in mouse models to infiltrate the tumor microenvironment and release chemotactic factors such as CXCL9, CXCL10, CCR9, and CXCR3, which stimulate immune cell trafficking to the tumor site (Routy et al., 2018; Tanoue et al., 2019). The relationship between antigens linked to tumors and microbes is another postulated mechanism. The gut microbiome's SCFAs can impact host immunity, enhancing cancer immunotherapy. Scientific advancements reveal that the microbiome influences the effectiveness of antineoplastic activity. Understanding interventional research methods and outcomes can improve immunotherapy interventions' effectiveness (Hegazy et al., 2017).

6.7 MECHANISMS OF MICROBIOME-INDUCED DRUG RESPONSE VARIABILITY

The human microbiome, composed of billions of microbes, significantly influences drug responses due to complex interactions between microbiota, host, and therapeutic drugs. The biotransformation of microorganisms is crucial for medication production, as different enzymes can metabolize medications, potentially enhancing therapeutic benefits. The composition and function of the microbiota influence drug biotransformation (Stearns et al., 2011; Wang et al., 2017). Microbiota affects the host's immune system, affecting drug toxicity and efficacy. Metabolites and biological factors can alter immunological responses, hindering host defense. Individuals with diverse microbiome profiles may experience varying degrees of success or adverse effects from immunomodulation treatment. Another way involves the microbiota influencing the pharmacokinetics of the medicine. The interactions between the microbiota, human enzymes, and transporters may affect drug absorption, biotransformation, distribution, and waste elimination. The treatment's effectiveness might be affected by variations in medication concentrations at the target region resulting from these unexpected systems. The gut–brain axis may be influenced by microbiota, potentially affecting drug response. The cardiovascular and central nervous systems interact, potentially affecting the pharmacological effects of medications, particularly those for neurological issues. Microbial metabolites and signaling molecules can alter neurotransmitter concentrations and receptor function, potentially affecting the central nervous system's response to drug treatment (Zhou et al., 2021; Cohen et al., 2021). The microbiota plays a crucial role in various therapeutic responses, necessitating a comprehensive understanding of these pathways to develop personalized medical treatments. The emerging field of microbiome research has the potential to uncover these intricate connections, enabling more targeted and efficient therapeutic methods and enhancing the effectiveness of pharmacological treatment (Hadrich, 2018).

6.7.1 GUT MICROBIOTA AND METABOLISM

The gut microbiota, comprised of billions of bacteria, plays a crucial role in human biotransformation, influencing energy management, nutrient absorption, and food component biotransformation through a delicate symbiotic interaction (Thursby and Juge, 2017). Digestive bacteria convert complex carbohydrates into soluble fatty acids during indigestible fiber fermentation, regulating lipid and glucose metabolism. The gut microbiota influences bile acid biotransformation, affecting the digestion and absorption of dietary lipids. Microbial enzymes change secondary bile acids, affecting lipid biotransformation, energy expenditure, and glucose homeostasis (Rowland et al., 2018; De Angelis et al., 2019). Gut microbes play a crucial role in the biotransformation of dietary ingredients like polyphenols and xenobiotics into beneficial metabolites. These medications affect host biotransformation, inflammation, and overall health through changes in metabolism and bioavailability. Understanding these interactions could lead to targeted interventions (Table 6.2) (Kumar Singh et al., 2019; Kasprzak-Drozd et al., 2021).

TABLE 6.2 A List of Medicines that the Gut Microbiome Biotransforms

Drugs Class	Drug	Effect on Medication	Microbial Metabolism Type	Bacterial Species Involved	References
Antibacterial	Prontosil	Prodrug activation	Azo reduction	Not known	Sun et al. (2019)
	Neoprontosil	Prodrug activation	Azo reduction	Not known	Wilson and Nicholson (2017)
Anti-inflammatory drugs	Sulfasalazine	Prodrug activation	Azo reduction	Not known	Crouwel et al. (2020)
	Balsalazide	Prodrug activation	Azo reduction	Not known	Crouwel et al. (2020)
	Olsalazine	Prodrug activation	Azo reduction	Not known	Zhang et al. (2021)
Analgesics	Acetaminophen	Toxicity	O-sulfation; C-S cleavage of acetaminophen-3-cysteine	*Clostridium difficile*	Jourova et al. (2016)
Cardiotonic	Digoxin	A reduction in heart activity	Reduction	*Eggerthella lenta*	Haiser et al. (2014)
Antipsychotics	Risperidone	Triggering Parkinson's disease symptoms	Hydroxylation or Isoxazole scission	Not known	Parashar and Udayabanu (2017)
Prebiotics	Lactulose	Promoting the development of helpful bacteria	Hydrolysis	Not known	Karakan et al. (2021)
Anthelmintics	Levamisole	Heightened activity	Thiazole ring opening	*Bacteroides* and *Clostridium* spp.	Li et al. (2016)
Hypnotics	Nitrazepam	Causing the teratogenicity	Nitro reduction	*Clostridium leptum*	Mousa et al. (2023)

6.7.2 ENZYMATIC MODIFICATION OF DRUGS BY MICROBES

Drug biotransformation in pharmaceuticals is influenced by microbes' enzymatic changes, particularly in the gut microbiome. These enzymes can accelerate drug biotransformation, potentially impacting certain medications' pharmacokinetics and therapeutic efficiency (Zhao et al., 2021; Pant et al., 2023). Bacterial biotransformation is crucial for drug production, with gut flora potentially increasing therapeutic activity. Understanding gut microbiota is essential for designing new medical treatments and drugs. Accurate treatment reactions require knowledge of specific enzymes and individual variations, and understanding complex interactions between medications and gut microbiota is crucial (Koppel et al., 2017).

6.8 CLINICAL IMPLICATIONS AND APPLICATIONS

The human microbiome plays a crucial role in various professions, and our understanding of its connection to health is expanding, enabling the development of innovative treatments (Morowitz et al., 2011). The gut microbiota is vital for digestion, nutrient absorption, and maintaining the gut barrier. Dysbiosis can lead to degenerative diseases like colon cancer and IBD. Targeted antibiotics like probiotics, prebiotics, and fecal microbiota transplantation are being used to treat digestive issues. Microbiome changes can also affect allergies, infections, and autoimmune illnesses. Researchers are exploring immunomodulatory therapies that optimize the microbiome (Vijay and Valdes, 2022). The knowledge of how viruses interact with hosts to influence an illness's susceptibility, response to therapy, and chance of recurrence has increased thanks to studies on microbiomes. It is crucial to alter antibiotic treatments to consider the microbiome to optimize harm to beneficial bacterial populations, thereby reducing potential harm. Novel methods for weight management and metabolic health have been made possible by the microbiome's function in metabolism and its correlation with illnesses like obesity and metabolic syndrome. Personalized nutrition regimens that include a person's microbiome profile are being investigated to maximize nutritional treatments. Furthermore, studies on the use of microbial therapies, such as fecal microbiota transplantation and microbial-based treatments, for metabolic diseases are still being conducted (Patangia et al., 2022). The gut–brain axis, which denotes the exchange of information between the stomach and the central nervous system, has drawn interest in mental health. Neurodegenerative illnesses, anxiety, and depression may be affected by the microbiome's impact on neuroinflammation and neurotransmitter synthesis. The study of adjuvant therapy for mental health issues explores probiotics and dietary interventions to promote healthy gut microbiota. This method provides tailored and optimized care, which may help different medical specialties. Knowledge of the microbiota can drastically alter prevention, diagnosis, and therapy (Clapp et al., 2017).

6.8.1 PERSONALIZED MEDICINE AND MICROBIOME PROFILING

Microbiome profiling is used in individualized therapy to optimize benefits and minimize adverse effects by studying microbial communities within the human body, considering an individual's genetic makeup and health (Behrouzi et al., 2019). Microbiota profiling is crucial for personalized treatment, particularly in medication biotransformation and response optimization. It correlates with drug bioavailability and efficacy, enabling cautious dosage adjustments, especially for stomach-affecting drugs. Microbiome studies are increasingly used in developing individualized treatment programs for gastrointestinal diseases, such as irritable bowel syndrome and IBD. Understanding these bacterial patterns allows for personalized treatment regimens (Li et al., 2016). Microbiota analysis is a promising approach for cancer treatment, as gut microbiome composition can impact immunotherapy responses and treatment effectiveness. Oncologists can personalize therapy based on microbiome patterns, increasing response rates. In preventive medicine, a microbiome-based diet is gaining popularity. Individuals' gut flora composition can influence their response to eating patterns and nutrient metabolism. Personalized meal suggestions can improve gut health, boost nutrient absorption, and potentially prevent or cure disorders like metabolic syndrome and obesity. This approach could improve cancer treatment outcomes (Gebrayel et al., 2022; Li et al., 2016). Despite the potential of personalized medicine and microbiome profiling in healthcare, there are challenges, such as the need for optimization methods, explanation of complex data, and ethical concerns about data privacy. As technology advances and our understanding of the microbiome deepens, this combination could further revolutionize healthcare (Cullen et al., 2020).

6.8.2 FUTURE DIRECTIONS AND RESEARCH OPPORTUNITIES

Microbiome research holds the potential for growth and optimization of pharmacological reactions. Studying the complex mechanisms underlying interactions between bacteria and pharmaceuticals is crucial for developing targeted pharmaceuticals. Research on microbiota's regulation of drug biotransformation, absorption, and effectiveness is crucial for developing targeted pharmaceuticals, necessitating further studies on metabolites and microbial enzymes (Aggarwal et al., 2023). Microbiome research is advancing personalized medicine by examining individual microbiome profiles. This allows medical professionals to modify treatment plans, increase doses, and reduce side effects. Combining genetic and microbiome data can help understand why people react differently to pharmaceuticals. Analyzing deliberate microbiome changes, such as fecal microbiota transplantation, can improve treatment results and create individualized microbial therapeutics (Berg et al., 2020). Researchers aim to understand gut bacteria's role in immunotherapy, particularly cancer treatment. Discovering microbiological fingerprints linked to positive responses could improve immunotherapy success. Future research should use longitudinal studies to monitor microbiome changes and understand microbial community resilience. Practical longitudinal approaches are crucial for long-term treatment outcomes (Cullen et al., 2020; Quigley, 2022). Research into microbiomes is crucial for developing effective treatments for diverse communities worldwide. Methodologies include immunotherapy optimization, long-term research, worldwide inclusion, microbial management, individualized healthcare, mechanical research, and study on mechanical systems, aiming for precise, individualized, and reliable treatment regimens (Allaband et al., 2019).

6.9 CONCLUSION

This chapter explores the relationship between the human microbiome and the chemical processes in the body, highlighting the numerous relationships between a person's unique microbiota and how they metabolize drugs.

It also highlights medications' reciprocal impacts on the microbiota, illustrating how these changes can influence drug biotransformation and alter the microbiome's makeup. It shows that pharmaceutical drugs affecting the gut microbiota can benefit and harm microbe communities. It also discusses the impact of stomach microbes on prescription medications, improving our understanding of the therapeutic responses that patients experience due to the microbiota's influence on medication biotransformation. The experimental implications and applications section focus on how microbiota research can be used to create tailored medications for specific people. It emphasizes the importance of informed consent, rigorous data confidentiality protection, and adaptive regulatory frameworks to guide the development of microbiome-based pharmaceuticals while maintaining patient safety. The chapter provides a foundation for further research, ethical considerations, and regulatory frameworks, paving the way for more personalized and efficient medication use.

KEYWORDS

- **microbiome**
- **pharmaceutical response**
- **pharmacokinetics**
- **host defensive system**
- **metabolic irregularities**

REFERENCES

Aggarwal, N., Kitano, S., Puah, G. R. Y., Kittelmann, S., Hwang, I. Y., Chang, M. W. (2023). Microbiome and human health: Current understanding, engineering, and eabling technologies. *Chemical Reviews*, *123*(1), 31–72. https://doi.org/10.1021/acs.chemrev.2c00431

Ahn, J., Hayes, R. B. (2021). Environmental influences on the human microbiome and implications for noncommunicable disease. *Annual Review of Public Health*, *42*, 277–292. https://doi.org/10.1146/annurev-publhealth-012420-105020

Allaband, C., McDonald, D., Vazquez-Baeza, Y., Minich, J. J., Tripathi, A., Brenner, D. A., Knight, R. (2019). Microbiome 101: Studying, analyzing, and interpreting gut microbiome data for clinicians. *Clinical Gastroenterology and Hepatology*, *17*(2), 218–230. https://doi.org/10.1016/j.cgh.2018.09.017

Bajaj, J. S., Acharya, C., Fagan, A., White, M. B., Gavis, E., Heuman, D. M., Gillevet, P. M. (2018). Proton pump inhibitor initiation and withdrawal affects gut microbiota and readmission risk in cirrhosis. *The American Journal of Gastroenterology*, *113*(8), 1177–1186. https://doi.org/10.1038/s41395-018-0085-9

Behrouzi, A., Nafari, A. H., Siadat, S. D. (2019). The significance of microbiome in personalized medicine. *Clinical and Translational Medicine*, *8*(1), 16. https://doi.org/10.1186/s40169-019-0232-y

Belkaid, Y., Hand, T. W. (2014). Role of the microbiota in immunity and inflammation. *Cell*, *157*(1), 121–141. https://doi.org/10.1016/j.cell.2014.03.011

Berg, G., Rybakova, D., Fischer, D., Cernava, T., Verges, M. C., Charles, T., Schloter, M. (2020). Microbiome definition re-visited: Old concepts and new challenges. *Microbiome*, *8*(1), 103. https://doi.org/10.1186/s40168-020-00875-0

Blaser, M. J. (2016). Antibiotic use and its consequences for the normal microbiome. *Science*, *352*(6285), 544–545. https://doi.org/10.1126/science.aad9358

Bull, M. J., Plummer, N. T. (2014). Part 1: The human gut microbiome in health and disease. *Integrative medicine (Encinitas)*, *13*(6), 17–22.

Chambers, E. S., Preston, T., Frost, G., Morrison, D. J. (2018). Role of gut microbiota-generated short-chain fatty acids in metabolic and cardiovascular health. *Current Nutrition Reports*, *7*(4), 198–206. https://doi.org/10.1007/s13668-018-0248-8

Chassaing, B., Raja, S. M., Lewis, J. D., Srinivasan, S., Gewirtz, A. T. (2017). Colonic microbiota encroachment correlates with dysglycemia in humans. *Cellular and Molecular Gastroenterology and Hepatology*, *4*(2), 205–221. https://doi.org/10.1016/j.jcmgh.2017.04.001

Clapp, M., Aurora, N., Herrera, L., Bhatia, M., Wilen, E., Wakefield, S. (2017). Gut microbiota's effect on mental health: The gut-brain axis. *Clinics and Practice*, *7*(4), 987. https://doi.org/10.4081/cp.2017.987

Cohen, I., Ruff, W. E., Longbrake, E. E. (2021). Influence of immunomodulatory drugs on the gut microbiota. *Translational Research*, *233*, 144–161. https://doi.org/10.1016/j.trsl.2021.01.009

Collado, M. C., Rautava, S., Aakko, J., Isolauri, E., Salminen, S. (2016). Human gut colonisation may be initiated in utero by distinct microbial communities in the placenta and amniotic fluid. *Scientific Reports*, *6*, 23129. https://doi.org/10.1038/srep23129

Crouwel, F., Buiter, H. J. C., de Boer, N. K. (2020). Gut microbiota-driven drug metabolism in inflammatory bowel disease. *Journal of Crohn's and Colitis*, *15*(2), 307–315. https://doi.org/10.1093/ecco-jcc/jjaa143

Cullen, C. M., Aneja, K. K., Beyhan, S., Cho, C. E., Woloszynek, S., Convertino, M., Rosen, G. L. (2020). Emerging priorities for microbiome research. *Frontiers in Microbiology*, *11*, 136. https://doi.org/10.3389/fmicb.2020.00136

D Hills Jr, R., Erpenbeck, E. (2018). Guide to popular diets, food choices, and their health outcome. *HealthCare: Current Reviews*, *6*(2). https://doi.org/10.4172/2375-4273.1000223

David, L. A., Maurice, C. F., Carmody, R. N., Gootenberg, D. B., Button, J. E., Wolfe, B. E., Turnbaugh, P. J. (2014). Diet rapidly and reproducibly alters the human gut microbiome. *Nature*, *505*(7484), 559–563. https://doi.org/10.1038/nature12820

De Angelis, M., Garruti, G., Minervini, F., Bonfrate, L., Portincasa, P., Gobbetti, M. (2019). The food-gut human axis: The effects of diet on gut microbiota and metabolome. *Current Medicinal Chemistry*, *26*(19), 3567–3583. https://doi.org/10.2174/0929867324666170428103848

DeGruttola, A. K., Low, D., Mizoguchi, A., Mizoguchi, E. (2016). Current understanding of dysbiosis in disease in human and animal models. *Inflammatory Bowel Disease*, *22*(5), 1137–1150. https://doi.org/10.1097/mib.0000000000000750

Dekaboruah, E., Suryavanshi, M. V., Chettri, D., Verma, A. K. (2020). Human microbiome: An academic update on human body site specific surveillance and its possible role. *Archives of Microbiology*, *202*(8), 2147–2167. https://doi.org/10.1007/s00203-020-01931-x

Doestzada, M., Vila, A. V., Zhernakova, A., Koonen, D. P. Y., Weersma, R. K., Touw, D. J. (2018). Pharmacomicrobiomics: A novel route towards personalized medicine? *Protein Cell*, *9*(5), 432–445. https://doi.org/10.1007/s13238-018-0547-2

Ejtahed, H. S., Hasani-Ranjbar, S., Larijani, B. (2017). Human microbiome as an approach to personalized medicine. *Alternative Therapies in Health and Medicine*, *23*(6), 8–9.

Falony, G., Joossens, M., Vieira-Silva, S., Wang, J., Darzi, Y., Faust, K. (2016). Population-level analysis of gut microbiome variation. *Science*, *352*(6285), 560–564. https://doi.org/10.1126/science.aad3503

Floris, I., Marc Jan, B., Arnau Vich, V., Jingyuan, F., Zlatan, M., Lisa, V., Ettje, F. T. (2016). Proton pump inhibitors affect the gut microbiome. *Gut*, *65*(5), 740. https://doi.org/10.1136/gutjnl-2015-310376

Forgacs, I., Loganayagam, A. (2008). Overprescribing proton pump inhibitors. *British Medical Journal*, *336*(7634), 2–3. https://doi.org/10.1136/bmj.39406.449456.BE

Forslund, K., Hildebrand, F., Nielsen, T., Falony, G., Le Chatelier, E., Sunagawa, S. (2015). Disentangling type 2 diabetes and metformin treatment signatures in the human gut microbiota. *Nature*, *528*(7581), 262–266. https://doi.org/10.1038/nature15766

Foster, J. A., McVey Neufeld, K. A. (2013). Gut-brain axis: How the microbiome influences anxiety and depression. *Trends in Neuroscience*, *36*(5), 305–312. https://doi.org/10.1016/j.tins.2013.01.005

Fuller, A. T. (1937). Is p-aminobenzenesulphonamide the active agent in prontosil therapy. *The Lancet*, *229*(5917), 194–198. https://doi.org/10.1016/s0140-6736(00)97447-6

Ge, X., Ding, C., Zhao, W., Xu, L., Tian, H., Gong, J. (2017). Antibiotics-induced depletion of mice microbiota induces changes in host serotonin biosynthesis and intestinal motility. *Journal of Translational Medicine*, *15*(1), 13. https://doi.org/10.1186/s12967-016-1105-4

Gebrayel, P., Nicco, C., Al Khodor, S., Bilinski, J., Caselli, E., Comelli, E. M., Egert, M. (2022). Microbiota medicine: Towards clinical revolution. *Journal of Translational Medicine*, *20*(1), 111. https://doi.org/10.1186/s12967-022-03296-9

Gopalakrishnan, V., Helmink, B. A., Spencer, C. N., Reuben, A., Wargo, J. A. (2018a). The influence of the gut microbiome on cancer, immunity, and cancer immunotherapy. *Cancer Cells*, *33*(4), 570–580. https://doi.org/10.1016/j.ccell.2018.03.015

Gopalakrishnan, V., Spencer, C. N., Nezi, L., Reuben, A., Andrews, M. C., Karpinets, T. V., Prieto, P. A. (2018b). Gut microbiome modulates response to anti-PD-1 immunotherapy in melanoma patients. *Science*, *359*(6371), 97–103. https://doi.org/10.1126/science.aan4236

Groer, M. W., Luciano, A. A., Dishaw, L. J., Ashmeade, T. L., Miller, E., Gilbert, J. A. (2014). Development of the preterm infant gut microbiome: A research priority. *Microbiome*, *2*, 38. https://doi.org/10.1186/2049-2618-2-38

Grosso, G., Marventano, S., Yang, J., Micek, A., Pajak, A., Scalfi, L. (2017). A comprehensive meta-analysis on evidence of Mediterranean diet and cardiovascular disease: Are individual components equal? *Critical Reviews in Food Science and Nutrition*, *57*(15), 3218–3232. https://doi.org/10.1080/10408398.2015.1107021

Guaraldi, F., Salvatori, G. (2012). Effect of breast and formula feeding on gut microbiota shaping in newborns. *Frontiers in Cellular and Infection Microbiology*, *2*, 94. https://doi.org/10.3389/fcimb.2012.00094

Hadrich, D. (2018). Microbiome research is becoming the key to better understanding health and nutrition. *Frontiers in Genetics*, *9*, 212. https://doi.org/10.3389/fgene.2018.00212

Haiser, H. J., Gootenberg, D. B., Chatman, K., Sirasani, G., Balskus, E. P., Turnbaugh, P. J. (2013). Predicting and manipulating cardiac drug inactivation by the human gut bacterium *Eggerthella lenta*. *Science*, *341*(6143), 295–298. https://doi.org/10.1126/science.1235872

Haiser, H. J., Seim, K. L., Balskus, E. P., Turnbaugh, P. J. (2014). Mechanistic insight into digoxin inactivation by *Eggerthella lenta* augments our understanding of its pharmacokinetics. *Gut Microbes*, *5*(2), 233–238. https://doi.org/10.4161/gmic.27915

Halmos, E. P., Gibson, P. R. (2019). Controversies and reality of the FODMAP diet for patients with irritable bowel syndrome. *Journal of Gastroenterology and Hepatology*, *34*(7), 1134–1142. https://doi.org/10.1111/jgh.14650

Handelsman, J. (2004). Metagenomics: Application of genomics to uncultured microorganisms. *Microbiology and Molecular Biology Reviews*, *68*(4), 669–685. https://doi.org/10.1128/mmbr.68.4.669-685.2004

Hegazy, A. N., West, N. R., Stubbington, M. J. T., Wendt, E., Suijker, K. I. M., Datsi, A. (2017). Circulating and tissue-resident CD4(+) T cells with reactivity to intestinal microbiota are abundant in healthy individuals and function is altered during inflammation. *Gastroenterology*, *153*(5), 1320–1337 e1316. https://doi.org/10.1053/j.gastro.2017.07.047

Imhann, F., Vich Vila, A., Bonder, M. J., Lopez Manosalva, A. G., Koonen, D. P. Y. (2017). The influence of proton pump inhibitors and other commonly used medication on the gut microbiota. *Gut Microbes*, *8*(4), 351–358. https://doi.org/10.1080/19490976.2017.1284732

Ipci, K., Altıntoprak, N., Muluk, N. B., Senturk, M., Cingi, C. (2017). The possible mechanisms of the human microbiome in allergic diseases. *European Archives of Oto-Rhino-Laryngology*, *274*(2), 617–626. https://doi.org/10.1007/s00405-016-4058-6

Isaac, S., Scher, J. U., Djukovic, A., Jimenez, N., Littman, D. R., Abramson, S. B. (2017). Short- and long-term effects of oral vancomycin on the human intestinal microbiota. *Journal of Antimicrobial Chemotherapy*, *72*(1), 128–136. https://doi.org/10.1093/jac/dkw383

Jackson, M. A., Verdi, S., Maxan, M. E., Shin, C. M., Zierer, J. (2018). Gut microbiota associations with common diseases and prescription medications in a population-based cohort. *Nature Communications*, *9*(1), 2655. https://doi.org/10.1038/s41467-018-05184-7

Jandhyala, S. M., Talukdar, R., Subramanyam, C., Vuyyuru, H., Sasikala, M., Nageshwar Reddy, D. (2015). Role of the normal gut microbiota. *World Journal of Gastroenterology*, *21*(29), 8787–8803. https://doi.org/10.3748/wjg.v21.i29.8787

Jourova, L., Anzenbacher, P., Anzenbacherova, E. (2016). Human gut microbiota plays a role in the metabolism of drugs. *Biomedical Papers of the Medical Faculty of the University Palacký, Olomouc, Czech Republic*, *160*(3), 317–326. https://doi.org/10.5507/bp.2016.039

Kadooka, Y., Sato, M., Ogawa, A., Miyoshi, M., Uenishi, H. (2013). Effect of *Lactobacillus gasseri* SBT2055 in fermented milk on abdominal adiposity in adults in a randomised controlled trial. *British Journal of Nutrition*, *110*(9), 1696–1703. https://doi.org/10.1017/s0007114513001037

Karakan, T., Tuohy, K. M., Janssen-van Solingen, G. (2021). Low-dose lactulose as a prebiotic for improved gut health and enhanced mineral absorption. *Frontiers in Nutrition*, *8*, 672925. https://doi.org/10.3389/fnut.2021.672925

Kashyap, P. C., Chia, N., Nelson, H., Segal, E., Elinav, E. (2017). Microbiome at the frontier of personalized medicine. *Mayo Clinic Proceedings*, *92*(12), 1855–1864. https://doi.org/10.1016/j.mayocp.2017.10.004

Kasprzak-Drozd, K., Oniszczuk, T., Stasiak, M., Oniszczuk, A. (2021). Beneficial effects of phenolic compounds on gut microbiota and metabolic syndrome. *International Journal of Molecular Sciences*, *22*(7). https://doi.org/10.3390/ijms22073715

Klingensmith, N. J., Coopersmith, C. M. (2016). The gut as the motor of multiple organ dysfunction in critical illness. *Critical Care Clinics*, *32*(2), 203–212. https://doi.org/10.1016/j.ccc.2015.11.004

Koppel, N., Maini Rekdal, V., Balskus, E. P. (2017). Chemical transformation of xenobiotics by the human gut microbiota. *Science*, *356*(6344). https://doi.org/10.1126/science.aag2770

Kumar Singh, A., Cabral, C., Kumar, R., Ganguly, R., Kumar Rana, H., Gupta, A., Pandey, A. K. (2019). Beneficial effects of dietary polyphenols on gut microbiota and strategies to improve delivery efficiency. *Nutrients*, *11*(9). https://doi.org/10.3390/nu11092216

Lamb, C. A., Saifuddin, A., Powell, N., Rieder, F. (2022). The future of precision medicine to predict outcomes and control tissue remodeling in inflammatory bowel disease. *Gastroenterology*, *162*(5), 1525–1542. https://doi.org/10.1053/j.gastro.2021.09.077

Lee, Y. M., Kim, K. S., Jacobs, D. R., Jr., Lee, D. H. (2017). Persistent organic pollutants in adipose tissue should be considered in obesity research. *Obesity Reviews*, *18*(2), 129–139. https://doi.org/10.1111/obr.12481

Lewis, B. B., Buffie, C. G., Carter, R. A., Leiner, I., Toussaint, N. C., Miller, L. C., Pamer, E. G. (2015). Loss of microbiota-mediated colonization resistance to *Clostridium difficile* infection with oral vancomycin compared with metronidazole. *The Journal of Infectious Diseases*, *212*(10), 1656–1665. https://doi.org/10.1093/infdis/jiv256

Li, G., Xie, C., Lu, S., Nichols, R. G., Tian, Y., Li, L., Gonzalez, F. J. (2017). Intermittent fasting promotes white adipose browning and decreases obesity by shaping the gut microbiota. *Cell Metabolism*, *26*(4), 672–685. https://doi.org/10.1016/j.cmet.2017.08.019

Li, H., He, J., Jia, W. (2016). The influence of gut microbiota on drug metabolism and toxicity. *Expert Opinion on Drug Metabolism & Toxicology*, *12*(1), 31–40. https://doi.org/10.1517/17425255.2016.1121234

Lloyd-Price, J., Arze, C., Ananthakrishnan, A. N., Schirmer, M., Avila-Pacheco, J., Poon, T. W., Huttenhower, C. (2019). Multi-omics of the gut microbial ecosystem in inflammatory bowel diseases. *Nature, 569*(7758), 655–662. https://doi.org/10.1038/s41586-019-1237-9

Maier, L., Pruteanu, M., Kuhn, M., Zeller, G., Telzerow, A., Anderson, E. E. (2018). Extensive impact of non-antibiotic drugs on human gut bacteria. *Nature, 555*(7698), 623–628. https://doi.org/10.1038/nature25979

Miclotte, L., Van de Wiele, T. (2020). Food processing, gut microbiota and the globesity problem. *Critical Reviews in Food Science and Nutrition, 60*(11), 1769–1782. https://doi.org/10.1080/10408398.2019.1596878

Momtaz, P., Postow, M. A. (2014). Immunologic checkpoints in cancer therapy: Focus on the programmed death-1 (PD-1) receptor pathway. *Pharmacogenomics and Personalized Medicine, 7*, 357–365. https://doi.org/10.2147/PGPM.S53163

Morgan, X. C., Huttenhower, C. (2012). Human microbiome analysis. *PLOS Computational Biology, 8*(12). https://doi.org/10.1371/journal.pcbi.1002808

Morowitz, M. J., Carlisle, E. M., Alverdy, J. C. (2011). Contributions of intestinal bacteria to nutrition and metabolism in the critically ill. *Surgical Clinics of North America, 91*(4), 771–785. https://doi.org/10.1016/j.suc.2011.05.001

Mousa, S., Sarfraz, M., Mousa, W. K. (2023). The interplay between gut microbiota and oral medications and its impact on advancing precision medicine. *Metabolites, 13*(5). https://doi.org/10.3390/metabo13050674

Nagata, N., Tohya, M., Fukuda, S., Suda, W., Nishijima, S., Takeuchi, F. (2019). Effects of bowel preparation on the human gut microbiome and metabolome. *Scientific Reports, 9*(1), 4042. https://doi.org/10.1038/s41598-019-40182-9

Nagpal, R., Tsuji, H., Takahashi, T., Nomoto, K., Kawashima, K., Nagata, S., Yamashiro, Y. (2017). Ontogenesis of the gut microbiota composition in healthy, full-term, vaginally born and breast-fed infants over the first 3 years of life: A quantitative bird's-eye view. *Frontiers in Microbiology, 8*, 1388. https://doi.org/10.3389/fmicb.2017.01388

Ogunrinola, G. A., Oyewale, J. O., Oshamika, O. O., Olasehinde, G. I. (2020). The human microbiome and its impacts on health. *International Journal of Microbiology, 2020*, 8045646. https://doi.org/10.1155/2020/8045646

Othman, F., Card, T. R., Crooks, C. J. (2016). Proton pump inhibitor prescribing patterns in the UK: A primary care database study. *Pharmacoepidemiology and Drug Safety, 25*(9), 1079–1087. https://doi.org/10.1002/pds.4043

Pant, A., Maiti, T. K., Mahajan, D., Das, B. (2023). Human gut microbiota and drug metabolism. *Microbial Ecology, 86*(1), 97–111. https://doi.org/10.1007/s00248-022-02081-x

Parashar, A., Udayabanu, M. (2017). Gut microbiota: Implications in Parkinson's disease. *Parkinsonism & Related Disorders, 38*, 1–7. https://doi.org/10.1016/j.parkreldis.2017.02.002

Pascal, M., Perez-Gordo, M., Caballero, T., Escribese, M. M., Lopez Longo, M. N., Luengo, O., Mayorga, C. (2018). Microbiome and allergic diseases. *Frontiers in Immunology, 9*, 1584. https://doi.org/10.3389/fimmu.2018.01584

Patangia, D. V., Anthony Ryan, C., Dempsey, E., Paul Ross, R., Stanton, C. (2022). Impact of antibiotics on the human microbiome and consequences for host health. *Microbiology Open, 11*(1), 1260. https://doi.org/10.1002/mbo3.1260

Petersen, J., Ciacchi, L., Tran, M. T., Loh, K. L., Kooy-Winkelaar, Y., Croft, N. P. (2020). T cell receptor cross-reactivity between gliadin and bacterial peptides in celiac disease. *Nature Structural & Molecular Biology*, *27*(1), 49–61. https://doi.org/10.1038/s41594-019-0353-4

Quigley, E. M. M. (2022). Clinical trials of probiotics in patients with irritable bowel syndrome: Some points to consider. *Journal of Neurogastroenterology and Motility*, *28*(2), 204–211. https://doi.org/10.5056/jnm22012

Routy, B., Le Chatelier, E., Derosa, L., Duong, C. P. M., Alou, M. T., Daillere, R. (2018). Gut microbiome influences efficacy of PD-1-based immunotherapy against epithelial tumors. *Science*, *359*(6371), 91–97. https://doi.org/10.1126/science.aan3706

Rowland, I., Gibson, G., Heinken, A., Scott, K., Swann, J., Thiele, I., Tuohy, K. (2018). Gut microbiota functions: Metabolism of nutrients and other food components. *European Journal of Nutrition*, *57*(1), 1–24. https://doi.org/10.1007/s00394-017-1445-8

Sherman, M. P., Zaghouani, H., Niklas, V. (2015). Gut microbiota, the immune system, and diet influence the neonatal gut-brain axis. *Pediatric Research*, *77*(1–2), 127–135. https://doi.org/10.1038/pr.2014.161

Shin, N. R., Lee, J. C., Lee, H. Y., Kim, M. S., Whon, T. W., Lee, M. S., Bae, J. W. (2014). An increase in the *Akkermansia* spp. population induced by metformin treatment improves glucose homeostasis in diet-induced obese mice. *Gut*, *63*(5), 727–735. https://doi.org/10.1136/gutjnl-2012-303839

Singh, R. K., Chang, H. W., Yan, D., Lee, K. M., Ucmak, D., Wong, K. (2017). Influence of diet on the gut microbiome and implications for human health. *Journal of Translational Medicine*, *15*(1), 73. https://doi.org/10.1186/s12967-017-1175-y

Skodje, G. I., Sarna, V. K., Minelle, I. H., Rolfsen, K. L., Muir, J. G. (2018). Fructan, rather than gluten, induces symptoms in patients with self-reported non-celiac gluten sensitivity. *Gastroenterology*, *154*(3), 529–539. https://doi.org/10.1053/j.gastro.2017.10.040

Skonieczna-Zydecka, K., Marlicz, W., Misera, A., Koulaouzidis, A., Łoniewski, I. (2018). Microbiome—the missing link in the gut-brain axis: Focus on its role in gastrointestinal and mental health. *Journal of Clinical Medicine*, *7*(12). https://doi.org/10.3390/jcm7120521

Sonnenburg, J. L., Backhed, F. (2016). Diet-microbiota interactions as moderators of human metabolism. *Nature*, *535*(7610), 56–64. https://doi.org/10.1038/nature18846

Stearns, J. C., Lynch, M. D., Senadheera, D. B., Tenenbaum, H. C., Goldberg, M. B., Cvitkovitch, D. G., Neufeld, J. D. (2011). Bacterial biogeography of the human digestive tract. *Scientific Reports*, *1*, 170. https://doi.org/10.1038/srep00170

Sun, C., Chen, L., Shen, Z. (2019). Mechanisms of gastrointestinal microflora on drug metabolism in clinical practice. *Saudi Pharmaceutical Journal*, *27*(8), 1146–1156. https://doi.org/10.1016/j.jsps.2019.09.011

Sun, L., Xie, C., Wang, G., Wu, Y., Wu, Q., Wang, X. (2018). Gut microbiota and intestinal FXR mediate the clinical benefits of metformin. *Nature Medicine*, *24*(12), 1919–1929. https://doi.org/10.1038/s41591-018-0222-4

Swanson, H. I. (2015). Drug metabolism by the host and gut microbiota: A partnership or rivalry? *Drug Metabolism and Disposition*, *43*(10), 1499–1504. https://doi.org/10.1124/dmd.115.065714

Tanoue, T., Morita, S., Plichta, D. R., Skelly, A. N., Suda, W., Sugiura, Y. (2019). A defined commensal consortium elicits CD8 T cells and anti-cancer immunity. *Nature*, *565*(7741), 600–605. https://doi.org/10.1038/s41586-019-0878-z

Thomas, A. M., Manghi, P., Asnicar, F., Pasolli, E., Armanini, F., Zolfo, M., Beghini, F. (2019). Metagenomic analysis of colorectal cancer datasets identifies cross-cohort microbial diagnostic signatures and a link with choline degradation. *Nature Medicine*, *25*(4), 667–678. https://doi.org/10.1038/s41591-019-0405-7

Thursby, E., Juge, N. (2017). Introduction to the human gut microbiota. *Biochemical Journal*, *474*(11), 1823–1836. https://doi.org/10.1042/bcj20160510

Trompette, A., Gollwitzer, E. S., Yadava, K., Sichelstiel, A. K., Sprenger, N. (2014). Gut microbiota metabolism of dietary fiber influences allergic airway disease and hematopoiesis. *Nature Medicine*, *20*(2), 159–166. https://doi.org/10.1038/nm.3444

Tropini, C., Moss, E. L., Merrill, B. D., Ng, K. M., Higginbottom, S. K. (2018). Transient osmotic perturbation causes long-term alteration to the gut microbiota. *Cell*, *173*(7), 1742–1754. https://doi.org/10.1016/j.cell.2018.05.008

Tsunoda, S. M., Gonzales, C., Jarmusch, A. K., Momper, J. D., Ma, J. D. (2021). Contribution of the gut microbiome to drug disposition, pharmacokinetic and pharmacodynamic variability. *Clinical Pharmacokinetics*, *60*(8), 971–984. https://doi.org/10.1007/s40262-021-01032-y

Ursell, L. K., Metcalf, J. L., Parfrey, L. W., Knight, R. (2012). Defining the human microbiome. *Nutrition Review*, *38*–44. https://doi.org/10.1111/j.1753-4887.2012.00493.x

Valdes, A. M., Walter, J., Segal, E., Spector, T. D. (2018). Role of the gut microbiota in nutrition and health. *British Medical Journal*, *361*. https://doi.org/10.1136/bmj.k2179

Vandeputte, D., Falony, G., Vieira-Silva, S., Tito, R. Y., Joossens, M., Raes, J. (2016). Stool consistency is strongly associated with gut microbiota richness and composition, enterotypes and bacterial growth rates. *Gut*, *65*(1), 57–62. https://doi.org/10.1136/gutjnl-2015-309618

Vandeputte, D., Kathagen, G., D'Hoe, K., Vieira-Silva, S. (2017). Quantitative microbiome profiling links gut community variation to microbial load. *Nature*, *551*(7681), 507–511. https://doi.org/10.1038/nature24460

Vemuri, R., Gundamaraju, R., Shastri, M. D., Shukla, S. D., Kalpurath, K. (2018). Gut microbial changes, interactions, and their implications on human lifecycle: An ageing perspective. *BioMed Research International*, 4178607. https://doi.org/10.1155/2018/4178607

Vetizou, M., Pitt, J. M., Daillere, R., Lepage, P., Waldschmitt, N. (2015). Anticancer immunotherapy by CTLA-4 blockade relies on the gut microbiota. *Science*, *350*(6264), 1079–1084. https://doi.org/10.1126/science.aad1329

Vila, A., Collij, V., Sanna, S., Sinha, T., Imhann, F. (2020). Impact of commonly used drugs on the composition and metabolic function of the gut microbiota. *Nature Communications*, *11*(1), 362. https://doi.org/10.1038/s41467-019-14177-z

Vila, A., Imhann, F., Collij, V., Jankipersadsing, S. A., Gurry, T. (2018). Gut microbiota composition and functional changes in inflammatory bowel disease and irritable bowel syndrome. *Science Translational Medicine*, *10*(472). https://doi.org/10.1126/scitranslmed.aap8914

Vijay, A., Valdes, A. M. (2022). Role of the gut microbiome in chronic diseases: A narrative review. *European Journal of Clinical Nutrition*, *76*(4), 489–501. https://doi.org/10.1038/s41430-021-00991-6

Vrieze, A., Out, C., Fuentes, S., Jonker, L., Reuling, I., Kootte, R. S. (2014). Impact of oral vancomycin on gut microbiota, bile acid metabolism, and insulin sensitivity. *Journal of Hepatology*, *60*(4), 824–831. https://doi.org/10.1016/j.jhep.2013.11.034

Walker, A. W., Ince, J., Duncan, S. H., Webster, L. M., Holtrop, G., Ze, X., Flint, H. J. (2011). Dominant and diet-responsive groups of bacteria within the human colonic microbiota. *The ISME Journal*, *5*(2), 220–230. https://doi.org/10.1038/ismej.2010.118

Wampach, L., Heintz-Buschart, A., Hogan, A., Muller, E. E. L., Narayanasamy, S., Laczny, C. C., Wilmes, P. (2017). Colonization and succession within the human gut microbiome by archaea, bacteria, and microeukaryotes during the first year of life. *Frontiers in Microbiology*, *8*, 738. https://doi.org/10.3389/fmicb.2017.00738

Wang, B., Yao, M., Lv, L., Ling, Z., Li, L. (2017). The human microbiota in health and disease. *Engineering*, *3*(1), 71–82. https://doi.org/10.1016/j.Eng.2017.01.008

Watson, H., Mitra, S., Croden, F. C., Taylor, M. (2018). A randomised trial of the effect of omega-3 polyunsaturated fatty acid supplements on the human intestinal microbiota. *Gut*, *67*(11), 1974–1983. https://doi.org/10.1136/gutjnl-2017-314968

Whiteside, S. A., Razvi, H., Dave, S., Reid, G., Burton, J. P. (2015). The microbiome of the urinary tract—a role beyond infection. *Nature Reviews Urology*, *12*(2), 81–90. https://doi.org/10.1038/nrurol.2014.361

Wilson, I. D., Nicholson, J. K. (2017). Gut microbiome interactions with drug metabolism, efficacy, and toxicity. *Translational Research*, *179*, 204–222. https://doi.org/10.1016/j.trsl.2016.08.002

Windey, K., De Preter, V., Verbeke, K. (2012). Relevance of protein fermentation to gut health. *Molecular Nutrition & Food Research*, *56*(1), 184–196. https://doi.org/10.1002/mnfr.201100542

Wu, H., Esteve, E., Tremaroli, V., Khan, M. T., Caesar, R. (2017). Metformin alters the gut microbiome of individuals with treatment-naive type 2 diabetes, contributing to the therapeutic effects of the drug. *Nature Medicine*, *23*(7), 850–858. https://doi.org/10.1038/nm.4345

Zhang, X., Han, Y., Huang, W., Jin, M., Gao, Z. (2021). The influence of the gut microbiota on the bioavailability of oral drugs. *Acta Pharmaceutica Sinica B*, *11*(7), 1789–1812. https://doi.org/10.1016/j.apsb.2020.09.013

Zhang, Y., Chen, R., Zhang, D., Qi, S., Liu, Y. (2023). Metabolite interactions between host and microbiota during health and disease: Which feeds the other? *Biomedicine & Pharmacotherapy*, *160*, 114295. https://doi.org/10.1016/j.biopha.2023.114295

Zhao, M., Ma, J., Li, M., Zhang, Y. (2021). Cytochrome P450 enzymes and drug metabolism in humans. *International Journal of Molecular Sciences*, *22*(23). https://doi.org/10.3390/ijms222312808

Zhernakova, A., Kurilshikov, A., Bonder, M. J., Tigchelaar, E. F., Schirmer, M. (2016). Population-based metagenomics analysis reveals markers for gut microbiome composition and diversity. *Science*, *352*(6285), 565–569. https://doi.org/10.1126/science.aad3369

Zhou, C. B., Zhou, Y. L., Fang, J. Y. (2021). Gut microbiota in cancer immune response and immunotherapy. *Trends in Cancer*, *7*(7), 647–660. https://doi.org/10.1016/j.trecan.2021.01.010

Zhou, W., Sailani, M. R., Contrepois, K., Zhou, Y., Ahadi, S. (2019). Longitudinal multi-omics of host-microbe dynamics in prediabetes. *Nature*, *569*(7758), 663–671. https://doi.org/10.1038/s41586-019-1236-x

Zitvogel, L., Daillere, R., Roberti, M. P., Routy, B., Kroemer, G. (2017). Anticancer effects of the microbiome and its products. *Nature Reviews Microbiology*, *15*(8), 465–478. https://doi.org/10.1038/nrmicro.2017.44

Zmora, N., Zeevi, D., Korem, T., Segal, E., Elinav, E. (2016). Taking it personally: Personalized utilization of the human microbiome in health and disease. *Cell Host & Microbe*, *19*(1), 12–20. https://doi.org/10.1016/j.chom.2015.12.016

PART III

Microbiology and Drug Development

CHAPTER 7

Microbes and Medicine: Revolutionizing Healthcare with Biotech and Pharma

TOHFA SIDDIQUI*, KOMAL GUPTA, and PRACHI ACHAL SHAHU

Galgotias College of Pharmacy, Greater Noida, Uttar Pradesh, India

*Corresponding author

ABSTRACT

This chapter outlines the significant contributions that pharmaceutical biotechnology and microbiology have made to medication development and healthcare. Using biological systems and living beings, biotechnology creates novel goods, particularly in the medical field. On the other hand, by examining microorganisms essential to manufacturing procedures, pharmaceutical microbiology guarantees the security and effectiveness of medications. Genetic engineering and other contemporary biotechnological techniques have completely changed how diseases are treated and prevented. The chapter emphasizes aseptic processing and contamination control for product safety while highlighting the use of microbes in the production of biopharmaceuticals and biofuels. It is imperative to continue studying microbial genetics since multidrug resistance illnesses are becoming more common. Biotechnology and pharmaceutical microbiology work together to create a symbiotic connection that might lead to revolutionary improvements in healthcare. Cutting-edge methods for managing disease, including gene editing and personalized therapy, provide revolutionary potential. The chapter highlights the critical role these domains play in modern medicine as well as their promise for innovation in the future.

Advances in Pharmaceutical Microbiology: From Bench to Bedside. Harpreet Singh, Arun Kumar Mishra, Jeyabalan Sangeetha, and Devarajan Thangadurai (Eds.)

DOI: 10.1201/9781779640918-10

7.1 INTRODUCTION

At the cutting-edge of innovation, biotechnology and pharmaceutical microbiology are two linked pillars that are driving revolutionary changes in medication development and healthcare systems. This chapter explores the dynamic interaction between these fields and their significant impact on the development of new treatment approaches and paradigms in healthcare. Through biotech applications, the world of colors and biotechnology are intricately connected. This has made the development of a color-based categorization system necessary. Biotechnology for industrial use (production of chemicals, paper, textiles, and food), environment (bioremediation, ecological diversity preservation), drugs (the development of new medications and treatments), farming (the growth of genetically engineered crops, biofuels, biological treatment), and other fields are developing advanced technologies and services (Scott, 2022). Within the pharmaceutical industry, biotechnology is a new and developing sector that applies biotechnology concepts to medication creation. The majority of pharmaceuticals on the market today, referred to as "bioformulations," consist of materials such as vaccinations, nucleic acid products, and antibodies (Schnurr and Addison, 2021). Nevertheless, biotechnology has advanced significantly in the medical field. Pharmaceutical biotechnology is a new and developing field that uses biotechnology principles to produce pharmaceuticals (Labrou, 2021). Vaccinations, nucleic acid products, and antibodies are examples of bioformulations that make up the majority of therapeutic medications available today. The pharmaceutical industry benefits from biotechnology by using it to develop new products, services, and processes, as well as to enhance existing ones. Pharmacological drug research and development now heavily relies on biotechnological techniques (Ranade, 2010). Currently, biopharmaceuticals make up 15% of all drug sales. The most prevalent indications include musculoskeletal disorders, metabolic diseases, and oncology. Future projections indicate that the significance of biopharmaceuticals will increase (Bartusik-Aebisher and Aebisher, 2020). Presently, approximately 25% of all compounds undergoing preclinical testing are biotechnology-based chemicals. The items with the highest rate of success are those for infectious diseases, metabolic disorders, and cancer. RNA interference is one of the novel therapeutic approaches that make up 1.5% of all biological preclinical medications, and it plays a small part in the present commercial drug research and development process (Agarwal et al., 2020).

The ethical ramifications of biotechnology should be taken into consideration as we investigate these advancements. The ability to control life at the molecular level brings up concerns about appropriate use, effects on the environment, and fair distribution of advantages. Maintaining equilibrium between scientific advancement and ethical deliberations is a crucial facet of the dynamic field of biotechnology. This chapter provides a thorough examination of the application of biotechnology to the creation of innovative pharmaceutical products. It also discusses how biotechnology is influencing research and innovation in a number of medical domains. Creating and purifying the molecules, evaluating product durability, stability, toxicity, and immunogenicity, investigating drug delivery systems, securing patents, conducting clinical trials, and comprehending the principles pertaining to health and disease are some of the stages involved in developing these bioformulations. As an essential and frequently unappreciated protector of public health and product quality, pharmaceutical microbiology plays a critical role in the pharmaceutical business. This particular area of microbiology is concerned with the careful monitoring and testing of microbes during the manufacturing of pharmaceuticals. The task of detecting and avoiding microbiological contamination in raw materials, production settings, and finished goods falls to experts in this sector. Another important component is the ongoing fight against microbial resistance, in which pharmaceutical microbiologists produce antimicrobial medicines and research resistance mechanisms to guarantee the continued effectiveness of vital pharmaceuticals. Another cornerstone of their work is sterility assurance, where they create plans to keep injectable medication and vaccine production environments sterile. Pharmaceutical microbiologists are at the forefront of vaccine development, carrying out studies to optimize growth conditions, guarantee purity, and evaluate stability. New technologies, such as molecular diagnostics and rapid microbiological testing procedures, are revolutionizing old processes with faster and more accurate results as technology develops. Essentially, pharmaceutical microbiology plays a crucial role in maintaining the highest standards of quality, safety, and efficacy in medications that have a significant influence on millions of people's lives.

7.2 PHARMACEUTICAL MICROBIOLOGY: ENSURING SAFETY AND QUALITY

The specialized field of pharmaceutical microbiology is committed to guaranteeing the safety and caliber of pharmaceutical products. It is essential to the creation and production of pharmaceuticals since it focuses on the study of microbes and how they affect pharmaceutical procedures and final products. Ensuring the safety of pharmaceutical products is one of pharmaceutical microbiology's main goals. Medication containing microorganisms, including bacteria, viruses, and fungi, may be dangerous. Therefore, in order to avoid contamination throughout the production process, pharmaceutical microbiologists seek to identify and manage these microbes. This complex objective includes a variety of actions and procedures intended to ensure that the medications generated are dependable, advantageous, and uphold the highest standards of quality (Mccormick and Sanders, 2022).

7.3 ASSURING EFFICIENCY, SAFETY, AND INTEGRITY OF PHARMACEUTICAL GOODS

Throughout the production process, pharmaceutical microbiologists constantly look to prevent and control microbial contamination. This is crucial because dangerous microbes have a chance to put at risk the safety of pharmaceuticals. Endotoxin detection is crucial because these chemicals possess the ability to trigger undesirable reactions in patients. A major component of the safety of pharmaceutical products is ensuring that their contents have no endotoxins (Chatterjee and Abraham, 2018). Rigorous testing of both raw materials and finished products is conducted to ensure that the pharmaceutical goods meet predetermined quality standards. This includes assessing the concentration of active ingredients to guarantee the intended therapeutic effect (Bulk et al., 2005). Pharmaceutical microbiologists play a role in supporting clinical trials, ensuring that the effectiveness of new drugs is thoroughly evaluated before reaching the market (Durrant, 2001).

7.3.1 QUALITY ASSURANCE

To preserve the quality and integrity of the products, aseptic methods have to be used when manufacturing sterile pharmaceuticals (WHO, 2011).

Pharmaceutical microbiologists analyze the shelf life and stability of pharmaceutical products to make sure that the effectiveness is sustained until their expiration date and to ensure their quality is maintained throughout time (Capen et al., 2012). Pharmaceutical microbiologists analyze the shelf life and stability of pharmaceutical products to make sure that the effectiveness is sustained until their expiration date and to ensure their quality is maintained throughout time (Vandivort et al., 2020).

Basically, pharmaceutical microbiologists collaborate in order to ensure that pharmaceutical drugs are safe to use, effective for the intended therapeutic purposes, and of the highest possible standard. They accomplish this by preventing contamination, conducting quality control tests, working with clinical trials, and looking at different aspects of product quality. The significance of pharmaceutical microbiology in the creation and production of medications that improve public health is highlighted by its dedication to safety, efficacy, and quality (Ratajczak et al., 2015).

Medicinal microbiology is equally concerned with preserving the quality of medicinal goods as it is with safety. This entails meticulous testing and observation of pharmaceuticals in their finished form, production settings, and raw ingredients to guarantee they adhere to specified criteria. Pharmaceutical microbiologists enhance the uniformity and efficacy of medications by putting in place stringent quality control procedures (Quality Assurance of Pharmaceuticals, 2020).

7.3.2 EMPHASIS ON ASEPTIC PROCESSING, STERILITY ASSURANCE, AND MICROBIAL CONTAMINATION CONTROL

Aseptic processing refers to the techniques and procedures used in the pharmaceutical industry to prevent microbial contamination and maintain a sterile environment during the production of sterile drug products. The goal is to ensure that the final pharmaceutical product is free from viable microorganisms that could compromise patient safety (Tanzini et al., 2023). Aseptic processing is conducted in cleanrooms with controlled environmental conditions. These include air filtration, temperature, humidity, and pressure control to minimize the presence of airborne contaminants (Schicht, 1998). All equipment and components coming into contact with the pharmaceutical product must be sterilized. This includes containers, closures, and manufacturing equipment (WHO, 2011). Strict hygiene protocols are enforced for personnel involved in aseptic processing. This includes gowning procedures, hand hygiene, and ongoing training to minimize the risk of introducing contaminants (Mathur, 2011). Advanced technologies such as isolators and restricted access barrier systems are employed to physically separate the product from the surrounding environment, reducing the risk of microbial contamination (Rauschnabel, 2007). Sterilization techniques such as autoclaving, gamma irradiation, and aseptic filtration are used to ensure the sterility of critical components and materials (Bernal-Chávez et al., 2021).

7.3.3 STERILITY ASSURANCE

The process of ensuring a pharmaceutical product is free of living microorganisms to maintain its safety, effectiveness, and compliance with legal requirements is known as sterility assurance (Lambert et al., 2021). Products undergo rigorous sterility testing to verify the absence of viable microorganisms. This testing is performed using validated methods in compliance with regulatory requirements. The sterilization processes used in manufacturing are thoroughly validated to ensure their effectiveness in eliminating or reducing microbial contamination to an acceptable level. Continuous monitoring of the manufacturing environment for microbial contamination is essential. This includes air and surface monitoring in critical areas to detect and address potential sources of contamination (Griffith, 2016). Validation of aseptic processing and sterilization procedures is crucial to demonstrate that the entire manufacturing process consistently produces sterile products (Schmidt et al., 1999).

7.3.4 MICROBIAL CONTAMINATION CONTROL

Microbial contamination control involves strategies and measures to prevent, detect, and eliminate microbial contaminants throughout the pharmaceutical manufacturing process (Baird et al., 1979). Strict adherence to Good Manufacturing Practice is fundamental for microbial contamination control. This includes maintaining clean facilities, proper personnel hygiene, and documentation of all processes (Maldonade et al., 2019). Regular monitoring and control of the microbial bioburden in raw materials and the manufacturing environment help prevent the introduction of contaminants into the production process (Drinkwater and Lucas, 2013).

Effective segregation of manufacturing processes and the use of dedicated equipment help prevent cross-contamination between different products (Dzerzhinskaya et al., 2022). Thorough cleaning and sanitization procedures are implemented to eliminate microbial residues and prevent the buildup of contaminants on equipment and surface (Schmidt, 2012). Adoption of rapid microbiological methods allows for quicker detection of microbial contaminants, enabling timely corrective actions and reducing the risk of product loss (Greb, 2010). By emphasizing aseptic processing, sterility assurance, and microbial contamination control, pharmaceutical manufacturers can produce high-quality, safe, and effective products that comply with regulatory standards and meet the expectations of healthcare providers and patients (Lambert et al., 2021).

The work of pharmaceutical microbiologists directly translates to the well-being of patients. Ensuring that pharmaceutical products are free from harmful microorganisms and meet stringent quality standards is crucial for the safety and efficacy of medications. This dedication to microbiological safety contributes to building trust in the pharmaceutical industry and safeguarding public health.

7.4 BIOTECHNOLOGICAL METHODS

Biotechnological methods have undergone a transformative evolution, paving the way for modern innovations that have revolutionized various industries. In the realm of scientific discovery and technological advancement, biotechnology stands at the forefront, with cutting-edge techniques to manipulate biological systems for the betterment of society. This interdisciplinary field seamlessly integrates principles from biology, chemistry, genetics, and engineering to develop novel solutions for challenges in medicine, agriculture, environmental conservation, and beyond (Chui et al., 2023). From gene editing tools like Clustered Regularly Interspaced Short Palindromic Repeats (CRISPR)-Cas to advanced fermentation processes and synthetic biology, these modern innovations exemplify the incredible potential of biotechnological methods to address complex issues and reshape the landscape of scientific possibilities. As researchers and practitioners continue to push the boundaries of what is achievable, the impact of biotechnology on our world is increasingly profound, offering unprecedented opportunities for sustainable development and improved quality of life (Zhu, 2022).

7.4.1 GENETIC ENGINEERING

Genetic engineering, also known as genetic modification or recombinant DNA technology, is a powerful set of techniques used to manipulate the genetic material (DNA) of organisms to achieve specific traits or outcomes. This field has wide-ranging applications in agriculture, medicine, industry, and environmental management. The fundamental goal is to introduce, alter, or delete specific genetic information within an organism's DNA to express desired traits or characteristics (Khan et al., 2016). Genetic material is the set of instructions encoded in an organism's DNA that governs its growth, development, and functioning (Shah, 2019). DNA consists of genes, which are segments of the DNA molecule that code for specific proteins or functional RNA molecules. Recombinant DNA technology involves the manipulation of DNA from different sources, combining them to create recombinant DNA molecules. Enzymes like restriction enzymes are used to cut DNA at specific points, and ligases are used to join DNA fragments together (Mandrich, 2013).

The process of making identical copies of a gene is known as gene cloning. This can be achieved by inserting a gene of interest into a vector, often a plasmid or a viral DNA, which is then introduced into a host organism, such as bacteria or yeast. Polymerase chain reaction (PCR) is a technique that allows the amplification of specific DNA sequences, enabling the production of large quantities of a particular gene for further study or manipulation.

7.4.2 SYNTHETIC BIOLOGY

Synthetic biology is an interdisciplinary field that combines principles from biology, chemistry, physics, engineering, and computer science to design and construct new biological entities or redesign existing biological systems for useful purposes. The goal of synthetic biology is to apply engineering principles to biology, allowing scientists to create, modify, and optimize biological systems in a predictable and controlled manner (Garner, 2021). In synthetic biology, researchers start by designing the desired biological system or entity on a computer. This involves specifying the genetic components, pathways, and overall structure of the biological system they want to create. Computer-aided design tools play a crucial role in this phase, helping scientists' model and simulate the behavior of the designed system (Marucci et al., 2020). Once the design is finalized, the next step is to physically construct the designed biological entity. This often involves synthesizing DNA sequences, which encode the genetic information for the desired system. Advances in DNA synthesis technologies have significantly facilitated this process, allowing researchers to order custom DNA sequences for specific genetic components (Wang et al., 2013). The synthesized DNA sequences are then assembled into functional genetic circuits or pathways. This can be done using various molecular biology techniques, such as PCR and DNA ligation. The assembled genetic constructs are then inserted into host organisms, such as bacteria or yeast, to express the desired traits (Hughes and Ellington, 2017). After construction and assembly, scientists rigorously characterize the behavior of the synthetic biological entity. This involves testing the system's functionality, efficiency, and stability under different conditions. Characterization helps researchers understand how well the designed biological system aligns with their initial goals and allows for iterative improvements (David et al., 2021). Based on the characterization results, the synthetic system can be optimized to enhance its performance or adapt it to specific applications. This iterative process of design, construction, characterization, and optimization is a key feature of synthetic biology (Anderson et al., 2019).

Synthetic biology has diverse applications, including the development of biofuels, the production of pharmaceuticals, the creation of biosensors, and the design of novel materials. It also has the potential to address various challenges in fields such as medicine, agriculture, and environmental science by providing tailored solutions through the engineering of biological systems.

7.5 BIOPROCESSING

Bioprocessing is a field within biotechnology that involves using biological systems, such as cells or microorganisms, to produce valuable compounds through a series of controlled and optimized processes (Damaso et al., 2014). The primary goal of bioprocessing is to harness the capabilities of living organisms to efficiently manufacture a wide range of products, including pharmaceuticals, biofuels, enzymes, chemicals, and food ingredients (Mitra and Murthy, 2022). This approach leverages the inherent biochemical and metabolic pathways within cells to conduct specific tasks for large-scale production. The choice of host organism is a critical aspect of bioprocessing. Commonly used organisms include bacteria, yeast, fungi, and mammalian cells. Each organism has unique characteristics that make it suitable for specific applications. For example, bacteria like *Escherichia coli* are often used for the production of proteins, while yeast, such as *Saccharomyces cerevisiae*, is employed for the production of biofuels and certain chemicals (Walker and Pretorius, 2018). Bioprocessing often involves fermentation, a controlled process where microorganisms, typically bacteria or yeast, are cultured in large bioreactors under optimized conditions. These conditions include nutrient availability, temperature, pH, and oxygen levels. The fermentation process allows the microorganisms to grow and produce the desired product, whether it's a therapeutic protein, biofuel, or other valuable compound (Unrean, 2016).

Advances in genetic engineering play a crucial role in optimizing host organisms for specific bioprocessing applications. Researchers modify the genetic makeup of the host cells to enhance their productivity, increase yield, and improve the quality of the desired product. This may involve introducing genes for the synthesis of specific enzymes or proteins, or modifying metabolic pathways to increase the production of target compounds (Pickens et al., 2011). Once the fermentation process is complete, the next step is downstream processing, where the product is separated and purified from the culture broth. This involves various techniques such as filtration, centrifugation, chromatography, and precipitation. Downstream processing is critical for obtaining the product in a pure and concentrated form suitable for commercial use. Bioprocessing often starts at a small laboratory scale and then transitions to larger industrial scales for commercial production (Khanra et al., 2018). Scaling up involves addressing challenges related to mass transfer, mixing, and maintaining optimal conditions in larger bioreactors. This step is crucial to ensure that the bioprocess remains efficient and economically viable. Bioprocessing has numerous applications, including the production of bio-based chemicals, therapeutic proteins, vaccines, enzymes, and biofuels (Ganeshan et al., 2021). It offers a sustainable and environmentally friendly approach to manufacturing by using renewable resources and reducing reliance on traditional chemical synthesis methods. The flexibility and versatility of bioprocessing make it a key technology in the growing field of industrial biotechnology.

The type of regulatory microbiological testing requirement is given in Table 7.1 (Wiltschi et al., 2020).

TABLE 7.1 Regulatory Microbiological Testing Requirement

Regulatory Body	Testing Requirement	References
FDA	Microbial limits testing, sterility testing, validation	Center for Drug Evaluation and Research (2018)
EMA	Bioburden testing, environmental monitoring	Hentz (2013)
WHO	Microbial quality control, aseptic processing	Aseptic Processing: A Primer: NIBRT's Ray O'Connor Provides an Overview of Aseptic Processing (2013)

7.5.1 IMPACT ON MEDICINE: REVOLUTIONIZING APPROACHES TO ILLNESS TREATMENT AND PREVENTION

The impact of bioprocessing and related biotechnological advances on medicine has been revolutionary, fundamentally transforming approaches to illness treatment and prevention (Barragán-Ocaña et al., 2020). Here are several key ways in which these technologies have influenced and continue to shape the field of medicine.

Bioprocessing plays a crucial role in the large-scale production of therapeutic proteins, such as monoclonal antibodies, insulin, and vaccines. By using genetically modified host organisms such as bacteria, yeast, or mammalian cells, biotechnologists can produce these proteins with high efficiency and precision (Tripathi and Shrivastava, 2019). Therapeutic proteins have become essential in treating various diseases, including cancer, autoimmune disorders, and infectious diseases. Advances in genetic engineering and bioprocessing have contributed to the development of personalized or precision medicine (Yu et al., 2023). Tailoring medical treatments to individual genetic profiles allows for more targeted and effective therapies. This is particularly evident in the field of cancer treatment, where specific genetic mutations or biomarkers can be targeted with precision drugs produced through bioprocessing techniques (Krzyszczyk et al., 2018). Bioprocessing plays a critical role in the development and production of vaccines. Traditional and emerging vaccines, including mRNA vaccines like those against COVID-2019, involve bioprocessing techniques to produce viral components or antigens.

The speed and flexibility of bioprocessing have been particularly important in responding to emerging infectious diseases by rapidly developing and scaling up vaccine production (Meade et al., 2023).

Bioprocessing is integral to the field of gene and cell therapies. Techniques such as CRISPR gene editing have enabled the modification of genes for therapeutic purposes. Bioprocessing is then employed to produce and deliver these modified cells to patients, offering potential cures for genetic disorders, certain cancers, and other diseases. Bioprocessing contributes to regenerative medicine by enabling the production of tissues and organs for transplantation. Techniques such as tissue engineering involve the cultivation and assembly of cells into functional tissues. Bioprocessing helps scale up these processes for clinical applications, holding promise for the treatment of organ failure and tissue damage (Petrosyan et al., 2022). Bioprocessing facilitates the high-throughput screening of potential drug candidates and the production of large quantities of biopharmaceuticals for preclinical and clinical trials. This accelerates the drug development pipeline and allows for more rapid translation of discoveries from the laboratory to the clinic (Szymański et al., 2012). The efficiency and scalability of bioprocessing contribute to reducing the costs associated with drug production. This can lead to more affordable medications and increased accessibility to advanced medical treatments, particularly in resource-limited settings (Mitra and Murthy, 2022).

The impact of bioprocessing on medicine is multifaceted, ranging from the production of essential drugs and vaccines to the development of cutting-edge therapies that hold the potential to revolutionize the treatment and prevention of various diseases. These advancements represent a paradigm shift toward more targeted, personalized, and effective medical interventions (Karathanasis, 2014).

7.6 APPLICATIONS OF BIOTECHNOLOGY IN MEDICINE

Biotechnology has made profound contributions to medicine, offering a diverse array of applications that have revolutionized diagnostics, treatment, and disease prevention. In diagnostics, biotechnology plays a pivotal role in the development of advanced molecular tools for detecting genetic markers, pathogens, and biomolecules, leading to more accurate and rapid diagnostic tests (Venkataraman and Hefferon, 2021). In therapeutics, the production of biopharmaceuticals using genetically engineered microbes or mammalian cells has enabled the creation of targeted and personalized medicines, including insulin, monoclonal antibodies, and vaccines (Kesik-Brodacka, 2018). Biopharmaceuticals are made by using microorganisms, such as yeast and bacteria, to produce medicinal medications. This procedure is essential to biotechnology and has greatly aided in the creation of numerous pharmaceuticals (Jozala et al., 2016). A popular bacterium for the synthesis of biopharmaceuticals is *E. coli*. It is a well-researched, manipulable organism. Bacterial systems could not have the cellular apparatus needed for intricate posttranslational changes, nevertheless (Baeshen et al., 2015).

The common yeast used in the manufacturing process of biopharmaceuticals is *S. cerevisiae*. Yeast cells are effective for manufacturing proteins like insulin because they can carry out certain posttranslational changes (Nielsen, 2013). Mammalian cells, such as Chinese Hamster Ovary cells, are used for the production of more complex proteins that require specific posttranslational modifications. Mammalian cell systems are often preferred for the production of therapeutic proteins with high biological activity (Gray, 1997). The genetic material of the chosen host organism is modified through genetic engineering to introduce the gene encoding the therapeutic protein of interest (Balabanova et al., 2015). This involves inserting the gene into the host organism's DNA and optimizing its expression. Once the modified organism contains the desired gene, it is cultured in large bioreactors under controlled conditions (Khan et al., 2016). The gene is expressed, leading to the synthesis of the therapeutic protein within the microbial cells. The cultivation of microbes in large-scale bioreactors is often referred to as fermentation. This process provides the necessary conditions for the growth and reproduction of the microbial cells, allowing them to produce the therapeutic protein (Jozala et al., 2016).

After fermentation, the next step is downstream processing, where the therapeutic protein is separated from the microbial culture and purified. This involves various techniques such as filtration, chromatography, and centrifugation to obtain a pure and concentrated biopharmaceutical product (Jungbauer, 2013). Microbial systems may lack certain post-translational modification capabilities found in higher eukaryotic cells. For more complex proteins that require specific modifications, such as glycosylation, mammalian cell systems are often preferred. Rigorous quality control measures are implemented throughout the entire process to ensure the safety, efficacy, and consistency of the biopharmaceutical product. This includes testing for purity, potency, and absence of contaminants (Wang et al., 2014).

7.6.1 BIOFUELS: USING BIOLOGICAL PROCESSES TO PRODUCE ENERGY SUSTAINABLY

Biofuels are clean, sustainable energy sources produced by biological processes from organic materials such as trash, algae, or plants. The purpose of biofuels is to offer conventional fossil fuels a more environmentally responsible and sustainable substitute. Biofuels come in two primary varieties: Biodiesel and bioethanol (Mahapatra et al., 2021). Often, crops high in sugar or starch, such as sugarcane, corn, or wheat, are used to make bioethanol. As an alternative, cellulosic feedstocks such as agricultural wastes or switchgrass can be employed. During the fermentation process, the feedstock's sugars are broken down by microorganisms—usually yeast—into carbon dioxide and ethanol (Bušić et al., 2018). This biological process produces bioethanol as the primary end product. Biodiesel is commonly produced from vegetable oils (e.g., soybean, canola) or animal fats. Nonfood sources like algae are also explored for their oil content. Biodiesel is produced through a chemical process called transesterification. In this process, triglycerides (fats) are reacted with an alcohol (usually methanol or ethanol) and a catalyst to yield biodiesel (fatty acid methyl or ethyl esters) and glycerol (Yang et al., 2021b).

Researchers are looking into the possibility of producing biofuels from microalgae. Lipids that algae accumulate can be transformed into biodiesel. High lipid content is provided by algae-based biofuels, which do not compete with food crops for arable land. Because the amount of carbon dioxide emitted during combustion is almost equivalent to the amount absorbed by the plants during growth, biofuels are regarded as carbon neutral. In contrast, fossil fuels contribute to the greenhouse effect by releasing stored carbon into the atmosphere (Khan et al., 2018).

7.6.2 LIMITATIONS AND IMPROVEMENT

Concerns regarding possible rivalry with food production have been raised by the use of food crops for the production of biofuel. These issues have been solved by technological advancements like the creation of second-generation biofuels from waste materials and nonfood crops. The main goals of ongoing research are to generate more resilient and fruitful crops or microbes, optimize feedstock selection, and increase the efficiency of biofuel production processes. Compared to conventional fossil fuels, biofuels have the potential to produce less greenhouse gases because of their carbon-neutral nature and renewable source. By using biofuels to harness biological processes for sustainable energy, we can lessen our reliance on finite fossil fuel supplies, counteract climate change, and promote a more environmentally friendly and sustainable energy industry. The goal of ongoing studies and technological breakthroughs is to improve the production of renewables' overall sustainability, cost-effectiveness, and efficiency.

7.7 BIOBASED PRODUCTS: DEVELOPING ENVIRONMENTALLY FRIENDLY PRODUCTS

Biobased products refer to items that are derived from renewable biological resources, such as plants, animals, and microorganisms, as opposed to traditional products derived from fossil fuels. The development of biobased products is driven by the desire to create environmentally friendly alternatives that are sustainable, reduce dependence on nonrenewable resources, and have a lower environmental impact throughout their life cycle (Dahiya et al., 2020). Biobased products use renewable feedstocks, such as crops (e.g., corn, sugarcane), forestry residues, agricultural by-products, or even microorganisms. These resources can be replenished, making them more sustainable than fossil fuels (Malode et al., 2021). Corn flour, sugarcane, or vegetable oils are examples of natural sources from which biobased plastics, also known as biopolymers, are made. They can be used to create things such as biodegradable goods, disposable cutlery, and packaging materials (Atiwesh et al., 2021).

These materials combine biobased polymers with natural fibers or particles, creating durable and environmentally friendly alternatives for applications such as construction materials and automotive components (Arumugam et al., 2022). Biobased products extend to biofuels, including biodiesel and bioethanol, which are used as renewable alternatives to traditional fossil fuels. Biofuels can be derived from crops, algae, or waste materials (Neupane, 2023). Everyday items such as cleaning products, textiles, and personal care items can be developed using biobased ingredients. These products often aim to reduce the environmental impact associated with the production and disposal of conventional alternatives. Biobased products generally have lower carbon footprints and can contribute to a reduction in greenhouse gas emissions. The production of these products often requires less energy compared to their petroleum-based counterparts. Many biobased products are designed to be biodegradable, reducing the persistence of waste in the environment. Additionally, the use of biobased materials supports the concept of a circular economy, where products are designed to be recycled or reused, minimizing waste (Atiwesh et al., 2021).

7.7.1 LIMITATIONS AND IMPROVEMENT

Challenges in the widespread adoption of biobased products include cost competitiveness, scalability of production, and potential competition with food production. Ongoing research and technological advancements aim to address these challenges and enhance the feasibility and efficiency of biobased manufacturing. Governments and regulatory bodies in various regions are increasingly supporting the development and use of biobased products through incentives, mandates, and sustainability certifications. Growing environmental awareness among consumers is driving demand for sustainable products (Scarlat et al., 2015). Companies are responding by incorporating biobased materials into their product lines, reflecting the shift toward more eco-friendly consumer choices (Jeong et al., 2021). In summary, the development of biobased products represents a sustainable and eco-friendly approach to manufacturing across various industries. The ongoing commitment to research, innovation, and regulatory support is crucial for further advancing the adoption of biobased materials and products in the global market.

7.8 ENSURING PRODUCT SAFETY: ASEPTIC PROCESSING AND STERILITY ASSURANCE

Ensuring product safety is a critical aspect of industries such as pharmaceuticals, biotechnology, and food production. Aseptic processing and sterility assurance are key principles and practices implemented to prevent microbial contamination and ensure the safety and efficacy of products. Here's an explanation of these concepts.

7.8.1 ASEPTIC PROCESSING

There are many techniques to prevent contamination during production. Aseptic processing refers to the method of handling and producing products in a way that prevents microbial contamination. It involves maintaining a sterile environment during the production and packaging of sensitive products, particularly those intended for medical use or human consumption. Aseptic processing requires a controlled and sterile environment. This is typically achieved in cleanrooms or isolators equipped with high-efficiency particulate air filters to remove airborne particles, including microorganisms. All components, including equipment, containers, and packaging materials, must be sterilized before use to prevent the introduction of contaminants (WHO, 2011). Strict aseptic techniques are employed during the entire manufacturing process. This includes the use of sterile gloves, gowns, and tools to avoid contamination.

7.8.2 STERILITY ASSURANCE

The set of measures and processes put in place to guarantee that a product is free from viable microorganisms. In industries such as pharmaceuticals and healthcare, ensuring sterility is crucial to prevent infections and ensure the efficacy of medical interventions. Products are subjected to rigorous sterility testing to verify the absence of viable microorganisms (Rutala and Weber, 2014). This involves taking samples from different batches and subjecting them to cultivation or other analytical methods to detect the presence of microbes. Sterility assurance involves the validation of processes, equipment, and environments to ensure that they consistently meet the required sterility standards. This includes routine monitoring and periodic revalidation. Equipment and component sterilization techniques that are often used include autoclaving and dry heat sterilization. The method of filtering liquids and gases via membranes with defined pore sizes eliminates germs. Certain heat-sensitive materials are sterilized using chemical agents like ethylene oxide or hydrogen peroxide. The type of sterilization assurance method and validation parameters are given in Table 7.2 (Phipps et al., 2017).

TABLE 7.2 Sterilization Assurance and Validation Parameters

Sterilization Assurance Method	Temperature Range	Duration	Validation Parameter	References
Autoclaving	121°C	15–20 min	Temperature, pressure, time	Garibaldi et al. (2017)
Dry heat sterilization	160–180°C	2–4 h	Temperature, time, uniformity	Shintani (2012)
Filtration	–	–	Pore size, integrity testing, microbial retention	McBurnie and Bardo (2004)

7.8.3 IMPORTANCE IN BIOPHARMACEUTICALS: CRITICAL FOR PRODUCT SAFETY AND EFFICACY

Aseptic processing and sterility assurance are crucial in the field of biopharmaceuticals because they guarantee the product's safety, effectiveness, and general quality (Lambert et al., 2021). Patient safety is the main priority in the manufacture of biopharmaceuticals. Biopharmaceutical products, including gene treatments, monoclonal antibodies, and vaccinations, are highly susceptible to microbial contamination, which can result in serious side effects or infections for patients. The guarantee of sterility guarantees that these items are devoid of living germs (Jozala et al., 2016). The biopharmaceutical business must meet strict regulations and norms imposed by regulatory bodies, including the US Food and Drug Administration (FDA) and the European Medicines Agency (EMA). Following these rules is necessary to obtain approval for new medications and ensure the ongoing quality of goods that are already on the market (Anderson et al., 2020). Microbial contamination can jeopardize the effectiveness of biopharmaceutical products in addition to posing dangers to patient safety. These products' proteins, nucleic acids, or active substances may be susceptible to microbial interactions, which could result in deterioration or changes to their medicinal qualities (Tropea, 2022).

Fermentation, the application of living cells, and laborious purification procedures are just a few of the sophisticated bioprocessing activities that are frequently involved in the creation of biopharmaceuticals. Because of the potential for microbiological contamination caused by these circumstances, aseptic processing is essential to preserving the product's integrity (Langer et al., 2018). Strict sterility testing is a crucial component of quality assurance in the production of biopharmaceuticals. This testing is done on various batches to make sure that no live bacteria remain in the finished product (Gebo and Lau, 2020). An entire batch may be rejected if any of the sterility tests are unsuccessful. The sterility assurance and aseptic processes help prolong the shelf life of biopharmaceutical products. These procedures assist in preserving the stability and effectiveness of the product throughout time by avoiding contamination during production and storage (von Woedtke and Kramer, 2008). Aseptic processing is even more important when it comes to gene and cell therapies, which involve giving patients living cells or genetic material. Contamination has the potential to affect the therapeutic outcome by compromising the integrity of genetic material or the survival of cells (Rafi, 2011).

To enable aseptic processing, biopharmaceutical businesses extensively invest in cutting-edge facilities furnished with cutting-edge technologies and cleanroom settings. This shows how dedicated the industry is to upholding the greatest standards of product quality and safety (Hole et al., 2021). The difficulty of maintaining sterile conditions, the possibility of human mistakes, and the requirement for ongoing monitoring and validation are some of the difficulties associated with implementing aseptic procedures and guaranteeing sterility. To sum up, in businesses where product safety is of utmost importance, aseptic processing and sterility assurance are essential procedures (WHO, 2011). These procedures are essential for guaranteeing the safety of medications, biotechnological products, and some foods by preventing microbial contamination. These procedures require constant validation in addition to strict adherence to aseptic procedures.

7.8.4 TACKLING MICROBIAL GENETICS AND ANTIMICROBIAL DEVELOPMENT ISSUES RELATED TO MULTI-DRUG RESISTANCE

The treatment of diseases becomes more challenging when certain germs acquire resistance to numerous medications, a condition known as multidrug resistance (MDR). The development of antimicrobials and microbial genetics are crucial elements of tactics meant to overcome this resistance (Yang et al., 2021a). The study of bacteria and other microbes' genetic makeup is the main focus of microbial genetics. Genetic mechanisms play a major role in many drug resistance cases in microorganisms. Comprehending the genetic underpinnings underlying resistance facilitates the development of focused approaches to surmount it (Hoffman, 2001). Resistance gene transmission can occur horizontally across microorganisms, especially bacteria, involving transposon movement and plasmid exchange. This serves an essential role in the quick spread of medication resistance. Investigating these genetic components aids in locating possible therapeutic targets. Tackling common microorganisms in pharmaceutical contamination is given in Table 7.3 (Bennett, 2008).

The monitoring of microbial genomes for the existence of resistance genes is made possible by developments in genomic technologies and bioinformatics. This makes it possible to identify new resistance patterns early on and helps with the development of successful treatment plans. Comprehending the genetics of microorganisms enables the logical creation of medications that target the genetic pathways responsible for treatment resistance (Uddin et al., 2021). By interfering with or inhibiting the genetic components that give resistance, this method seeks to render the microorganism receptive to therapeutic intervention.

TABLE 7.3 Tackling Common Microorganisms in Pharmaceutical Contamination

Microorganism	Source	Potential Impact	References
Bacteria	Air, water	Product spoilage, disease	Russell and Houlihan (2003)
Fungi	Air, raw materials	Contamination, allergies	Adhikari et al. (2020)
Viruses	Contaminated surfaces	Infections, product loss	Aregbesola et al. (2019)
Endotoxins	Cell walls of bacteria	Pyrogenic reactions	Heinrich et al. (2022)

The creation of novel medications to fight bacteria that are resistant to existing medications is known as antimicrobial development. The unique modes of action of next-generation antibiotics are intended to overcome the resistance mechanisms found in current medications. Combining several antimicrobial drugs with various modes of action can increase effectiveness and lower the chance of developing resistance. This strategy is very helpful for treating MDR, as a single medication might not be enough. As a potential treatment for bacterial illnesses, phage therapy makes use of bacteriophages, viruses that infect and kill bacteria (Reygaert, 2018). Phages are a highly targeted and dynamic countermeasure that can be developed or selected to target certain drug-resistant bacteria (Lin et al., 2017).

Antimicrobial stewardship programs aim to optimize the use of antimicrobial agents to prevent resistance. This involves appropriate prescribing practices, dosage optimization, and duration of treatment to minimize the selective pressure for resistance development. Developing vaccines against drug-resistant pathogens can prevent infections, reducing the need for antimicrobial treatments. Additionally, strategies such as infection prevention and control measures in healthcare settings play a crucial role in minimizing the spread of drug-resistant microbes (Ahmad et al., 2020).

7.9 FUTURE AND CHALLENGES: SYNERGY FOR REVOLUTIONARY HEALTHCARE IMPROVEMENTS

Revolutionary advancements in healthcare are anticipated in the future, fueled by the convergence of technology, medicine, and healthcare systems. But before these developments can be widely and fairly implemented, a number of issues need to be resolved. Precision medicine is becoming possible thanks to developments in genomics, proteomics, and other omics technologies. This means that a person's treatment can be customized based on their genetic composition. Treatment regimens that are tailored to each patient's particular needs may result in more focused and efficient interventions. The requirement for substantial genetic and molecular data, ethical issues, and guaranteeing accessibility and affordability for all people are some of the implementation obstacles. Improved access to healthcare services is made possible by the combination of telemedicine and remote patient monitoring technologies, particularly in underserved or distant locations. Remote patient monitoring on a regular basis can help with early detection and treatment (Natarajan et al., 2023). To ensure the fair adoption of telemedicine, it is necessary to address infrastructure restrictions, differences in access to technology, and legislative considerations. Enhanced cooperation between academics, engineers, data scientists, and healthcare practitioners can result in creative answers and comprehensive strategies for dealing with healthcare issues. Multidisciplinary collaboration can promote a more thorough comprehension of intricate medical problems. It can be difficult to create efficient channels of communication and dismantle disciplinary silos. In order to overcome disciplinary barriers, healthcare education and practice must undergo a cultural transformation (Johnson et al., 2021). Cooperating on global health initiatives and improving pandemic preparedness can help healthcare systems be more resilient to emerging threats. Investing in research, surveillance, and international cooperation is crucial. Global health initiatives confront numerous challenges, such as handling geopolitical concerns and overcoming disparities in developed and developing countries' healthcare infrastructure and access (Madhav et al., 2017). Information sharing with patients, promotion of health literacy, and patient autonomy over treatment choices can lead to improved health outcomes and more efficient healthcare systems. To ensure that patients are active participants in their care and to attain widespread health literacy, coordinated initiatives in healthcare education and communication are required to remove language and cultural barriers. It is critical to carefully navigate the concerns surrounding genetic testing, emerging technologies, and data privacy to sustain moral and equitable healthcare practices. Developing precise legal frameworks, handling ownership and use of patient data concerns, and striking a balance between innovation and moral standards are never easy tasks. Future healthcare gains will largely depend on how well patient-centered care, multidisciplinary teamwork, and technological advancements are integrated. To fully realize the promise of these revolutionary advances in healthcare, however, concerns about ethics, equity, and global injustices must be addressed. Legislators, researchers, and healthcare professionals must collaborate in order to solve these challenges and build a patient-centered, cost-effective, and accessible healthcare system in the future.

7.10 CONCLUSION

To sum up, the convergence of biotechnology and pharmaceutical microbiology proves to be a powerful driving force behind ground-breaking discoveries in modern medicine and drug discovery. Because of this symbiotic interaction, genetic engineering and microbial fermentation have revolutionized bioprocessing technologies, causing a paradigm shift. Thanks to the remarkable precision provided by gene editing technologies, medicine is now able to customize treatment methods with unparalleled accuracy, ushering in an era of personalized interventions. The combination of these fields has not only ushered in the era of customized healthcare but has also revealed novel treatments based on a thorough comprehension of the microbiome. This collaborative endeavor has the potential to tackle contemporary medical issues and uncover innovative remedies for an extensive range of ailments. But as we venture into these unknown waters, careful monitoring and a diligent adherence to moral principles are still necessary. The combined efforts of pharmaceutical microbiology and biotechnology not only build upon the revolutionary successes of the past but also create the groundwork for a future in which medicine is highly precise, dynamic, and intricately linked to the workings of microbial systems. The intersection of these fields continues to influence the direction of healthcare in this dynamic environment, pointing to a time when scientific innovation will be properly used to improve patient outcomes and increase medical knowledge.

KEYWORDS

- **biotechnology**
- **pharmaceutical microbiology**
- **personalized medicine**
- **microbiome**
- **therapies**
- **advanced bioprocessing**
- **gene editing**

REFERENCES

Adhikari, M., Isaac, E. L., Paterson, R. R. M., Maslin, M. A. (2020). A review of potential impacts of climate change on coffee cultivation and mycotoxigenic fungi. *Microorganisms*, *8*(10), 1625.

Agarwal, G., Carcache, P. J. B., Addo, E. M., Kinghorn, A. D. (2020). Current status and contemporary approaches to the discovery of antitumor agents from higher plants. *Biotechnology Advances*, *38*, 107337.

Ahmad, N., Althemery, A., Haseeb, A., Yusuf, R., Hassali, A., Khan, A. (2020). Inclining trend of the researchers interest in antimicrobial stewardship: A systematic review. *Journal of Pharmacy and Bioallied Sciences*, *12*(1), 11.

Anderson, D. A., Jones, R. D., Arkin, A. P., Weiss, R. (2019). Principles of synthetic biology: A MOOC for an emerging field. *Synthetic Biology*, *4*(1), ysz010.

Anderson, N. M., Benyathiar, P., Mishra, D. K. (2020). Aseptic processing and packaging. In: Demirci, A., Feng, H., Krishnamurthy, K. (Eds.), *Food Engineering Series* (pp. 661–692), Springer: Cham..

Aregbesola, O. Z., Legg, J. P., Sigsgaard, L., Lund, O. S., Rapisarda, C. (2019). Potential impact of climate change on whiteflies and implications for the spread of vectored viruses. *Journal of Pest Science*, *92*, 381–392.

Arumugam, S., Kandasamy, J., Venkatesan, S., Murugan, R., Narayanan, V. L., Sultan, M. T. H., Shahar, F. S., Shah, A. U. M., Khan, T., Sebaey, T. A. (2022). A review on the effect of fabric reinforcement on strength enhancement of natural fiber composites. *Materials*, *15*(9), 3025.

Atiwesh, G., Mikhael, A., Parrish, C. C., Banoub, J., Le, T. A. T. (2021). Environmental impact of bioplastic use: A review. *Heliyon*, *7*(9), e07918.

Baeshen, M. N., Al-Hejin, A. M., Bora, R. S., Ahmed, M. M. M., Ramadan, H. A. I., Saini, K. S., Baeshen, N. A., Redwan, E. M. (2015). Production of biopharmaceuticals in *E. coli*: Current scenario and future perspectives. *Journal of Microbiology and Biotechnology*, *25*(7), 953–962.

Baird, R. M., Crowden, C. A., O'farrell, S. M., Shooter, R. A. (1979). Microbial contamination of pharmaceutical products in the home. *Journal of Hygiene*, *83*(2), 277–283.

Balabanova, L., Golotin, V., Podvolotskaya, A., Rasskazov, V. (2015). Genetically modified proteins: Functional improvement and chimeragenesis. *Bioengineered*, 6(5), 262–274.

Barragán-Ocaña, A., Silva-Borjas, P., Olmos-Peña, S., Polanco-Olguín, M. (2020). Biotechnology and bioprocesses: Their contribution to sustainability. *Processes*, *8*(4), 436.

Bartusik-Aebisher, D., Aebisher, D. (2020). Biopharmaceuticals: Perspectives. *An Essential Guide to Biopharmaceuticals* (pp. 111–134), Nova Science Publishers, Inc.: Hauppauge, NY, USA.

Bennett, P. M. (2008). Plasmid encoded antibiotic resistance: Acquisition and transfer of antibiotic resistance genes in bacteria. *British Journal of Pharmacology*, *153*(S1), S347–S357.

Bernal-Chávez, S. A., Del Prado-Audelo, M. L., Caballero-Florán, I. H., Giraldo-Gomez, D. M., Figueroa-Gonzalez, G., Reyes-Hernandez, O. D., González-Del Carmen, M., González-Torres, M., Cortés, H., Leyva-Gómez, G. (2021). Insights into terminal sterilization processes of nanoparticles for biomedical applications. *Molecules*, *26*(7), 2068.

Bulk, G. D., Materials, G., Continuous, Q. (2005). WHO good manufacturing practices: Water for pharmaceutical use. *WHO Technical Report Series*, *929*, 67–89.

Bušić, A., Mardetko, N., Kundas, S., Morzak, G., Belskaya, H., Šantek, M. I., Komes, D., Novak, S., Šantek, B. (2018). Bioethanol production from renewable raw materials and its separation and purification: A review. *Food Technology and Biotechnology*, *56*(3), 289–311.

C Reygaert, W. (2018). An overview of the antimicrobial resistance mechanisms of bacteria. *AIMS Microbiology*, *4*(3), 482–501.

Capen, R., Christopher, D., Forenzo, P., Ireland, C., Liu, O., Lyapustina, S., O'Neill, J., Patterson, N., Quinlan, M., Sandell, D., Schwenke, J., Stroup, W., Tougas, T. (2012). On the shelf life of pharmaceutical products. *AAPS PharmSciTech*, *13*(3), 911–918.

Center for Drug Evaluation and Research. (2018). Drug Quality Sampling and Testing Programs. *U.S. Food and Drug Administration*, *11*(2), 215–222.

Chatterjee, A., Abraham, J. (2018). Microbial contamination, prevention, and early detection in food industry. *Microbial Contamination and Food Degradation* (pp. 21–47), Academic Press.

Chui, M., Evers, M., Manyika, J., Zheng, A., Nisbet, T. (2023). The bio revolution: Innovations transforming economies, societies, and our lives. *Augmented Education in the Global Age*, *1*, 48–74.

Dahiya, S., Katakojwala, R., Ramakrishna, S., Mohan, S. V. (2020). Biobased products and life cycle assessment in the context of circular economy and sustainability. *Materials Circular Economy*, *2*(1), 7.

Damaso, M. C. T., Machado, C. M. M., Rodrigues, D. de S., Belem, S. G., Salum, T. F. C. (2014). Bioprocesses for biofuels: An overview of the Brazilian case. *Chemical and Biological Technologies in Agriculture*, *1*, 1–8.

David, F., Davis, A. M., Gossing, M., Hayes, M. A., Romero, E., Scott, L. H., Wigglesworth, M. J. (2021). A perspective on synthetic biology in drug discovery and development—current impact and future opportunities. *SLAS Discovery*, *26*(5), 581–603

Drinkwater, J., Lucas, R. (2013). Bioburden control in bioprocessing using hydrogen peroxide vapor. *BioProcessing Journal*, *12*(1), 14–19.

Durrant, C. (2001). The responsibility of the pharmaceutical industry. *Clinical Microbiology and Infection*, *7*(6), 2–4.

Dzerzhinskaya, A. A., Spiridonova, A. A., Khomutova, E. G. (2022). Systematic approach to cross-contamination risk management in the production of medicinal products. *Drug Development and Registration*, *11*(1), 149–158.

Ganeshan, S., Kim, S. H., Vujanovic, V. (2021). Scaling-up production of plant endophytes in bioreactors: Concepts, challenges and perspectives. *Bioresources and Bioprocessing*, *8*(1), 63.

Garibaldi, B. T., Reimers, M., Ernst, N., Bova, G., Nowakowski, E., Bukowski, J., Ellis, B. C., Smith, C., Sauer, L., Dionne, K., Carroll, K. C., Maragakis, L. L., Parrish, N. M. (2017). Validation of autoclave protocols for successful decontamination of category a medical waste generated from care of patients with serious communicable diseases. *Journal of Clinical Microbiology*, *55*(2), 545–551.

Garner, K. L. (2021). Principles of synthetic biology. *Essays in Biochemistry*, *65*(5), 791–811.

Gebo, J. E. T., Lau, A. F. (2020). Sterility testing for cellular therapies: What is the role of the clinical microbiology laboratory? *Journal of Clinical Microbiology*, *58*(7), e01492–e01519.

Gray, D. (1997). Overview of protein expression by mammalian cells. *Current Protocols in Protein Science*, *10*(1), 591–5918.

Greb, E. (2010). An overview of rapid microbial-detection methods. *Pharmaceutical Technology*, *34*, 46–50.

Griffith, C. (2016). Surface sampling and the detection of contamination. In: *Handbook of Hygiene Control in the Food Industry* (pp. 673–696). Woodhead Publishing.

Heinrich, M. A., Mangia, M., Prakash, J. (2022). Impact of endotoxins on bioengineered tissues and models. *Trends in Biotechnology*, *40*(5), 532–534.

Hentz, N. G. (2013). Pharmaceutical bioburden testing. In: *Encyclopedia of Industrial Biotechnology* (pp. 757–774). Wiley.

Hoffman, S. B. (2001). Mechanisms of antibiotic resistance. *Compendium on Continuing Education for the Practicing Veterinarian*, *23*(5), 464–472.

Hole, G., Hole, A. S., McFalone-Shaw, I. (2021). Digitalization in pharmaceutical industry: What to focus on under the digital implementation process?*International Journal of Pharmaceutics: X*, *3*, 100095.

Hughes, R. A., Ellington, A. D. (2017). Synthetic DNA synthesis and assembly: Putting the synthetic in synthetic biology. *Cold Spring Harbor Perspectives in Biology*, *9*(1), a023812.

Jeong, D., Park, H., Jang, B. K., Ju, Y. Bin, Shin, M. H., Oh, E. J., Lee, E. J., Kim, S. R. (2021). Recent advances in the biological valorization of citrus peel waste into fuels and chemicals. *Bioresource Technology*, *323*, 124603.

Johnson, K. B., Wei, W. Q., Weeraratne, D., Frisse, M. E., Misulis, K., Rhee, K., Zhao, J., Snowdon, J. L. (2021). Precision medicine, AI, and the future of personalized health care. *Clinical and Translational Science*, *14*(1), 86–93.

Jozala, A. F., Geraldes, D. C., Tundisi, L. L., Feitosa, V. de A., Breyer, C. A., Cardoso, S. L., Mazzola, P. G., de Oliveira-Nascimento, L., Rangel-Yagui, C. de O., Magalhães, P. de O., de Oliveira, M. A., Pessoa, A. (2016). Biopharmaceuticals from microorganisms: From production to purification. *Brazilian Journal of Microbiology*, *47*, 51–63.

Jungbauer, A. (2013). Continuous downstream processing of biopharmaceuticals. *Trends in Biotechnology*, *31*(8), 479–492.

Karathanasis, S. K. (2014). Regenerative medicine: Transforming the drug discovery and development paradigm. *Cold Spring Harbor Perspectives in Medicine*, *4*(8), a014084.

Kesik-Brodacka, M. (2018). Progress in biopharmaceutical development. *Biotechnology and Applied Biochemistry*, *65*(3), 306–322.

Khan, M. I., Shin, J. H., Kim, J. D. (2018). The promising future of microalgae: Current status, challenges, and optimization of a sustainable and renewable industry for biofuels, feed, and other products. *Microbial Cell Factories*, *17*(1), 36.

Khan, S., Ullah, M. W., Siddique, R., Nabi, G., Manan, S., Yousaf, M., Hou, H. (2016). Role of recombinant DNA technology to improve life. *International Journal of Genomics*, *2016*.

Khanra, S., Mondal, M., Halder, G., Tiwari, O. N., Gayen, K., Bhowmick, T. K. (2018). Downstream processing of microalgae for pigments, protein and carbohydrate in industrial application: A review. *Food and Bioproducts Processing*, *110*, 60–84.

Krzyszczyk, P., Acevedo, A., Davidoff, E. J., Timmins, L. M., Marrero-Berrios, I., Patel, M., White, C., Lowe, C., Sherba, J. J., Hartmanshenn, C., O'Neill, K. M., Balter, M. L., Fritz, Z. R., Androulakis, I. P., Schloss, R. S., Yarmush, M. L. (2018). The growing role of precision and personalized medicine for cancer treatment. *Technology*, *6*(3 and 4), 79–100.

Labrou, N. E. (2021). The role of pharmaceutical biotechnology in the fight against viral pandemics. *Current Pharmaceutical Biotechnology*, *22*(1), 1–3.

Lambert, B. J., Hansen, J. M., Bryans, T. D., Lam, S. (2021). Sterility assurance across-sectors—new paradigms and tools. *Frontiers in Medical Technology*, *3*, 622710.

Langer, E., Rader, A., Shevitz, J., Fenge, C., Chotteau, V., Eckerle, S., DeJongh, A., Whitford, W., Bisschops, M., Sinclair, A., Johnson, T. (2018). *Continuous Bioprocessing—Industry Best Practices* (pp. 1–163). Repligen.

Lin, D. M., Koskella, B., Lin, H. C. (2017). Phage therapy: An alternative to antibiotics in the age of multi-drug resistance. *World Journal of Gastrointestinal Pharmacology and Therapeutics*, *8*(3), 162.

Madhav, N., Oppenheim, B., Gallivan, M., Mulembakani, P., Rubin, E., Wolfe, N. (2017). Pandemics: Risks, impacts, and mitigation. In: Jamison D. T., Gelband, H,. Horton, S., et al., (Eds.), *Disease Control Priorities: Improving Health and Reducing Poverty* (pp. 315–345). The International Bank for Reconstruction and Development/The World Bank: Washington, DC.

Mahapatra, S., Kumar, D., Singh, B., Sachan, P. K. (2021). Biofuels and their sources of production: A review on cleaner sustainable alternative against conventional fuel, in the framework of the food and energy nexus. *Energy Nexus*, *4*, 100036.

Maldonade, I. R., Ginani, V. C., Riquette, R. F. R., Gurgel-Gonçalves, R., Mendes, V. S., Machado, E. R. (2019). Good manufacturing practices of minimally processed vegetables reduce contamination with pathogenic microorganisms. *Revista Do Instituto de Medicina Tropical de Sao Paulo*, *61*.

Malode, S. J., Prabhu, K. K., Mascarenhas, R. J., Shetti, N. P., Aminabhavi, T. M. (2021). Recent advances and viability in biofuel production. *Energy Conversion and Management X*, *10*.

Mandrich, L. (2013). DNA Cloning: The history of the future. *Mandrich L*, *2*, 106.

Marucci, L., Barberis, M., Karr, J., Ray, O., Race, P. R., de Souza Andrade, M., Grierson, C., Hoffmann, S. A., Landon, S., Rech, E., Rees-Garbutt, J., Seabrook, R., Shaw, W., Woods, C. (2020). Computer-aided whole-cell design: Taking a holistic approach by integrating synthetic with systems biology. *Frontiers in Bioengineering and Biotechnology*, *8*, 942.

Mathur, P. (2011). Hand hygiene: Back to the basics of infection control. *Indian Journal of Medical Research*, *134*(11), 611–620.

McBurnie, L., Bardo, B. (2004). Validation of sterile filtration. *Pharmaceutical Technology*, 13–23.

Mccormick, K., Sanders, J. H. (2022). Pharmaceutical microbiology. *Quality*, 299–325.

Meade, E., Rowan, N., Garvey, M. (2023). Bioprocessing and the production of antiviral biologics in the prevention and treatment of viral infectious disease. *Vaccines*, *11*(5), 992.

Mitra, S., Murthy, G. S. (2022). Bioreactor control systems in the biopharmaceutical industry: A critical perspective. *Systems Microbiology and Biomanufacturing*, *2*(1), 91–112.

Natarajan, R., Lokesh, G. H., Flammini, F., Premkumar, A., Venkatesan, V. K., Gupta, S. K. (2023). A novel framework on security and energy enhancement based on internet of medical things for healthcare 5.0. *Infrastructures*, *8*(2), 22.

Neupane, D. (2023). Biofuels from renewable sources, a potential option for biodiesel production. *Bioengineering*, *10*(1), 29.

Nielsen, J. (2013). Production of biopharmaceutical proteins by yeast. *Bioengineered*, *4*(4), 207–211.

Petrosyan, A., Montali, F., Peloso, A., Citro, A., Byers, L. N., La Pointe, C., Suleiman, M., Marchetti, A., Mcneill, E. P., Speer, A. L., Ng, W. H., Ren, X., Bussolati, B., Perin, L., Di

Nardo, P., Cardinale, V., Duisit, J., Monetti, A. R., Savino, J. R., Asthana, A., Orlando, G. (2022). Regenerative medicine technologies applied to transplant medicine. An update. *Frontiers in Bioengineering and Biotechnology, 10.*

Phipps, A., Vaynshteyn, E., Kowalski, J. B., Ngo, M. D., Merritt, K., Osborne, J., Chnari, E. (2017). Chemical sterilization of allograft dermal tissues. *Cell and Tissue Banking, 18*(4), 573–584.

Pickens, L. B., Tang, Y., Chooi, Y. H. (2011). Metabolic engineering for the production of natural products. *Annual Review of Chemical and Biomolecular Engineering, 2,* 211–236.

Quality Assurance of Pharmaceuticals. (2020). *Encyclopedia of Pharmaceutical Science and Technology* (pp. 2885–2894).

Rafi, M. A. (2011). Gene and stem cell therapy: Alone or in combination?*BioImpacts*, *1*(4), 213–218.

Ranade, V. V. (2010). Biotechnology: Pharmaceutical aspects. *American Journal of Therapeutics*, *17*(1), 121.

Ratajczak, M., Kubicka, M. M., Kamińska, D., Sawicka, P., Długaszewska, J. (2015). Microbiological quality of non-sterile pharmaceutical products. *Saudi Pharmaceutical Journal*, *23*(3), 303–307.

Rauschnabel, J. (2007). The advantages of restricted-access barrier systems. *Pharmaceutical Technology*, *31*(3), 80–92.

Russell, J. B., Houlihan, A. J. (2003). Ionophore resistance of ruminal bacteria and its potential impact on human health. *FEMS Microbiology Reviews*, *27*(1), 65–74.

Rutala, W. A., Weber, D. J. (2014). Disinfection, sterilization, and control of hospital waste. *Mandell, Douglas, and Bennett's Principles and Practice of Infectious Diseases*, *2*, 3294–3309.

Scarlat, N., Dallemand, J. F., Monforti-Ferrario, F., Nita, V. (2015). The role of biomass and bioenergy in a future bioeconomy: Policies and facts. *Environmental Development*, *15*, 3–34.

Schicht, H. H. (1998). International cleanroom standards and their impact on the pharmaceutical industry. In: *Institute of Environmental Sciences—Proceedings, Annual Technical Meeting* (pp. 110–114).

Schmidt, M., Krutzfeldt, R., Ross, A. (1999). Validation of a separator CSA8 regarding sterilization for aseptic processes. *Process Biochemistry*, *34*(8), 769–776.

Schmidt, R. H. (2012). Basic elements of equipment cleaning and sanitizing in food processing and handling operations 1. *IFAS Extension,* University of Florida, 1–11.

Schnurr, M. A., Addison, L. (2021). Biotechnology. *Handbook of Critical Agrarian Studies*, 427–437.

Scott, D. (2022). Biotechnology. *The Routledge Companion to Environmental Ethics*, 481–491.

Shah, N. J. (2019). Recombinant DNA technology. *Introduction to Basics of Pharmacology and Toxicology: Volume 1: General and Molecular Pharmacology: Principles of Drug Action*, 413–417.

Shintani, H. (2012). Validation study and routine control monitoring of moist heat sterilization procedures. *Biocontrol Science*, *17*(2), 57–67.

Szymański, P., Markowicz, M., Mikiciuk-Olasik, E. (2012). Adaptation of high-throughput screening in drug discovery-toxicological screening tests. *International Journal of Molecular Sciences*, *13*(1), 427–452.

Tanzini, A., Ruggeri, M., Bianchi, E., Valentino, C., Vigani, B., Ferrari, F., Rossi, S., Giberti, H., Sandri, G. (2023). Robotics and aseptic processing in view of regulatory requirements. *Pharmaceutics*, *15*(6), 1581.

Tripathi, N. K., Shrivastava, A. (2019). Recent developments in bioprocessing of recombinant proteins: Expression hosts and process development. *Frontiers in Bioengineering and Biotechnology*, *7*.

Tropea, A. (2022). Microbial contamination and public health: An overview. *International Journal of Environmental Research and Public Health*, *19*(12), 7441.

Uddin, T. M., Chakraborty, A. J., Khusro, A., Zidan, B. R. M., Mitra, S., Emran, T. Bin, Dhama, K., Ripon, M. K. H., Gajdács, M., Sahibzada, M. U. K., Hossain, M. J., Koirala, N. (2021). Antibiotic resistance in microbes: History, mechanisms, therapeutic strategies and future prospects. *Journal of Infection and Public Health*, *14*(12), 1750–1766.

Unrean, P. (2016). Bioprocess modelling for the design and optimization of lignocellulosic biomass fermentation. *Bioresources and Bioprocessing*, *3*(1). https://doi.org/10.1186/s40643-015-0079-z

Vandivort, T. C., Horton, D. B., Johnson, S. B. (2020). Regulatory and strategic considerations for addressing immunogenicity and related responses in biopharmaceutical development programs. *Journal of Clinical and Translational Science*, *4*(6), 547–555.

Venkataraman, S., Hefferon, K. (2021). Application of plant viruses in biotechnology, medicine, and human health. *Viruses*, *13*(9), 1697.

von Woedtke, T., Kramer, A. (2008). The limits of sterility assurance. *GMS Krankenhaushygiene Interdisziplinar*, *3*(3).

Walker, R. S. K., Pretorius, I. S. (2018). Applications of yeast synthetic biology geared towards the production of biopharmaceuticals. *Genes*, *9*(7).

Wang, Y. C., Peterson, S. E., Loring, J. F. (2014). Protein post-translational modifications and regulation of pluripotency in human stem cells. *Cell Research*, *24*(2), 143–160.

Wang, Y. H., Wei, K. Y., Smolke, C. D. (2013). Synthetic biology: Advancing the design of diverse genetic systems. *Annual Review of Chemical and Biomolecular Engineering*, *4*, 69–102.

WHO. (2011). Annex 6 WHO good manufacturing practices for sterile pharmaceutical products. *WHO Technical Report Series*, *961*, 45–47.

Wiltschi, B., Cernava, T., Dennig, A., Galindo Casas, M., Geier, M., Gruber, S., Haberbauer, M., Heidinger, P., Herrero Acero, E., Kratzer, R., Luley-Goedl, C., Müller, C. A., Pitzer, J., Ribitsch, D., Sauer, M., Schmölzer, K., Schnitzhofer, W., Sensen, C. W., Soh, J., Steiner, K., Winkler, C. K., Winkler, M., Wriessnegger, T. (2020). Enzymes revolutionize the bioproduction of value-added compounds: From enzyme discovery to special applications. *Biotechnology Advances*, *40*, 107520.

Yang, X., Ye, W., Qi, Y., Ying, Y., Xia, Z. (2021a). Overcoming multidrug resistance in bacteria through antibiotics delivery in surface-engineered nano-cargos: Recent developments for future nano-antibiotics. *Frontiers in Bioengineering and Biotechnology*, *9*, 696514.

Yang, Y., Tian, Z., Lan, Y., Wang, S., Chen, H. (2021b). An overview of biofuel power generation on policies and finance environment, applied biofuels, device and performance. *Journal of Traffic and Transportation Engineering*, *8*(4), 534–553.

Yu, M., Peng, Y., Wang, X., Ran, F. (2023). Emerging design strategies toward developing next-generation implantable batteries and supercapacitors. *Advanced Functional Materials*, *33*(37), 2301877.

Zhu, Y. (2022). Advances in CRISPR/Cas9. *BioMed Research International, 2022*.

CHAPTER 8

Advances in Benchside Microbial Testing Techniques for Pharmaceuticals

BHARTI SHARMA and ARCHANA KAPOOR*

Department of Pharmaceutical Sciences, Guru Jambheshwar University of Science and Technology, Hisar, Haryana, India

*Corresponding author

ABSTRACT

The invasion and proliferation of microbes that are not ordinarily found inside the body, such as bacteria, viruses, fungi, and parasites, is referred to as microbial infection. The presence of harmful microbes in pharmaceutical products can lead to toxic and infectious effects in humans. Microbial testing methods are generally employed to assess the total number of active bacteria or certain pathogens present in pharmaceutical products, including injectables, tablets, ophthalmic solutions, capsules, nasal sprays, oral suspensions, and other healthcare products. Microbial limit test (bioburden testing), microbial identification, bacterial endotoxin testing, growth promotion test, sterility testing, environmental monitoring, and water microbiological analysis are some major examples of conventional methods. The limitations of classical methods used in the pharmaceutical industry include lower sensitivity, time-consuming, labor-intensive, low accuracy, inefficiency, specialized equipment required, and environmental contamination. As a result, researchers are very curious about the development of rapid and automated techniques used in the pharmaceutical sector for microbiological testing. The majority of the rapid methods in microbiology are from the branch of biotechnology, such as real-time reverse transcriptase-polymerase chain reaction (RT-PCR),

Advances in Pharmaceutical Microbiology: From Bench to Bedside. Harpreet Singh, Arun Kumar Mishra, Jeyabalan Sangeetha, and Devarajan Thangadurai (Eds.)

DOI: 10.1201/9781779640918-11

multiplex PCR, impedance method, enzyme-linked immunosorbent assay, biosensors, and adenosine triphosphate bioluminescence, etc. Moreover, advances in pharmaceutical microbiological fields will become clearer and more effective in the forthcoming years.

8.1 INTRODUCTION

Microorganisms have consistently been vital to human existence, and yeasts, bacteria, and molds have been linked to both positive and negative effects (Bisen et al., 2012). Microbial infection is the invasion and growth of microbes that are not normally found inside the body, such as bacteria, viruses, fungi, and parasites. Microorganisms' propensity to flourish in food, pharmaceutical, and cosmetic goods has been come in existence from many years and has been the topic of discussion. The presence of pathogenic bacteria in pharmaceutical products makes them dangerous and would be unacceptable from an infectious perspective (Kobayashi and Rittmann, 1982). Organisms that appear in pharmaceutical products include *Staphylococcus aureus*, *Escherichia coli. Coli*, *Pseudomonas aeruginosa*, and *Salmonella* sp., and their arrival is considered to be a sign of contamination, which ultimately resulted in pharmaceutical product disapproval (Denyer et al., 2004). Microbial infections can potentially modify the biological as well as physicochemical characteristics of active chemicals, making them hazardous (Garrett et al., 2008). The toxins released by microbes cause disorders such as diarrhea, acute gastroenteritis, and abdominal pain. However, according to the individual's tolerance to the poison, signs may include minor distress to gastrointestinal mortality (Ratajczak et al., 2015). Microbial methods are frequently employed in various industries, including pharmaceutical, cosmetic, biopharmaceutical, food, and water, to detect, quantify, and identify the different species of bacteria, yeasts, and molds discovered in samples (Henriques et al., 2019). Microbial testing techniques are used to determine the total number of viable bacteria or pathogens present in pharmaceutical products such as injectables, tablets, ophthalmic solutions, capsules, nasal sprays, oral suspensions, and other healthcare products. The presence of microbial contaminants demonstrates a lack of process control measures and good developing techniques (Ashutosh, 2008). There are several classical techniques for identifying and diagnosing such marker pathogens in the pharmaceutical industry for quality assessment of ingredients and final products in various pharmacopoeias that have certain advantages as well as some drawbacks too (Ayurvedic Pharmacopoeia Committee, 2001; British Pharmacopoeia Commission, & Great Britain, 2000; European Pharmacopoeia Commission, 1980). Examples include microbial limit testing (bioburden testing), microbial identification, limulus amebocyte lysate (LAL) test, also known as the bacterial endotoxin test, growth promotion testing, sterility testing, environmental monitoring, and water microbiological analysis (Indian Pharmacopoeia, 1996, 2018).

8.2 IDENTIFICATION OF MICROORGANISMS: A HISTORICAL EVOLUTION

Over the past 10 years, researchers have looked for quicker and more accurate ways to identify microorganisms. The sole identification method available for a number of years was the phenotypic categorization, even though this methodology consistently produced analytical uncertainties and challenges. Several reports have shown that phenotype-based evolution of microbial strains is inaccurate. In another example, Yeung et al. (2002) used phenotype-based methods to describe various taxonomical mismatches in *Lactobacillus casei* and *Lactobacillus acidophilus* groups. Some important investigations of the phenotype-based identification approach were explored by Lagier et al. (2015), who previously frequently used, including enzyme profiles, cellular fatty acid detection, carbon source utilization, pH-based reactions, and acid detection. Phenotypic procedures were often determined by dichotomous keys, with Gram's staining being the initial test, followed by oxidase and catalase tests coming next. Initially, the end products (CO_2, lactate, and acetate) and acid production analysis (pH) were used to assess the metabolism of carbohydrates. Enzyme tests (galactosidase, glucosidase, glucuronidase, and fucosidase) came into use later on. Protein and amino acid metabolism tests, other tests which included measuring the production of indole and H_2S, the digestion of gelatin and casein, the decarboxylation of arginine dihydrolase, arginine, ornithine, phenylalanine deaminase, lysine, and urease, have some advantages over the phenotype-based testing. There are several tests based on cell wall receptors, such as optochin, bile solubility, and lysozyme susceptibility tests, which were widely employed for distinguishing Gram-positive cocci. Additional phenotypic tests covered the digestion of tween along with enzymes for lipid metabolism, for example, lecithinase and lipase on egg yolk agar (Franco-Duarte et al., 2019). These days, a variety of phenotypic traits can be independently confirmed in 4–48 hours using commercial kits and/or automatic phenotypic tools. As initially detailed by Skerman (1959), the tests are arranged logically, and each result suggests the next test in the sequence. Consequently, sequence databases and molecular tools appeared in the latter half of the 20th century. The power of microbiology was enhanced to a significant level by these techniques, which also led to an increase in the number of recognized microbial species (1971 in 1980, 8168 in 2007, and 12,391 in 2013). The discovery of DNA as the genetic material in 1941 initially unlocked the era of molecular biology, according to Madigan et al. (2012) (although bacterial genetics was later found in 1946). The invention of the PCR in 1985 marked the beginning of the role of genetics as a useful method for identifying microorganisms. Since then, a variety of techniques (both culture-dependent and culture-independent) have been introduced using various underlying theories, including hybridization, 16S rRNA sequencing as well and DNA sequencing. Metagenomics, metabolomics, transcriptomics, lipidomics, and proteomics are examples of omics technologies that work toward a high-throughput characterization and quantification of biological molecular pools that are indicative of an organism or an organism's function, structure, and dynamics (Franco-Duarte et al., 2019). These methods are widely exploited by researchers nowadays as they exhibit important applications (e.g., functional genome analysis, phylogeny, microbial ecology, and transcriptional profiling).

According to this strategy, molecular techniques by themselves are typically unable to establish precise boundaries between phylogenetically related species, even though phenotypic traits commonly overlap with genetically diverse species. As a result, a reorganized plan for accurate identification urged to concentrate on its genetic profile, biochemical, physiological, as well as morphological characteristics (Franco-Duarte et al., 2019).

8.2.1 TECHNIQUES OF IDENTIFICATION USING CHROMOGENIC MEDIA

The primary goal of these techniques is to identify microorganisms through cultivation in order to obtain pure cultures. There are several methods for getting a pure culture of a single kind of microbe from enrichment cultures. In this pipeline, liquid dilution, deep seeding in solid media, and dewatering are common isolation techniques. The most expedient and convenient way of seeding through exhaustion is for organisms that colonize solid medium plates. One can obtain a pure culture by repeatedly collecting and fertilizing an isolated colony. It is feasible to employ the seeding method by depletion to clean both aerobic as well as anaerobic organisms in solid medium plates with the help of a proper incubation apparatus. The technique is completely dependent on the medium's reaction with the released metabolites. It is also crucial to note that during cultivation, the microorganism can be identified through the formation of particular metabolites, that are generated in the medium with lactic acid and others. However, it could be challenging to identify microorganisms based solely on cultivation-dependent biodiversity due to enrichment distortion. Microbial ecologists believe that the current representation of phylotypes in laboratory cultures is less than 0.1% of those found through community genetic analysis (Franco-Duarte et al., 2019).

8.2.2 MICROSCOPY METHODS

To identify microorganisms found in a natural sample, a microscope is a crucial tool. Images captured by microscopy allow researchers to classify biological items, perform motion tracking, and perform shape analysis. In both clinical and scientific settings, the use of a microscope to enquire morphological distinctions is still common for defining the characteristics of desirable bacteria, including streptococci, staphylococci, bacilli (e.g., *Listeria monocytogenes*, *E. coli*, or *Salmonella* spp.), and *Vibrio*. Automatic segmentation remains an obstacle for many commonly used nonfluorescence, interference-based microscopy imaging modalities, despite its importance (e.g., contrast microscopy). However, here are a few reasons why microscopy on its alone is insufficient for identifying microorganisms: small cells are typically difficult to identify; prokaryotes mainly vary in size, and some cells are near the optical microscope's resolution limits; these cells can easily be overlooked when observing natural samples, particularly if the sample consists of a lot of particulate matter or a lot of larger cells; and it can be challenging to distinguish living cells from dead cells or inanimate materials found in natural samples (Franco-Duarte et al., 2019). Microscopic analysis, however, becomes more promising when combined with other instruments. Some of the other electron microscopy methods that become effective tools for identifying microorganisms are scanning electron microscopy, transmission electron microscopy, confocal microscopy, and atomic force microscopy. As these techniques are beneficial in identifying bacteria within biofilms, electron microscopy becomes highly valuable (Franco-Duarte et al., 2019).

8.3 CONVENTIONAL MICROBIAL TESTING METHODS

8.3.1 MICROBIAL LIMIT TEST METHOD (BIOBURDEN TESTING)

Bioburden is an abundance of live microorganisms on a product or in its packaging. It can also be stated that bioburden is the total amount of microbiological inputs from various sources, such as initial supplies, manufacturing ingredients, assembly methods, manufacturing environment, assembly/manufacturing assists (including water, lubricants, and compressed gases, cleaning procedures, and packaged products). Therefore, validation and revalidation of sterilization operations are the primary utilities for bioburden's versatility. This technique can also be used on surgical blades, medical equipment, and other similar products.

8.3.2 MICROBIAL IDENTIFICATION

The process of identification involves comparing an organism's traits, either phenotypic or genotypic, to a recognized reference or standard, like a specific species. Many pharmacopoeias recommend the detection and identification of these indicator infections to evaluate the quality of raw materials and final products. They involve cultivating the isolates and characterizing them morphologically and biochemically (Sandle, 2013; Sutton et al., 2004).

8.3.3 BACTERIAL ENDOTOXIN TESTING

The basis of this method is the LAL reagent's ability to clot when endotoxins are present. The labeled adaptability of the LAL reagent is the amount of endotoxin needed to get the lysate to clot during ordinary circumstances. This technique can be used to analyze injectables, dialysis water, and water for injection.

8.3.4 STERILITY TESTING

Using this technique, a sample carrying microbes is aseptically injected into diluents, filtered using filter paper with a 0.45-μm size, followed by their inoculation in two media. As the organisms develop throughout the incubation period, turbidity is produced as endpoint. Nonparenteral preparations, aqueous solutions, parenteral preparations (such as Intravenous [IV] and Intramuscular [IM] injectables), ophthalmic preparations (which included eye-drops, lotions, and ointments), other oils or oily solutions, suspensions, antibiotics, solids, creams and ointments, bulks or mixes; surgical supplies, cotton balls, swabs, gauze, scalpels catheters, syringes, blades, and needles can be analyzed using this methodology (Chauhan and Jindal, 2020).

8.3.5 ENVIRONMENTAL MONITORING

Environmental monitoring often includes the monitoring of compressed gases, steam systems, and water systems. Since almost all manufacturing procedures include the use of air, aerobic monitoring is the main focus of typical environmental monitoring activities. Further, evaluating the microbiological quality of the critical and controlled areas in a sterile product manufacturing plant is the goal of the feasible environmental monitoring plan. When starting an environmental monitoring system, one task that is often overlooked is creating real test data to validate the growth media choices and the optimal incubation conditions that guarantee organism recovery. A written document that outlines the full environmental monitoring strategy is required by regulatory expectations. At least three distinct techniques are used to monitor the air in aseptic areas: passive air sampling, nonviable particulate monitoring, and active air sampling method (Moldenhauer, 2021).

In general, the pharmaceutical and drug industries generate high-quality medications that are meant to benefit people and society through controlled manufacturing processes. Various microbiological safety measurement steps can be taken through suitable microbial testing to ensure the purity and safety of pharmaceutical products (Table 8.1) (Chauhan and Jindal, 2020; Grove and Randall, 1955).

TABLE 8.1 Enumeration of Microbiological Safety Indicators that are Typically Suggested for the Examination of Various Pharmaceutical Products

Microbial Testing Methods	Pharmaceutical Products
Biochemical identification, like calcium pantothenate, biotin, and vitamin B12	Tablets, vitamin capsules, syrups/liquids, and granular powder.
Sterility testing	Nonparenteral preparations, aqueous solutions, and parenteral preparations (such as IV and IM injectables), ophthalmic preparations (which included eye-drops, lotions, and ointments) among others oils or oily solutions, suspensions, antibiotics solid, creams and ointments, bulks or mixes; surgical supplies, cotton balls, swabs, gauze, scalpels catheters, syringes, blades, and needles.
Microbial limit test	Ayurvedic as well as homoeopathic preparations, pills, syrup, raw materials, water for injection, antibiotics, dialysis water, oral suspension, and other related items.
Bacterial endotoxin test	Dialysis water, injectable water, and other substances.
Biochemical identification, such as Lactic acid bacteria	Probiotics, pills, raw materials, and other relevant materials.
Bioburden test	Medical equipment, surgical blades, and related materials.
Antibiotic assay	Antibiotics: Doxycycline, Amikacin, Kanamycin B, Framycetin, Streptomycin, Kanamycin Sulphate, Amphotericin B, Carbenicillin, Tetracycline, Erythromycin, Neomycin, Nystatin, Oxytetracycline, Bacitracin, Polymyxin B, Gentamicin, Rifampicin, Bleomycin, Novobiocin, other related antibiotic drugs.
Specific microbial identification, like *C. albicans*, *E. coli*, *Shigella* spp., *Salmonella* spp., *Clostridia* spp., *S. aureus*, and *P. aeruginosa*	Additional products include raw ingredients, pills, syrup, oral suspension, ayurvedic, and homeopathic preparations.

8.4 ADVANCEMENTS IN MICROBIOLOGICAL TESTING METHODS

Conventional techniques utilized in the pharmaceutical sector have low sensitivity, are time-consuming, labor-intensive, have low precision, are inefficient, need specialized equipment, and moreover pollute the environment. As a result, researchers are highly interested in the development of rapid and automated microbiological testing techniques, which should be explored in the pharmaceutical industry. The key priority parameters for pharmaceutical microbiological screening are drug safety and purity. The main issue with the old technique is the excessive time required to obtain microbiological data. Rapid techniques are advantageous to the pharmaceutical and medical companies. The use of rapid microbiological technologies in medical fields began in the mid-1960s, surged in the 1970s, and continues to grow to the present (Fung, 1994a, 1994b, 2002). The increasing desire for rapid outcomes prompted advancements in microbiological testing technologies for pharmaceutical products. Rapid microbiological methods (RMMs) are a huge class of analytical microbiological techniques that have the advantage of producing results in less time as compared with conventional, Pasteurian, highly laborious methods (Duguid et al., 2011; Green and Randell, 2016). The majority of RMMs outperform traditional, growth-based approaches in terms of sensitivity, precision, exactness, and durability. Besides, RMMs can be completely automated, have higher sample capacity, work in an uninterrupted data-collection mode that results in significantly decreased time to get valuable outcomes (e.g., from weeks or days to hours or minutes), and, in some cases, may perform real-time collection of data and tracking (Miller, 2019). Rapid methods in microbiology are part of the biotechnology branch and such as RT-PCR, impedance method, multiplex PCR (mPCR), enzyme-linked immunosorbent assay (ELISA), adenosine triphosphate (ATP) bioluminescence, and biosensors. These methods eliminated certain barriers faced by traditional methods via offering sensitive, simple-to-use, time-saving, accurate, and repeatable results.

The RMMs can be further divided into two categories: (1) the type of determination (which is directly related to the test objective) and (2) the detection principle. An RMM's determination type can be (1) qualitative, (2) quantitative, or (3) identification method. Qualitative RMM determines the existence or lack of live microbes, whereas quantitative RMM counts microbes in an actual sample. In contrast to these, identification tests classify them according to their taxonomic group. In addition, these methods commonly necessitate a preliminary colony purifying phase. The three primary detecting approaches are: (1) growth detection, (2) direct analysis, and (3) cell component analysis.

Growth detection depends upon the detection of byproducts of metabolism (e.g., CO_2) or heat generation via catabolic action. Direct analysis method detects the entire bacteria, whereas cell component analysis detects only specific sections of the cell, like ATP, fatty acids, or nucleic acids. Some approaches might involve the growth (i.e., enrichment) stage, during a result to be quantifiable outcome yet lacking the use of growth markers (e.g., metabolic by-products) for the purpose of detection (Henriques et al., 2019). Table 8.2 offers a broad overview of the available RMMs, their principles, the sort of analysis for which the RMM is employed, and knowledge on sensitivity as well as time in delivering a result.

8.5 ENUMERATION METHODS

The quantity of alive microbes found in pharmaceutical samples is an essential measurement to describe the product's microbiological quality. The number of microbial colonies is represented by the colony-forming unit (CFU). So far, numerous approaches for total viable cell count have been built and implemented. For many years, "standard plate count" has been the primary and most widely used approach in applied microbiology. Shortly after the cell culture preparation and dilution stages, the material is combined with standard agar medium, left to develop (at 35°C or 25°C incubation temperature), and colonies are counted 48 hours later (Fung, 1994a, 1994b, 2002; Sarker et al., 2007). Despite its simplicity and ease of use, this technique has certain limitations. This technique takes time along with the consumption of a huge amount of culture fluid as well as lots of sterile test items (including tubes, pipettes, and sterile plates) and broad incubation areas (Andon, 2006; Glasson et al., 2008; Sarker et al., 2007). Several efforts have been executed to improve the semiautomation and ease of use of the standard approach, including physical dispersing of the material on the outer shell of an agar plate (Glasson et al., 2008), the use of pores to isolate living organisms, followed by standard plate culture (Maruyama et al., 2000) and approaches involving nutrients held in films or strips (Fung, 1994a, 1994b, 2002). These approaches were built as alternative options for counting viable cells in the pharmaceutical sector. One of the most popular techniques in the food industry is the use of the most probable number (MPN) methodology. In 2007, a mechanized and automated method for the operation of the live cell count process was

TABLE 8.2 Broad Overview of the Rapid Microbiological Methods

Advanced Microbial Testing Methods	Testing Method	Testing Principle	Type of Determination	Resulting Time	References
ATP bioluminescence	Direct analysis	The analysis of bioluminescence in the ATP reaction in alive cells using luciferase.	Quantitative and qualitative	Sterility testing takes 4 to 7 days 1 hour	Miller and Miyashita (2012); Miller (2019)
Biochemical assays	Direct analysis	Detects bacteria's response to specific biochemical compounds (such as sugars). A strain purification process is required.	Identification	Depending on the test, the type of microorganism, and the strain purification process	Miller (2019)
Autofluorescence	Direct analysis	After blue light exposure of filtered colonies, fluorescence is detected. Incubation may be necessary to get colonies of a required size.	Quantitative	3 hours for detection	London et al. (2010)
CO_2 detection	Detection of growth	The release of CO_2 (as determined by a colorimetric reaction) indicates microbial development.	Qualitative	Sterility testing takes 24–72 hours	Parveen et al. (2011)
Direct laser scanning	Direct analysis	A laser is used to scan the filter surface after it has been filtered.	Quantitative	Few days	Miller (2019)
DEFT	Direct analysis	In order to distinguish living from inactive cells, a double staining technique with DAPI and 6CFDA is employed.	Quantitative and qualitative	<1 hour	Nakajima et al. (2005)
Flow cytometry	Direct analysis	A flow cytometer is used for the detection of fluorophore-labeled microorganisms.	Quantitative and qualitative	Few minutes	Pane et al. (2018)

TABLE 8.2 *(Continued)*

Advanced Microbial Testing Methods	Testing Method	Testing Principle	Type of Determination	Resulting Time	References
Fatty acid profile	Cell component analysis	When comparing the analysis with a database, it uses extremely stable fatty acid content along the taxonomic class. A strain purification process is required.	Identification	24–48 hours	Stead et al. (1992)
Fourier transform infrared	Direct analysis	Utilizes the IR area of the entire microbe. All microbes must be in the same stage of development.	Identification	6–8 hours (not including the culture step)	Maquelin et al. (2003)
Headspace pressure	Growth analysis	Bacterial gas generation or expenditure influences the gas component and pressure in a clogged media vial.	Qualitative	72 hours	Becherucci et al. (2016)
Mass spectrometry	Direct analysis and cell component analysis	The production of ions (via the comparative abundance and mass/charge proportion, respectively) is compared with a database.	Identification	<40 minutes	Thouvenot et al. (2018)
Solid phase cytometry	Direct analysis	Bacterial identification following filtration and labeling using an internally converted fluorophore.	Quantitative and qualitative	Sterility testing takes 3 hours	Smith et al. (2010)
Microcalorimetry	Detection of growth	Heat emitted by microbial catabolic action is measured.	Qualitative	24–72 hours	Brueckner et al. (2017)
Turbidimetry	Direct analysis	The existence of microbes (whether living or nonliving) alters the optical density of the media.	Qualitative	In accordance with the growth period	Miller (2019)

TABLE 8.2 *(Continued)*

Advanced Microbial Testing Methods	Testing Method	Testing Principle	Type of Determination	Resulting Time	References
Phage-based analysis	Direct analysis and cell component analysis	Gene appearance or intracellular content detection following phage contamination. Because phages might be unique for an established host, the approach can be employed to identify them.	Identification and qualitative	48 hours	Stanley et al. 2007)
Immunological methods	Cell component analysis	ELISA: Particular antibodies attached to a well-defined bacterial binding site. A labeled secondary antibody is used for detection.	Identification	Depending on the identification method	Miller (2019)
		IMS: Bacterial separation employing particular antibodies labeled with paramagnetic particles. Using a moving magnetic field facilitates the bacteria that are important to be separated. A linked detector is required.		Sterility testing takes 14–24 hours	
Genotypic methods	Cell component analysis	PCR: Enhancement of a specific or globally preserved nucleic acid sequence.	Qualitative, quantitative, and identification	<2 hours	Miller (2019); Saulnier et al. (2017)
		Restriction endonuclease analysis: Mapping genetic information employing restraint enzymes and matching the fragments to a database. It is necessary to have a pure colony.		Few hours	

introduced in the market. It consisted of a hands-free 16-tube system for the MPN method that was later used throughout the recognized pharmaceutical and food laboratories all over the world (Fung, 1994a, 1994b, 2002; Irwin et al., 2000). In recent years, several techniques that involve real-time alive cell counting have also been investigated. Such real-time studies rely on the application of "vital" dyes to stain "live" organisms in order to quantify fluorescing living organisms with the help of a magnifying device, resulting in extremely fast methods. Within an hour or less, a viable number of cells can be determined by eye or via an automated method. Viable bacterial cells (mostly RNA) are colored red using acridine orange in direct epifluorescent filter technique (DEFT), while dead cells (primarily DNA) are colored green. The major drawback of this approach is that RNA may be persistent in heat-damaged or preservative-treated cells and, therefore, stain red even in dead cells.

Newby (1991) published an improved DEFT approach called the microcolony technique. In the improved method, cells are initially filtered through a membrane, followed by preparation of several microcolonies, and then labelled as well as counted. Nakajima et al. (2005) used 6-carboxyfluorescein diacetate (CFDA) and 4′,6-diamidino-2-phenylindole (DAPI) to investigate a fluorescence staining approach for assessing the microbiological purity of herbal remedies. The outcomes were disclosed in relation to the standard colony count test. Their findings revealed that the usual colony-measuring test failed to detect the majority of physiologically active bacteria in medical samples. Based on its simplicity and rapid time (less than one hour) for labeling and enumeration, the authors stated that the 6CFDA-DAPI double-stained approach may be implemented in order to regular bacteriological monitoring (Nakajima et al., 2005). Another technique in this field is the detection of ATP in living cells confined in specific membranes. Viable cell counts can be obtained in one to four hours (Fung, 1994a, 1994b) using ATP detection techniques. In general, ATP detection tools measure the amount of light released throughout the enzymatic reaction (bioluminescence mechanism) (Turner et al., 2010). ATP bioluminescence established on the luciferine/luciferase response has gathered a lot of attention in the area of rapid microorganism identification (Figure 8.1). The finding of ATP with ATP-luminescence innovation is thus a preferred way to replace older methods and considerably reduce detection time without sacrificing reliability (Beckers et al., 1985; Girotti et al., 2001; Mafu et al., 1991; Squirrell et al., 2002).

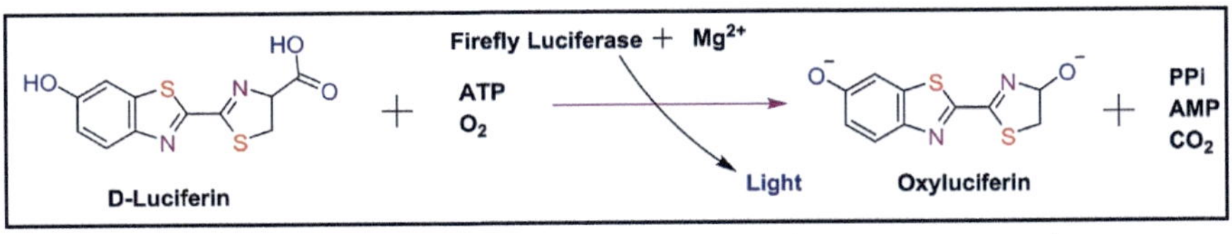

FIGURE 8.1 ATP bioluminescence derived from luciferine/luciferase reaction.

Impedance microbiology is a key field of rapid techniques that can be utilized for both qualitative as well as quantitative microbe tracing of microorganisms by monitoring fluctuations in electrical conductivity. Impedance technology is classified into two types: direct and indirect. In a direct impedance innovation, the change in the electric field of a liquid culture medium serves as a quantitative indicator, while the change in the electrostatic impedance of a reaction mixture is monitored in the indirect one (Cady et al., 1978; Wawerla et al., 1999). Connolly et al. (1993) investigated three quick microbial identification techniques for employing them in pharmaceuticals and cosmetic goods (such as dextrose, magnesium phosphate heptahydrate, potassium dihydrogen phosphate, and ammonium sulphate) toward *Aspergillus niger*, *P. aeruginosa*, *S. aureus*, and *Candida albicans*. Their findings revealed that neither the DEFT nor the ATP bioluminescence approaches provided a good dose/response line; however, the impedance approach did (Connolly et al., 1993).

8.6 DIAGNOSTIC METHODS

In pharmaceutical microbiology, various diagnostic technologies are currently utilized to get accurate results in a short period of time. The PCR, miniaturized diagnostic kits, microarray, Immunomagnetic separation (IMS), ELISA tests, and biochip innovations have become extensively employed in recent decades as diagnostic systems capable of handling numerous samples at a single time (Fritzler, 2006; Fung, 1994a, 1994b, 2002; Garcia-Cruz et al., 2012; Yakub and Stadterman-Knauer, 2004). Miniaturized devices are designed primarily to lower the volume of chemicals and media used in microbiological assays. Microtiter plates, containers for liquid and solid media, and a sterilized multiple inoculation device comprise a miniaturized setup. Diagnostic kits make it possible to promptly and properly identify pathogens, saving many lives.

A diagnostic kit reads each well's color reaction before identifying the microbe (key-out) using a manual recognition code. Recently, automatic detectors that can fast and accurately identify foreign cultures have also been developed (Fung, 1994a, 1994b). In medical and pharmaceutical microbiology, immunological techniques that make use of antigen and antibody interactions have long been used to detect microorganisms. The most popular immunological assay is the ELISA test. In ELISA assays, overnight incubation is required to achieve an acceptable amount of the target organism. This is the primary approach for identifying microbes such as *Salmonella, Listeria monocytogenes*, and *E. coli*. Nowadays, some completely automated ELISA devices have come into force (Fung, 1994a, 1994b, 2002; Hui et al., 2008; Nollet and Toldra, 2008), with test times ranging from 45 minutes to 2 hours (after the overnight incubation). PCR is frequently applied to identify microbes (like Salmonella) via the proliferation of the target DNA and recognition of the specific PCR results. Gel electrophoresis, unique stains, fluorescent sensors, and molecular beacons are all useful tools to detect PCR outcomes. Multiplexing is a method that allows various PCR-based approaches to screen four separate targets in a single sample (Adzitey et al., 2013; Amani et al., 2015; Fung, 2002). Quantitative real-time PCR is a fast method to afford precise and accurate DNA quantification, which can subsequently be used in the detection of microbes. This technique detects nucleic acids accurately in a mixture of substances, even if the initial concentration of the nucleic acid is low. The RT-PCR approach was employed for microbiological analysis of Amikacin against *S. aureus*. The outcomes indicated that the applied RT-PCR approach was correct and precise across the entire concentration range, while the manual turbidimetric approach demonstrated precision throughout the entire concentration range, except that correctness was limited to the middle and minimal concentrations. However, the RT-PCR method revealed certain drawbacks in contrast to turbidimetric techniques, including the fact that it operates as an indirect approach of identifying amikacin and requires expensive equipment along with time-consuming procedures (Lotfipour et al., 2015).

In another investigation, a research group implemented the mPCR method to regulate the microbiological purity of pharmaceutical products (Farajnia et al., 2009). Furthermore, the mPCR method was developed to detect and identify four hazardous bacterial species in a single reaction (<8 hour): *S. aureus*, *Salmonella*, *E. coli*, and *P. aeruginosa*. The application of specific primers targeting the marker bacteria was reported, followed by the measurement of both the specificity and sensitivity of every pair of primers. Specific bands for matched microorganisms were found concurrently via PCR of mixed DNA specimens. The mPCR assay detected a small amount of bacterial contamination that is below 10 cfu per milliliter or gram of sample. The mPCR assay may be employed to deliver cost-effective and fast microbiological testing of nonsterile pharmaceutical items in the pharmaceutical sector (Nemati et al., 2016). Paramagnetic particles coated with several substances (such as DNA, antigens, and antibodies) are used in IMS methods to capture desired cells (e.g., *E. coli* O157, *Listeria*). After that, the beads are covered in agar. This technique may also be employed in combination with an ELISA assay or a PCR method. This type of combination may result in shortening the incubation period while simultaneously increasing overall process sensitivity (Cho et al., 2008; Ricke and Jones, 2010). A biosensor is a type of analyzer that utilizes a biological element and a physicochemical detector to detect a chemical (Buhl et al., 2007; De Castro and Herrera, 2003). It may be a biological molecule or a set of molecules coupled to a signal identification substance. Any interaction that occurs between the substance being studied and the biosensor generates a detection signal, which is monitored through a device. Toxins, microbes, sugars, herbicides and pesticides, and ATPs are some examples of analytes. Optical, electrochemical, and other transducers are all utilized to produce indications for better recognition. Biochip and microchip technology are also employed for recognizing several kinds of molecules, consisting of pathogens like *E. coli*, *Listeria* sp., *Salmonella* sp., *S. aureus*, and others (Buhl et al., 2007; Cady et al., 1978; De Castro and Herrera, 2003; Fung, 2002). Table 8.3 summarizes the benefits and drawbacks of the discussed approaches.

8.7 CONCLUSION

The key priority parameters for pharmaceutical microbiological screening are drug safety and purity. The arrival of any infectious bacteria, molds, yeasts, or bacterial toxins is strictly monitored to ensure that no harm occurs. In this context, antibiotics are microbiology's most significant contribution to the pharmaceutical industry. There are numerous methods for microbial testing in the pharmaceutical companies that are constantly

TABLE 8.3 Benefits and Drawbacks of the Different Approaches

Techniques	Type of Method	Analytes	Benefits and Drawbacks Reported	References
Mechanized and automated MPN techniques	Enumeration method	Pharmaceutical and food items	Accuracy and automation in testing, with fewer human interventions and impurities.	Fung (1994a, 1994b, 2002)
Fluorescent staining	Enumeration method	Herbal medicines	Benefits: Easy and quick staining and enumeration.	Nakajima et al. (2005)
ATP bioluminescence and impedance techniques	Enumeration method	Pharmaceuticals and cosmetic items	Neither DEFT nor ATP bioluminescence approaches provided an acceptable dose/response curve, but the impedance technique produced a reasonable dose/response outcome.	Connolly et al. (1993)
RT-PCR technique	Diagnostic method	Pharmaceutical items	Benefits: A reliable and precise approach capable of detecting nucleic acids having a small concentration of starting material. Drawbacks: It acts as an indirect approach to detect Amikacin. It also involves a sophisticated process that requires expensive equipment and time-consuming operations.	Nemati et al. (2016)
Multiplex PCR technique	Diagnostic method	Pharmaceutical items	Possibility of detecting a small concentration of bacterial contamination of fewer than 10 cfu per milliliter or gram of sample. In the pharmaceutical sector, microbiological quality monitoring of nonsterile pharmaceutical samples may be accomplished cost-effectively and timely manner.	Nemati et al. (2016)

being used. Rapid microbial identification and automation have become a crucial subject in the pharmaceutical industry. The utilization of miniaturized systems, RT-PCR, mPCR, impedance method, ELISA, ATP bioluminescence processes, biosensors, and other technologies leads to several significant advancements in microbial testing methods. Additionally, the ease of implementation and adaptability of these tools overcomes the drawbacks of traditional approaches by possessing significant labor and time savings characteristics. These methods deal with the limitations of traditional methods by producing sensitive, easy-to-use, time-saving, exact, and reproducible results. Biochips and microarrays for the identification of bacteria in pharmaceuticals are a promising topic, but additional research is necessary to make the methods more relevant in microbiology. This area of study may be more relevant in genomics, which requires a large amount of data to gather useful knowledge. In the approaching years, advancements in the pharmaceutical microbiological sectors will become more evident and effective. As stepping alongside the automation and improvement in traditional testing facilities, this chapter affords the idea to researchers working in the field of microbiology regarding recent microbiological techniques with keen emphasis on their utilities.

KEYWORDS

- **adenosine triphosphate bioluminescence**
- **biosensors**
- **direct epifluorescent filter technique**
- **enzyme-linked immunosorbent assay**
- **impedance method**
- **labor-intensive**
- **limulus amebocyte lysate**
- **microbes**
- **multiplex polymerase chain reaction**
- **reverse transcriptase-polymerase chain reaction**

REFERENCES

Adzitey, F., Huda, N., Ali, G. R. R. (2013). Molecular techniques for detecting and typing of bacteria, advantages and application to foodborne pathogens isolated from ducks. *3 Biotech, 3*, 97–107.

Amani, J., Mirhosseini, S. A., Fooladi, A. A. I. (2015). A review approaches to identify enteric bacterial pathogens. *Jundishapur Journal of Microbiology, 8*(2), e17473.

Andon, B. M. (2006). Active air vs. passive air (settle plate) monitoring in routine environmental monitoring programs. *PDA Journal of Pharmaceutical Science and Technology, 60*(6), 350–355.

Ashutosh, K. *Pharmaceutical Microbiology* (pp. 1–240). New Age International (P) Ltd: New Delhi, 2008.

Ayurvedic Pharmacopoeia Committee. (2001). *The ayurvedic pharmacopoeia of India.* Government of India, Ministry of Health and Family Welfare. *New Delhi, India: Department of AYUSH, 1*(1) 144–145.

Becherucci, V., Gentile, F., Ceccantini, R., Gori, V., Piccini, L., Bisin, S., Allegrao, E., Brugnolo, F., Bindi, B., Pavan, P., Cunial, V., Ermini, S., Bambi, F. (2016). Validation of rapid sterility test with BacT/ALERT 3D on human mesenchymal stem cells as cell therapy product inside an hospital cell factory. *International Journal of Microbiology and Allied Sciences, 2*, 13–21.

Beckers, B., Lang, H. R. M., Schimke, D., Lammers, A. (1985). Evaluation of a bioluminescence assay for rapid antimicrobial susceptibility testing of mycobacteria. *European Journal of Clinical Microbiology, 4*, 556–561.

Bisen, P. S., Debnath, M., Prasad, G. B. (2012). *Microbes: Concepts and Applications* (pp. 65–121). John Wiley & Sons: Canada.

British Pharmacopoeia Commission, & Great Britain. (2000). Medicines commission. In: *British Pharmacopoeia* (Vol. 1). Bernan Press (PA): London.

Brueckner, D., Krähenbühl, S., Zuber, U., Bonkat, G., Braissant, O. (2017). An alternative sterility assessment for parenteral drug products using isothermal microcalorimetry. *Journal of Applied Microbiology, 123*(3), 773–779.

Buhl, A., Metzger, J. H., Heegaard, N. H., Von Landenberg, P., Fleck, M., Luppa, P. B. (2007). Novel biosensor–based analytic device for the detection of anti-double-stranded DNA antibodies. *Clinical Chemistry, 53*(2), 334–341.

Cady, P., Dufour, S. W., Shaw, J., Kraeger, S. J. (1978). Electrical impedance measurements: Rapid method for detecting and monitoring microorganisms. *Journal of Clinical Microbiology, 7*(3), 265–272.

Chauhan, A., Jindal, T. (2020). *Microbiological Methods for Environment, Food and Pharmaceutical Analysis* (pp. 303–423), Springer Nature: Switzerland.

Cho, K., Wang, X. U., Nie, S., Chen, Z., Shin, D. M. (2008). Therapeutic nanoparticles for drug delivery in cancer. *Clinical Cancer Research, 14*(5), 1310–1316.

Connolly, P., Bloomfield, S. F., Denyer, S. P. (1993). A study of the use of rapid methods for preservative efficacy testing of pharmaceuticals and cosmetics. *Journal of Applied Bacteriology, 75*(5), 456–462.

De Castro, M. L., Herrera, M. C. (2003). Enzyme inhibition-based biosensors and biosensing systems: Questionable analytical devices. *Biosensors and Bioelectronics, 18*(2–3), 279–294.

Denyer, S., Hodges, N., Gorman, S. (2004). *Introduction to Pharmaceutical Microbiology*. Hugo and Russell's, 7th edition.

Duguid, J., Balkovic, E., du Moulin, G. C. (2011). RMM-rapid microbiological methods: Where are they now. *American Pharmaceutical Review*, *14*(7), 18.

European Pharmacopoeia Commission. (1980). *European Pharmacopoeia* (Vol. 2). Maisonneuve.

Farajnia, S., Hassan, M., Hallaj Nezhadi, S., Mohammadnejad, L., Milani, M., Lotfipour, F. (2009). Determination of indicator bacteria in pharmaceutical samples by multiplex PCR. *Journal of Rapid Methods and Automation in Microbiology*, *17*(3), 328–338.

Franco-Duarte, R., Černáková, L., Kadam, S., Kaushik, K. S., Salehi, B., Bevilacqua, A., Corbo, M. R., Antolak, H., Dybka-Stępień, K., Leszczewicz, M., Tintino, S. R., Cintia, V., de Souza, A., Sharifi-Rad, J., Coutinho, H. D. M., Martins, N. Rodrigues, C. F. (2019). Advances in chemical and biological methods to identify microorganisms—from past to present. *Microorganisms*, *7*(5), 130.

Fritzler, M. J. (2006). Advances and applications of multiplexed diagnostic technologies in autoimmune diseases. *Lupus*, *15*(7), 422–427.

Fung, D. Y. C. (1994a). Rapid methods and automation for seafood microbiology. In: Martin, A. M. (Ed.), *Fisheries Processing* (pp. 18–50). Springer: New York.

Fung, D. Y. (1994b). Rapid methods and automation in food microbiology: A review. *Food Reviews International*, 10(3), 357–375.

Fung, D. Y. (2002). *Rapid methods and automation in microbiology*. In: *Workshop MRAMA* (No. I).

Garcia-Cruz, C., Aguilar, M. N., Arroyo-Helguera, O. (2012). Fungal and bacterial contamination on indoor surfaces of a hospital in Mexico. *Jundishapur Journal of Microbiology*, *5*(3), 460–464.

Garrett, T. R., Bhakoo, M., Zhang, Z. (2008). Bacterial adhesion and biofilms on surfaces. *Progress in Natural Science, 18*(9), 1049–1056.

Girotti, S., Ferri, E. N., Bolelli, L., Sermasi, G., Fini, F. (2001). Applications of bioluminescence in analytical chemistry. In: Garcia-Campana, A. M., Baeyens, W. R. G. (Ed.), *Chemiluminescence in Analytical Chemistry* (pp. 247–284). Dekker: Switzerland.

Glasson, J. H., Guthrie, L. H., Nielsen, D. J., Bethell, F. A. (2008). Evaluation of an automated instrument for inoculating and spreading samples onto agar plates. *Journal of Clinical Microbiology*, *46*(4), 1281–1284.

Green, S., Randell, C. (2016). Rapid microbiological methods explained. In: *Microbiological Contamination Control in Pharmaceutical Clean Rooms* (pp. 169–192). CRC Press.

Grove, D. C., Randall, W. A. (1955). *Assay Methods of Antibiotics* (pp. 48–65). Medical Encyclopedia Incorporated: New York.

Henriques, J., Cardoso, C., Vitorino, C. (2019). Rapid microbiological methods. They are rapid! Are they fast. http://meddocsonline.org/

Hui, Y., Nollet, L. M., Toldra, F. (2008) *Advances in Food Diagnostics*. John Wiley & Sons: New York.

Indian Pharmacopoeia. (1996). *Ministry of Health and Family Welfare* (Vol. 2). Government of India.

Indian Pharmacopoeia. (2018). Government of India, Ministry of Health and Family Welfare: New Delhi, India

Irwin, P., Tu, S., Damert, W., Phillips, J. (2000). A modified gauss-newton algorithm and ninety-six well micro-technique for calculating MPN using excel spreadsheets 1. *Journal of Rapid Methods and Automation in Microbiology, 8*(3), 171–191.

Kobayashi, H., Rittmann, B. E. (1982). Microbial removal of hazardous organic compounds. *Environmental Science and Technology, 16*(3), 170A–183A.

Lagier, J. C., Hugon, P., Khelaifia, S., Fournier, P. E., La Scola, B., Raoult, D. (2015). The rebirth of culture in microbiology through the example of culturomics to study human gut microbiota. *Clinical Microbiology Reviews, 28*(1), 237–264.

London, R., Schwedock, J., Sage, A., Valley, H., Meadows, J., Waddington, M., Straus, D. (2010). An automated system for rapid non-destructive enumeration of growing microbes. *PLoS One, 5*(1), e8609.

Lotfipour, F., Yeganeh, F., Tamizi, E., Zahedi, A., Asefi, M. (2015). Study of the efficacy of real time-PCR method for amikacin determination using microbial assay. *Advanced Pharmaceutical Bulletin, 5*(2), 181–188.

Madigan, M.T., Martinko, J.M., Bender, K.S., Buckley, D.H., Stahl, D.A. (Eds.) (2012). *Brock Biology of Microorganisms*, 13th edn. (p. 1032), Pearson: London, UK.

Mafu, A. A., Roy, D., Savoie, L., Goulet, J. (1991). Bioluminescence assay for estimating the hydrophobic properties of bacteria as revealed by hydrophobic interaction chromatography. *Applied and Environmental Microbiology, 57*(6), 1640–1643.

Maquelin, K., Kirschner, C., Choo-Smith, L. P., Ngo-Thi, N. A., Van Vreeswijk, T., Stammler, M., Endtlz, H. P., Bruining, H. A., Naumann, D., Puppels, G. J. (2003). Prospective study of the performance of vibrational spectroscopies for rapid identification of bacterial and fungal pathogens recovered from blood cultures. *Journal of Clinical Microbiology, 41*(1), 324–329.

Maruyama, A., Sunamura, M. (2000). Simultaneous direct counting of total and specific microbial cells in seawater, using a deep-sea microbe as target. *Applied and Environmental Microbiology, 66*(5), 2211–2215.

Miller, M. J. (2019). Rapid microbiological methods. In: *Pharmaceutical Microbiological Quality Assurance and Control: Practical Guide for Non-Sterile Manufacturing* (pp. 429–458).

Miller, M. J., Miyashita, N. (2012). Rapid micro methods and the next generation in ATP bioluminescence. *European Pharmaceutical Review, 17*, 14–16.

Moldenhauer, J. (2021). Environmental monitoring. In: *Handbook of Validation in Pharmaceutical Processes*, 4th edn. (pp. 503–516), CRC Press.

Nakajima, K., Nonaka, K., Yamamoto, K., Yamaguchi, N., Tani, K., Nasu, M. (2005). Rapid monitoring of microbial contamination on herbal medicines by fluorescent staining method. *Letters in Applied Microbiology, 40*(2), 128–132.

Nemati, M., Hamidi, A., Dizaj, S. M., Javaherzadeh, V., Lotfipour, F. (2016). An overview on novel microbial determination methods in pharmaceutical and food quality control. *Advanced Pharmaceutical Bulletin, 6*(3), 301–308.

Newby, P. J. (1991). Analysis of high-quality pharmaceutical grade water by a direct epifluorescent filter technique microcolony method. *Letters in Applied Microbiology, 13*(6), 291–293.

Nollet, L. M., Toldra, F. (2008). *Handbook of Muscle Foods Analysis*. CRC Press: New York.

Pane, M., Allesina, S., Amoruso, A., Nicola, S., Deidda, F., Mogna, L. (2018). Flow cytometry: Evolution of microbiological methods for probiotics enumeration. *Journal of Clinical Gastroenterology, 52*, S41–S45.

Parveen, S., Kaur, S., David, S. A. W., Kenney, J. L., McCormick, W. M., Gupta, R. K. (2011). Evaluation of growth based rapid microbiological methods for sterility testing of vaccines and other biological products. *Vaccine, 29*(45), 8012–8023.

Ratajczak, M., Kubicka, M. M., Kamińska, D., Sawicka, P., Długaszewska, J. (2015). Microbiological quality of non-sterile pharmaceutical products. *Saudi Pharmaceutical Journal, 23*(3), 303–307.

Ricke, S. C., Jones, F. T. (2010). *Perspectives on Food-safety Issues of Animal-derived Foods*. University of Arkansas Press: USA.

Sandle, T. (2013). Automated microbial identification: A comparison of USP and EP approaches. *American Pharmaceutical Review, 16*(4).

Sarker, S. D., Nahar, L., Kumarasamy, Y. (2007). Microtitre plate-based antibacterial assay incorporating resazurin as an indicator of cell growth, and its application in the *in vitro* antibacterial screening of phytochemicals. *Methods, 42*(4), 321–324.

Saulnier, D., De Decker, S., Tourbiez, D., Travers, M. A. (2017). Development of a duplex Taqman real-time PCR assay for rapid identification of *Vibrio splendidus*-related and *V. aestuarianus* strains from bacterial cultures. *Journal of Microbiological Methods, 140*, 67–69.

Skerman, V. (1959). *A Guide to the Identification of the Genera of Bacteria, with Methods and Digests of Generic Characteristics*, 2nd edn., Williams & Wilkins Co.: Philadelphia, PA, USA.

Smith, R., Von Tress, M., Tubb, C., Vanhaecke, E. (2010). Evaluation of the ScanRDI® as a rapid alternative to the pharmacopoeial sterility test method: Comparison of the limits of detection. *PDA Journal of Pharmaceutical Science and Technology, 64*(4), 356–363.

Squirrell, D. J., Price, R. L., Murphy, M. J. (2002). Rapid and specific detection of bacteria using bioluminescence. *Analytica Chimica Acta, 457*(1), 109–114.

Stanley, E. C., Mole, R. J., Smith, R. J., Glenn, S. M., Barer, M. R., McGowan, M., Rees, C. E. (2007). Development of a new, combined rapid method using phage and PCR for detection and identification of viable *Mycobacterium paratuberculosis* bacteria within 48 hours. *Applied and Environmental Microbiology, 73*(6), 1851–1857.

Stead, D. E., Sellwood, J. E., Wilson, J., Viney, I. (1992). Evaluation of a commercial microbial identification system based on fatty acid profiles for rapid, accurate identification of plant pathogenic bacteria. *Journal of Applied Bacteriology, 72*(4), 315–321.

Sutton, S. V., Cundell, A. M. (2004). Microbial identification in the pharmaceutical industry. *Pharmacopeial Forum, 30*(5), 1884–1894.

Thouvenot, P., Vales, G., Bracq-Dieye, H., Tessaud-Rita, N., Maury, M. M., Moura, A., Lecuit, M., Leclercq, A. (2018). MALDI-TOF mass spectrometry-based identification of *Listeria* species in surveillance: A prospective study. *Journal of Microbiological Methods, 144*, 29–32.

Turner, D. E., Daugherity, E. K., Altier, C., Maurer, K. J. (2010). Efficacy and limitations of an ATP-based monitoring system. *Journal of the American Association for Laboratory Animal Science, 49*(2), 190–195.

Wawerla, M., Stolle, A., Schalch, B., Eisgruber, H. (1999). Impedance microbiology: Applications in food hygiene. *Journal of Food Protection, 62*(12), 1488–1521.

Yakub, G. P., Stadterman-Knauer, K. L. (2004). Immunomagnetic separation of pathogenic organisms from environmental matrices. In: *Public Health Microbiology: Methods and Protocols* (pp. 189–197).

Yeung, P. S. M., Sanders, M. E., Kitts, C. L., Cano, R., Tong, P. S. (2002). Species-specific identification of commercial probiotic strains. *Journal of Dairy Science, 85*(5), 1039–1051.

PART IV

Regulatory Compliance and Future Perspectives

CHAPTER 9

Microbial Surveillance and Outbreak Investigation: A Global Necessity

ARCHANA SHAHA*, YOGITA SHINDE, and DIPALI TALELE

Department of Pharmacy, Vishwakarma University, Pune, Maharashtra, India

*Corresponding author

ABSTRACT

The major challenge faced by the medical fraternity in today's era is the increasing emergence of resistant and mutant variants of microorganisms. The emergence of superbugs, resistant strains of bacteria, ever mutating viruses like COVID-19, and many other incidents have made it imperative for the researchers and the governments to be vigilant and search for new antimicrobial. The major reason for microbial infections to spread across the globe is their presence in food, air, hospital acquired infections, and other areas. People migrating and travelling across continents usually spread the infections. Due to this reason, it is important for having a surveilling system that will monitor the infections and outbreak. This helps in establishing methods and protocols to keep the infection in control and minimize their spread. This chapter gives an in-depth data regarding the surveillance methodologies and investigations of microbial outbreak.

9.1 INTRODUCTION

The increase in communication and traveling of population across continents has led to an unprecedented rise in infectious diseases that

Advances in Pharmaceutical Microbiology: From Bench to Bedside. Harpreet Singh, Arun Kumar Mishra, Jeyabalan Sangeetha, and Devarajan Thangadurai (Eds.)

DOI: 10.1201/9781779640918-13

transcends across borders. Population growth, urbanization, globalization, changing climatic, and environmental conditions are the major key factors that contribute toward rise of life-threatening microbial outbreaks that severely affect the quality of life of a person. The major challenge faced by mankind today is the emergence of antibiotic-resistant microorganisms in the form of "Superbugs" that cannot be treated by the conventionally available antibiotics. Hence the need for a robust and sound microbial surveillance technology can help not only to monitor the infections but also help the countries across the globe to prepare for the outbreak and prevent it. This has led to initiatives that are being undertaken by the government agencies to ensure good health of people globally and has enabled them to respond to epidemics and pandemics like Severe Acute Respiratory Syndrome-Corona virus (SARS-CoV), Middle East Respiratory Syndrome (MERS), COVID-19, and other such infections (Heymann and Rodier, 2004; Kaiser, 2008; Knobler et al., 2006; Otten, 2000) in controlled manner. The emergence of microbial outbreaks has led to a collaborated effort by Government and International health authorities to update the International Health Regulations (IHR, 2005) in response to these outbreaks (World Health, 2004, 2008). As per IHR (2005), it is essential that all the countries be able to identify and control the outbreak of any infectious diseases. Regardless of where the emergency occurs, any country that becomes aware of a disease outbreak of international concern is required to report it to the World Health Organization (WHO) within 24 hours (Baker and Fidler, 2006; Racaniello, 2004). These significant policy changes are essential for the prompt identification and efficient containment of outbreaks of illness of international public health significance, but they might not be enough, and the threat still remains about global containment. An infectious disease outbreak requires a multistep, intricate approach for its prompt containment with the help of surveillance technologies. Typically, it starts with the monitoring system when an unexpected disease outbreak is identified and reported. The affected countries must confirm claims of outbreaks that seem plausible and could be significant for global public health (Mostashari and Hartman, 2003). The following are the fundamental elements of monitoring and response programs:

1. Surveillance: It involves a methodical observation for the occurrence of an uncommon disease or odd cluster of ailments or symptoms, which serves as the catalyst for the first reported case of an outbreak.

2. Reporting: It involves a description of the original disease epidemic, which includes a credible and potential public health relevance assessment.
3. Verification: It involves contacting the impacted nation and conducting a preliminary investigation to confirm the epidemic or outbreak.
4. Reaction: It involves intervention and active steps taken toward the containment of the outbreak.

In the fields of public health and policymaking, infectious disease surveillance refers to a broad range of ideas, approaches, and activities (Hopkins et al., 1985; Green and Kaufman, 2002; Lober et al., 2002). The Global Influenza Surveillance Network of the WHO is one example of an infectious disease surveillance program that tracks an illness over time, while the US Department of Defense's Biological Threat Reduction Program aims to identify and monitor particular viruses (Hitchcock et al., 2007). Still others provide information on odd cases of infection or disease outbreaks that the infectious disease society should be concerned about, according to specialists (Hutwagner et al., 2003). Public health officials are frequently notified when a physician, infection management nurse, or a clinical laboratory technician discovers an uncommon disease or an unusually high number of cases of an unusual disease. Clinicians were the ones who first identified staphylococcal toxic shock syndrome and eosinophilia-myalgia syndrome (Hertzman et al., 1990). Local newspapers or television news can occasionally inform public health officials about illness epidemics (Nakase, 2000). These systems though conventional help in surveillance of the outbreak and at the same time by creating awareness amongst masses helps in its containment.

9.2 MICROBIAL SURVEILLANCE METHODS

9.2.1 ENVIRONMENTAL SAMPLING TECHNIQUES

There are two types of sampling techniques: direct and indirect. Direct techniques do not require additional processing and are self-contained, like contact plates. For the removal of the sample from the collecting equipment, an extraction step is necessary for indirect procedures like swabs. Convex agar plates, or contact plates, can be applied straight to a surface in order to collect a quantitative sample. The target organism's recovery can vary depending on whether specific or not specific agar is used, as well as if a neutralizing agent is added or not. The primary benefit of contact plates is their ability to produce semiquantitative data, such as colony counts, that can be used to identify patterns (Getchell-White et al., 1989). Similar to contact plates, dip slides use a direct contact technique that is contained inside a container made of plastic to lower the danger of contamination and agar drying. The paddle-shaped dip slides can hold two distinct selective or nonselected agars on their two distinct surfaces. The two sides can be used to collect two samples using two different media types or two distinct samples utilizing two different media types. Dip slides typically have two sides: one with a nonspecific agar and one with a specific agar. Because of their flexibility, dip slides may be a preferable choice over contact plates since they are capable of sampling uneven surfaces without incurring additional processing losses that come with nondirect contact techniques like swabs. The majority of losses happen during processing, like vortexing (Buttner et al., 2007). These additional losses can be eliminated by using direct contact techniques like contact plates and dip slides. Swabs are indirect sampling tools that come in a variety of materials, such as rayon, cotton, polyester, calcium alginate, or macrofoam. Depending on how they are designed, there are many different ways to treat them. Swabs can be worked around challenging or uneven surfaces like bed rails, faucets, and door handles. Sponges are an indirect sampling tool that are easy to work with on uneven surfaces, allow for the easy sampling of a larger surface area, and allow for the application of pressure while sampling. If handling is not done properly during the sampling process, there could be a higher chance of contamination. Wipe procedures entail wiping a surface and gathering a sample with sterile gauze or cloth. For this procedure to prevent sample contamination, excellent aseptic technique is required. For additional processing, the wipe is put into a stomacher bag or sterile container.

9.2.2 CLINICAL SPECIMEN COLLECTION AND PROCESSING

Following sampling, direct plating on agar, enrichment, or molecular processing are the alternatives accessible when employing an indirect sample method. The organisms under investigation, the available funds, and the amount of time all influence the processing method selection. To be processed further, swab, sponge, and wipe samples must be extracted—that is, the target must be taken out of the swab. Phosphate-buffered saline, Tween, Butterfield's buffer, and maximum recovery solution are examples of extraction solutions (Downey et al., 2012). The choice of extraction solvent was discovered to have the second-biggest effect on extraction efficiency, after the target organism (Lutz et al., 2013). Reducing related losses requires ensuring the sample is extracted as optimally as possible. Three techniques (vortexing, agitation, or sonication) for the swab or sponge could promote healing. The process of enrichment is dropping the sample straight into a broth and letting it grow there for a while. It can be helpful for selecting the organism of choice from a swab or nonspecific sample, slower-growing organisms, or stressed cells. Aliquots are incubated, subcultured, and streaked out over a variety of selective and nonselective mediums. Broth infused with brain heart is commonly used (Roelofsen et al., 1999). The literature reported a range of incubation times and temperatures, including 18–48 hours or a general "overnight" (Dancer, 2004; Pinto et al., 2009; Rabuza et al., 2012; Rose et al., 2004). Because the temperatures needed to grow one organism may restrict the growth of another, the choice of incubation temperature may affect the growth or recovery of an organism. Temperatures between 25°C and 45°C were necessary for clinical pathogens (Lagier et al., 2015).

9.2.3 GENOMIC SURVEILLANCE AND SEQUENCING TECHNOLOGIES

Genomic surveillance and sequencing technologies play a crucial role in microbial surveillance by enabling scientists to monitor and understand the genetic makeup of microorganisms. The Seeliger and Hohne approach was used for the process of serotyping. AscI and ApaI restriction endonucleases were used for pulsed-field gel electrophoresis (PFGE) subtyping in compliance with the PulseNet standard procedure (Neves et al., 2008). Genomic surveillance involves studying the genetic material (genome) of microbes to identify and track pathogens responsible for diseases. It helps in monitoring changes in microbial populations, including mutations or the emergence of new strains, which could impact their virulence or resistance to treatments. By analyzing the genetic sequences of pathogens, scientists can trace outbreaks, identify the source of infections, and understand transmission patterns.

9.2.3.1 SEQUENCING TECHNOLOGIES

Sequencing technologies are like decoding machines for the language of life found in our cells. They help scientists read and understand the tiny instructions written in our DNA or RNA. The evolution of sequencing technologies has been marked by a relentless pursuit of innovation, driving the development of novel approaches such as long-read sequencing, single-cell sequencing, and metagenomics. These methodologies have not only expanded the horizons of genetic exploration and illuminated the complex dynamics of microbial communities.

9.2.3.1.1 Next-Generation Sequencing (NGS)

This technology revolutionized genomic surveillance by enabling quick and economic method of sequencing the genetic material such as DNA and RNA. Methods like Illumina sequencing, Ion Torrent sequencing, and others allow the simultaneous sequencing of millions of DNA fragments.

9.2.3.1.2 Long-Read Sequencing

Unlike short-read technologies, long-read sequencing (e.g., PacBio, Oxford Nanopore) produces longer sequences, aiding in resolving complex genomic structures and identifying genomic rearrangements or repetitive regions more accurately.

9.2.3.1.3 Metagenomics

This approach involves sequencing genetic material directly from environmental samples (e.g., soil, water) or complex microbial communities (e.g., gut microbiota) without the need for isolation and culture. It helps in understanding diverse microbial populations and identifying unknown pathogens (Kulski, 2016).

9.3 TYPES OF MICROBIAL OUTBREAKS

Classifying microbial outbreaks often involves considering their scale, severity, transmission modes, and the affected population. Outbreaks can range from sporadic incidents affecting a handful of individuals to epidemics that spread across communities or regions, and in severe cases, to pandemics that impact populations worldwide. Understanding these diverse types of outbreaks is fundamental for public health officials, researchers, and policymakers as it helps in tailoring appropriate response strategies, implementing preventive measures, and allocating resources effectively. By delineating these different outbreak types, we gain insights into the dynamics of infectious diseases, their patterns of transmission, and the impact they can have on societies and global health systems (Fenton and Pedersen, 2005).

9.3.1 FOODBORNE ILLNESSES

Diseases caused by agents that go into the body via the consumption of food are known as foodborne illnesses. These agents are typically either toxic or infectious in nature. Foodborne illness is a risk for everyone. As per the WHO (2021), a foodborne illness is a condition that people get from consuming tainted food that contains chemical, physical, or pathogenic microorganisms. Symptoms like nausea, vomiting, diarrhea, dehydration, headaches, and fever are frequently experienced by the victims. Depending on the variety of pathogen present in food, the quantity of contaminated food consumed, and the health status of the individual, different types and severity of manifestations can occur. Foodborne illness can be categorized as toxin-mediated infection, infection, or intoxication. Biological hazards can cause foodborne infections when consumed with food. Frequent signs of infection include fever, diarrhea, nausea, and abdominal pain. Eating food containing a toxic chemical can lead to intoxication. Microbes are the source of some toxins. Consuming toxic plants, seafood, or food contaminated with chemicals like pesticides or cleaning supplies can also result in food intoxications. Eating food contaminated by dangerous microorganisms that release toxins into the body can lead to a toxin-mediated infection. Toxin of toxin-mediated infection differs from intoxication in that it is produced within the human body (Frumkin, 2016). Foodborne illnesses are primarily brought on by physical, chemical, and biological hazards. Microscopic organisms like bacteria, viruses, and parasites are considered biological hazards. Since viruses and bacteria are the most prevalent sources of foodborne illness, reducing these biological risks is a top priority in all food safety programs.

9.3.1.1 BACTERIA

Pathogenic bacteria are harmful microbes that often do not change the color, taste, or smell of food, making it hard for people to detect contamination. This category of food, termed "potentially hazardous," must be handled and stored properly to prevent bacterial growth and toxin production, which can lead to foodborne illnesses. Bacteria causing such illnesses fall into two main types: spore-forming and nonspore-forming bacteria. Spore-forming bacteria, like *Clostridium perfringens*, can form spores, inactive or dormant bacterial forms that survive in harsh conditions like extreme temperatures or insufficient food. They commonly contaminate soil, vegetables, spices, and raw animal products. *C. perfringens* causes food poisoning by producing toxins in the human gut, resulting in severe abdominal cramps and diarrhea. Meats and poultry are often associated with this illness, especially when cooked or stored improperly within the temperature danger zone (5°C–57°C), allowing rapid spore growth. *Clostridium botulinum*, another anaerobic bacterium, causes botulism in improperly canned meats. Widely found in soil, water, and animal intestines, it produces a neurotoxin affecting the nervous system. Symptoms include dizziness, fatigue, double vision, and difficulty in breathing and swallowing. Heat destroys the toxin when food is boiled for around 20 minutes. Nonspore-forming bacteria, such as *Escherichia coli*, *Listeria*, *Salmonella*, and *Staphylococcus*, exist solely as vegetative cells and are easily destroyed by heat. *E. coli*, often found in meat, produces shiga toxins causing severe symptoms like abdominal pain, nausea, vomiting, and diarrhea. *Listeria monocytogenes*, capable of growing at refrigerator temperatures, contaminates meat and can lead to fever, muscle aches, and diarrhea. Salmonella, widely found in raw meat and poultry, causes symptoms like fever, stomach pain, diarrhea, and nausea. *Staphylococcus aureus*, commonly found in meat, eggs, and poultry, produces enterotoxins leading to symptoms like nausea, vomiting, and abdominal cramping. Workers' hands are a common source of contamination in food production (Zhan et al., 2014).

9.3.1.2 VIRUSES

Viruses, much smaller than bacteria, differ significantly as they cannot survive outside a living host, be it a human or animal. Among the notable viruses causing foodborne illness are Hepatitis A and noroviruses. Hepatitis A virus is commonly transmitted through infected workers' unwashed hands and can result in severe liver disease. This virus can survive for several hours in favorable conditions and may not exhibit symptoms for up to 6 weeks. Common symptoms include fatigue, loss of appetite, abdominal pain, diarrhea, and fever. Noroviruses are a group of viruses responsible for causing gastroenteritis in humans. People often get infected by consuming contaminated food or drinks, particularly after food handlers handle raw meat, especially poultry. Symptoms of norovirus illness typically include nausea, diarrhea, vomiting, and stomach cramps. This illness commonly affects the very young, elderly, and those with weakened immune systems (Pitchai et al., 2014).

9.3.1.3 PARASITES

Parasites, small creatures that live on or inside hosts, also pose a risk of foodborne illness. Two examples from pork are Toxoplasma and Trichinella. *Toxoplasma gondii*, found in improperly handled fresh pork sausage, can persist for extended periods and spread through various means such as wind, insects, or earthworms. It resides in the intestines and muscle tissue of animals. While it can endure refrigeration temperatures between 1°C and 4°C, freezing below −12°C or heat above 67°C can destroy it. *Trichinella* is a nematode parasite occurring in meat. Its infective larvae are ingested through meat consumption, mature in the intestine, and start a new cycle. While they can survive for years, they often die within 6–12 months (Robertson et al., 2014).

9.3.1.4 CHEMICAL HAZARDS

Chemical hazards in food can originate naturally or be improperly added during agricultural production, food processing, or by consumers. Naturally occurring toxins and food allergens produced by organisms fall under this category. Human-induced chemical contaminants include pesticides, fertilizers, food additives, metals, and residues from industrial processes. Heavy metals like arsenic, cadmium, mercury, and others are commonly found in nature and can contaminate food. Improper storage or polluted water sources containing mercury compounds may lead to heavy metal poisoning, resulting in symptoms such as numbness or weakness in the legs. Other chemical residues, such as detergents or sanitizers used for food handling, can cause illness if they enter food due to improper cleaning practices (Zhan et al., 2014).

9.3.1.5 PHYSICAL HAZARDS

Physical hazards, like foreign materials such as glass, stones, wood, or bone fragments, can enter food during processing, poor handling, or in retail establishments, posing risks if ingested. Glass, often used as packing material, must be handled carefully to prevent fragments from contaminating food. To address these hazards, commercial food manufacturers employ devices like X-ray machines and metal detectors to detect foreign materials. Additionally, ensuring quality control in raw materials and production environments helps minimize risks (Zhan et al., 2014). Foodborne illnesses are a significant global health issue and a major cause of economic losses. According to the WHO, approximately 1 billion cases of foodborne illnesses occur annually, affecting both developed and developing countries. These illnesses incur significant costs, with about 1/3 of people in developed countries experiencing foodborne illness. Tragically, foodborne microbial contamination leads to the deaths of approximately 1.7 million children aged 0–15 due to diarrhea. Given the widespread impact of foodborne illness, it is crucial to prioritize its prevention as it significantly affects human health and life (Charalambous et al., 2018).

9.3.2 WATERBORNE DISEASES

Waterborne diseases stem from pathogenic microbes transmitted through contaminated water, often used for drinking, food preparation, and sanitation. Many developing regions, especially rural areas, lack proper water treatment facilities, making water purification challenging due to scarce resources. Children are disproportionately affected by these diseases due to weaker immunity and poor hygiene practices. The emergence of various waterborne pathogens has gained prominence in global discussions over recent decades, spurring extensive research in this field. A staggering 844 million people lack access to basic drinking water services, with approximately 159 million relying on potentially contaminated surface water, according to the WHO (Moe, 2007). Moreover, about 2 billion individuals use drinking water sources tainted with fecal matter, contributing to approximately 502,000 annual deaths from waterborne diseases, primarily diarrheal illnesses. Waterborne diseases encompass a range of conditions, including cholera, diarrhea, typhoid, amebiasis, hepatitis, gastroenteritis, giardiasis, campylobacteriosis, scabies, and various worm infections, caused by pathogenic microorganisms and contaminants. Diarrhea, a prevalent waterborne disease, predominantly impacts children under five, leading to symptoms like dizziness, dehydration, pale skin, and in severe cases, loss of consciousness. Without treatment, it can be fatal. Cholera, caused by *Vibrio cholerae* bacteria through contaminated food or water, results in symptoms like diarrhea, vomiting, fever, and abdominal cramps. It poses a high mortality risk, especially among malnourished individuals or those with compromised immunity, such as HIV-infected individuals. Typhoid fever, caused by *Salmonella typhi* bacteria found in contaminated water, brings prolonged fever, appetite loss, nausea, headaches, constipation, and weight loss. Swift treatment is crucial to both cure the patient and prevent its contagious spread (Leclerc et al., 2002). Amoebiasis, caused by the parasite *Entamoeba histolytica*, transmits through unwittingly ingesting cysts in food, affecting the intestines. This parasite thrives in contaminated soil and fecal matter, leading to symptoms like abdominal cramps and watery stools. Hepatitis A, primarily impacting the liver due to the Hepatitis A virus, spreads orally or through contact with an infected person. Its common symptoms include fever, nausea, and vomiting, but without timely treatment, severe complications may arise (Wang and Doyle, 1998). Transmission of these waterborne diseases is influenced significantly by climate change, especially during heavy precipitation events like rains or snowfall, which heightens the risk. Natural disasters like floods can lead to sewage treatment plant overflows, presenting immediate risks requiring containment. Conversely, drought-affected areas pose risks due to a concentration of pathogens in limited water sources. Environmental changes post-natural disasters, like earthquakes or cyclones, can foster favorable conditions for specific pathogens to flourish, rendering untreated water unsafe for regular use due to increased microbial burden. Negligence in water treatment plant cleaning can greatly impact communities, particularly in towns lacking household water purifiers. Continuous use of contaminated water for agriculture can also result in pathogen colonization in soil, posing risks to residents consuming crops from these areas (Craun, 1990).

9.3.3 HEALTH-ASSOCIATED INFECTIONS (HAIS)

HAIs are infections that patients acquire, while receiving medical treatment in healthcare facilities, including hospitals, clinics, nursing homes, and other settings. These infections are not present or incubating at the time of admission and can be caused by various pathogens, including bacteria, viruses, fungi, and other microbes (Horan et al., 2008). Factors contributing to the occurrence of HAIs are discussed in the following sections:

9.3.3.1 MICROBIAL TRANSMISSION

Pathogens can spread through direct contact with infected individuals or contaminated surfaces, medical equipment, or healthcare workers' hands. Some infections, like tuberculosis or certain respiratory viruses, can spread through tiny airborne droplets when an infected person coughs or sneezes. Larger droplets produced when an infected person talks, coughs, or sneezes can directly land on nearby individuals, causing infections like flu or meningitis (Chinn and Sehulster, 2003).

9.3.3.2 INVASIVE MEDICAL PROCEDURES

Surgical procedures carry the risk of introducing pathogens into the body, especially if preventive measures like sterile techniques are not strictly followed. The use of medical devices like catheters, ventilators, or central lines can introduce bacteria into the body or provide a pathway for infections.

9.3.3.3 COMPROMISED IMMUNE SYSTEMS

Patients with weakened immune systems due to underlying illnesses, chemotherapy, or immunosuppressive medications are more susceptible to infections. Both the very young (neonates, infants) and the elderly have weaker immune responses, making them more vulnerable to infections.

9.3.3.4 EXTENDED HOSPITAL STAYS

Longer periods in healthcare facilities increase the risk of exposure to infectious agents, leading to higher chances of acquiring an HAI.

9.3.3.5 HAND HYGIENE

Poor hand hygiene among healthcare workers, including inadequate hand washing or improper use of gloves, can contribute significantly to the transmission of infections. Improper sterilization or disinfection of medical equipment and surfaces can facilitate the spread of infections.

9.3.3.6 ANTIBIOTIC RESISTANCE

Misuse or overuse of antibiotics can lead to the emergence of antibiotic-resistant bacteria, making infections more challenging to treat.

9.3.3.7 HOSPITAL ENVIRONMENT

Environmental contamination in healthcare settings, such as contaminated surfaces, ventilation systems, or water sources, can contribute to the spread of infections. HAIs have various types of infections that patients can acquire during medical care. These infections pose a significant risk to patients in healthcare settings and require vigilant preventive measures to reduce their occurrence and transmission. Different types of HAIs are discussed in the following sections.

9.3.3.7.1 Surgical Site Infections (SSIs)

These occur at the site of a surgical incision and can involve the skin, tissues, or organs. SSIs can range from superficial infections to more severe infections affecting deeper tissues.

9.3.3.7.2 Urinary Tract Infections (UTIs)

Typically linked to the use of urinary catheters, UTIs affect the bladder or kidneys. Catheterization provides a direct route for bacteria to enter the urinary system.

9.3.3.7.3 Central Line-Associated Bloodstream Infections

Infections that enter the bloodstream through central lines or catheters, which are tubes placed in large veins, commonly for medication or fluid administration.

9.3.3.7.4 Ventilator-Associated Pneumonia

This type of pneumonia develops in individuals who are on mechanical ventilation. Bacteria can enter the lungs through the breathing tube.

9.3.3.7.5 Clostridium Difficile Infections

An infection of the colon caused by the bacterium *C. difficile*, often associated with antibiotic use, leading to severe diarrhea and colitis (Pulvirenti et al., 2002).

9.3.3.7.6 Bloodstream Infections

Infections that travel through the bloodstream can originate from a variety of sources, including surgical wounds, catheters, or other medical devices.

9.3.3.7.7 Gastrointestinal Infections

These can occur due to contaminated food or water, leading to gastrointestinal issues such as nausea, vomiting, diarrhea, and abdominal pain.

9.3.3.7.8 Respiratory Tract Infections

Infections affecting the lungs or airways, including pneumonia or bronchitis, which can be acquired during hospitalization.

9.3.3.7.9 Skin and Soft Tissue Infections

Infections involving the skin, muscles, or underlying tissues can occur due to surgical procedures, wounds, or contaminated medical devices (Siegel et al., 2007). Preventive control measures are pivotal in curbing the incidence and impact of HAIs within medical facilities. These strategies encompass various approaches aimed at reducing the risk of infections and ensuring patient safety. Rigorous hand washing by healthcare workers is critical in preventing the spread of infections. Proper cleaning and sterilization of medical equipment and surfaces reduce the risk of contamination. Isolating patients with contagious infections help prevent the spread of pathogens. Responsible use of antibiotics helps combat the rise of antibiotic-resistant bacteria. Vaccination of healthcare workers and patients against preventable diseases reduces the risk of infection. Implementing comprehensive infection prevention and control strategies is crucial in minimizing the incidence of HAIs, and protecting both patients and healthcare workers within healthcare settings (Haque et al., 2018).

9.3.4 ZOONOTIC DISEASE OUTBREAKS

Zoonoses encompass diseases that transfer naturally between humans and vertebrate animals. These diseases are categorized into various types: epidemic zoonoses, occurring sporadically; endemic zoonoses, prevalent in multiple regions; and surfacing or re-occurrence zoonoses, either emerging in populations, which is new or resurging rapidly in terms of occurrence or geographical distribution (Di Bari et al., 2023). For instance, notable cases include the H1N1 pandemic of influenza strain in 2019; recently MERS-CoV. Zoonotic infections account for about 60% of the total infectious and life-threatening diseases, presenting significant concerns due to their high mortality and morbidity rates and the paucity of specialized drug therapy including vaccines to restrict their emergence and thereby reducing their escalation globally. As interactions between humans and animals increase, driven by factors like habitat destruction and population growth, new outbreaks of these diseases persistently arise. Studies show a correlation between declining forest cover, especially in biodiverse regions, and increased disease incidences. Additionally, climate change contributes to the spread of zoonotic diseases like the West Nile virus, which are caused by vectors, posing a threat to human health (Stephens et al., 2021). Previously confined zoonoses now transcend geographical boundaries, propelled by global trade and heightened travel. Stephens et al. (2022) examined major zoonotic outbreaks, revealing key drivers linked to factors such as abundance of vector, densely populated countries, climate change or global warming, and contamination of natural resources like soil, air, and water. Interestingly, the microbes behind these extensive epidemics or pandemics usually tend to be viral and are vector transmitted.

Recognizing this urgency, the WHO puts the stress on the need for cohesive global efforts for combating the emergence of infection causing organism and thereby aid in prevention of globally afflicting pandemics or epidemics. Its proactive measures have played pivotal roles in containing recent outbreaks, including those of the Swine flu, Ebola virus, Bird flu, and SARS-CoV-2. The COVID-19 pandemic starkly illustrated the catastrophic toll of zoonotic diseases (Holmes, 2022). Till date more than 600 million cases and greater than 6.5 million fatal incidents worldwide, it underscored the enduring presence of zoonotic illnesses, emphasizing the continual exchange of viruses among various kinds of races of humans and animals alike. For example, during the SARS-CoV-2, bats, humans, pangolins/raccoon and dogs served as reservoir, novel, and intermediate hosts, respectively. Despite numerous barriers—genetic, immunological, ecological, and epidemiological—that typically hinder inter-species transmission, SARS-CoV-2 managed to infect a range of animals, including mink, cats, lions, dogs, tigers in the US. Notably, in some animal populations, the virus reached high prevalence levels. The evolutionary history of the sarbecoviruses, including SARS-CoV-2, involves intricate genomic recombination events fostering genetic diversity and giving rise to virus variants adept at infecting humans. Shifting to Ebola, Ebola Virus Disease is a lethal condition caused by one of five Ebola virus strains. Its first recorded outbreak occurred in 1976 near the Ebola River in the Democratic Republic of the Congo, and since then, periodic outbreaks have persisted across Africa. The Ebola virus is believed to originate from bats, although this theory is yet to be conclusively proven. Its highly contagious nature primarily exposes individuals to the virus through direct contact with an infected person's bodily fluids, such as blood. Additionally, transmission can occur by handling contaminated objects, like clothing or syringes, from an infected patient. Although less common, Ebola may be transmitted with help of bat or coming in contact with meat which is infected because of animals. The manifestation of symptoms generally occurs about 21 days after being exposed to the virus; symptoms like elevated body temperature, diarrhea, headaches, and hemorrhaging were observed.

The unprecedented Ebola outbreak in West Africa in 2014 was the largest on record, affecting Liberia, Sierra Leone, and Guinea. This outbreak was particularly concerning as it hit urban areas, unlike previous instances that were confined to remote villages, making containment more challenging. Approximately 26,000 cases and nearly 10,000 deaths were reported in these countries within a year, highlighting the virus's severe impact. To control the virus, robust surveillance, prompt reporting of new cases, and educating the public on proper handling of infected patients and items are critical measures (Bell, 2016). On another front, the avian influenza strain H5N1, highly pathogenic to birds, was detected amongst the Asian and Middle Eastern poultry in 1990s. Though rare, usually infection to the humans happens if and when they come in contact with the bird that has been infected. In year 1997, Hong Kong reported first cases of Humans being infected. Over 650 H5N1, human cases have been documented in more than 15 countries, its fatality rate remains high at around 60% since 2003. Although H5N1 has not yet spread among humans, the virus's potential for mutation and its lethal impact in birds raises concerns. Scientists worry that a mutated strain might become transmissible among humans, causing a global epidemic, emphasizing the need for vigilance and continued monitoring (Baker and Wisely, 2023).

9.4 KEY PLAYERS IN OUTBREAK INVESTIGATION

Outbreak investigations are complex endeavors that require a coordinated effort from a diverse array of professionals, each playing a crucial role in identifying, understanding, and containing the spread of diseases. These key players form an intricate web of expertise, encompassing epidemiologists, laboratory scientists, healthcare workers, public health officials, and various other specialists. Their collective efforts are essential in every stage of outbreak response, from the early detection and assessment of potential threats to the implementation of targeted interventions and the dissemination of crucial information to the public. Individually, each of these professionals brings a unique set of skills, knowledge, and experience to the table, working synergistically to unravel the mysteries of disease outbreaks and protect communities from the impact of infectious diseases. This collaborative network forms the backbone of outbreak investigations, underscoring the significance of a multidisciplinary approach in tackling public health emergencies (Arias, 2000).

9.4.1 EPIDEMIOLOGISTS

Epidemiologists are pivotal figures in the intricate landscape of outbreak investigations, employing specialized skills to detect, analyze, and mitigate disease outbreaks. Their multifaceted roles encompass a broad spectrum of activities, commencing with meticulous surveillance and data analysis to discern unusual disease patterns. Once a potential outbreak surfaces, these professionals meticulously trace its origins by conducting comprehensive interviews, analyzing data, and utilizing statistical methods to unveil the outbreak's source (Polonsky et al., 2019). This meticulous detective work extends to assessing risk factors associated with the outbreak, aiding in the formulation of effective intervention strategies. Often working hands-on in the field, epidemiologists collaborate closely with various healthcare professionals, conducting surveys, collecting samples, and inspecting affected areas (Rasmussen and Goodman, 2018). Their contributions extend beyond fieldwork as they employ mathematical models to forecast outbreak trajectories and communicate findings to diverse stakeholders in understandable terms. Their proactive stance involves recommending and implementing control measures, while continuous learning and adaptation are integral to refining response strategies for future outbreaks. These professionals are the linchpin in safeguarding public health during outbreaks, consistently contributing invaluable insights and actions for disease control and prevention (Polonsky et al., 2019).

9.4.2 PUBLIC HEALTH OFFICIALS AND AGENCIES

Public health officials and agencies constitute the backbone of outbreak investigations, spearheading efforts to detect, assess, and manage infectious disease outbreaks. These entities, often at local, national, and international levels, are responsible for an array of critical functions essential to understanding, controlling, and mitigating the impact of outbreaks on populations. At the forefront, these officials are tasked with disease surveillance and monitoring (Brownson and Petitti, 1998).

They continuously track and analyze health data from various sources, including hospitals, laboratories, and community health centers. Through robust surveillance systems, they identify patterns, clusters, or anomalies in disease occurrences, enabling early detection of potential outbreaks or unusual trends in illnesses. When an outbreak is identified or suspected, rapid response becomes paramount. Public health officials mobilize swiftly, activating emergency response teams and coordinating with healthcare providers, laboratories, and other relevant stakeholders. They establish incident command structures, deploy field teams for contact tracing, and implement control measures like quarantine or isolation protocols to limit disease spread. Effective communication is a cornerstone of outbreak management (World Health Organization, 2018). Public health officials liaise with multiple stakeholders, including government agencies, healthcare providers, the media, and the public. Clear and transparent communication disseminates accurate information about the outbreak, preventive measures, symptoms, and recommended actions, reducing misinformation and panic within communities. Collaboration is fundamental in outbreak investigations. These officials work closely with epidemiologists, laboratory scientists, healthcare workers, and international bodies such as the WHO (Cassola et al., 2022). This multidisciplinary approach fosters a comprehensive understanding of the outbreak's origin, transmission dynamics, and effective response strategies. Public health officials contribute to policy development and implementation. They assist in formulating guidelines for disease prevention, surveillance systems, and emergency response protocols. These policies are crucial in guiding local, regional, and national efforts in managing outbreaks efficiently (Ortiz and Clancy, 2003).

9.4.3 LABORATORY PERSONNEL

Laboratory personnel play an important role in outbreak investigations by providing essential support in identifying, confirming, and characterizing infectious agents responsible for outbreaks. These skilled professionals, including microbiologists, virologists, and other specialists, operate sophisticated diagnostic tools and techniques to detect and analyze pathogens quickly and accurately. Their expertise in culturing, isolating, and sequencing microbial specimens obtained from affected individuals or environments is fundamental in determining the causative agent behind an outbreak. In the initial stages of an outbreak investigation, laboratory personnel collaborate closely with epidemiologists and public health officials to establish diagnostic criteria and testing protocols. They develop and validate specific assays or tests to detect the suspected pathogen efficiently. These assays might include polymerase chain reaction (PCR), serological tests, or genomic sequencing, allowing for rapid and accurate identification of the infectious agent. Laboratory personnel maintain stringent quality control measures to ensure the reliability and accuracy of test results. They adhere to established laboratory safety protocols while handling potentially hazardous materials, preventing accidental exposure and ensuring the safety of themselves and their colleagues. Their work extends beyond identification; they also contribute to understanding the characteristics and behavior of the pathogen. Through genome sequencing and analysis, they help trace the origin of the outbreak, study the genetic diversity of the pathogen, and track its transmission patterns, providing valuable information crucial for containing and managing the outbreak effectively. The insights and data generated by laboratory personnel are instrumental in guiding public health responses, informing healthcare providers about appropriate treatment strategies, and supporting decision-making processes for implementing control measures and preventive interventions (Nelson and Williams, 2014).

9.4.4 MEDICAL PERSONNEL

Medical professionals, including doctors, nurses, and healthcare staff, are pivotal in outbreak investigations. They play a crucial role in recognizing unusual symptoms or patterns of illness that might signal an outbreak. Their expertise helps in diagnosing and managing affected individuals, collecting patient data, and providing clinical specimens for laboratory analysis (Morgantini et al., 2020). They collaborate closely with epidemiologists to define cases, monitor new instances, and refine treatment strategies. Additionally, they educate the public, implement preventive measures, and support public health interventions to contain the outbreak's spread. Their expertise is fundamental in guiding responses and offering crucial care during outbreaks.

9.4.5 COMMUNICATION SPECIALISTS

Communication specialists are integral in outbreak investigations, ensuring effective dissemination of critical information to the public, healthcare professionals, and relevant stakeholders (Longfield). They craft clear, accurate, and timely messages to educate communities about the outbreak, preventive measures, and available resources. Through various communication channels like media releases, social media, and public service announcements, they help to manage panic, reduce misinformation, and encourage appropriate actions. Their role in crisis communication aids in maintaining transparency, building trust, and facilitating coordinated responses among different sectors involved in managing the outbreak (Tumpey et al., 2018).

9.4.6 ENVIRONMENTAL HEALTH

Environmental health experts play a crucial role in outbreak investigations by assessing the environmental factors contributing to the spread of diseases. They examine water quality, sanitation systems, air quality, and other environmental elements that might impact public health. These specialists collaborate with epidemiologists and public health officials to identify potential sources of contamination or vectors transmitting diseases. Their assessments contribute to developing preventive strategies, improving sanitation practices, and implementing measures to mitigate environmental risks, thereby safeguarding communities from further outbreaks (Dancer, 2014).

9.4.7 DATA ANALYSTS AND STATISTICIANS

Data analysts and statisticians are integral in outbreak investigations, utilizing their expertise to process, analyze, and interpret large volumes of data collected during outbreaks. They employ statistical models, data visualization tools, and mathematical techniques to identify patterns, trends, and correlations within the outbreak data (Kulldorff et al., 2005). By crunching numbers and assessing epidemiological data, they help in understanding the disease transmission dynamics, identifying affected populations, and predicting the outbreak's trajectory. Their analyses provide valuable insights for public health officials and policymakers to make informed decisions and implement targeted interventions to control and prevent further spread of the disease (Haining, 2003).

9.4.8 LOCAL COMMUNITIES AND NONGOVERNMENTAL ORGANIZATIONS (NGOS)

Local communities and NGOs play a crucial role in outbreak investigations by providing on-the-ground support, community engagement, and essential resources. They serve as liaisons between health authorities and the affected populations, facilitating communication and promoting health education and preventive measures (Teljeur, 2002). These organizations often contribute by offering healthcare services, disseminating vital information about disease prevention, and mobilizing resources to assist affected communities. Their involvement ensures that the response strategies align with the cultural, social, and economic contexts of the affected areas, fostering trust and collaboration for effective outbreak control and community resilience (Abiddin et al., 2022).

9.4.9 RESEARCHERS AND ACADEMIA

Researchers and academia are instrumental in outbreak investigations, lending their expertise to understand the pathogens, transmission dynamics, and potential interventions. They conduct in-depth studies on the outbreak's origin, spread, and behavior of the infectious agent, aiding in the development of diagnostic tools, treatments, and vaccines. Academics contribute by sharing research findings, scientific insights, and evidence-based recommendations to inform public health responses and policies (Hebebci et al., 2020).

9.4.10 INTERNATIONAL PARTNERSHIPS

International partnerships are critical in outbreak investigations, fostering collaboration among countries, organizations, and experts worldwide. These partnerships enable shared resources, expertise, and data, facilitating a coordinated response to contain and manage outbreaks.

International organizations like the WHO play a central role, offering technical support, guidelines, and frameworks for effective outbreak control (World Health, 2021). Collaborative efforts also involve sharing information, best practices, and research findings across borders, aiding in early detection, rapid response, and the implementation of preventive measures. By pooling resources and expertise, these partnerships enhance surveillance, strengthen healthcare systems, and bolster preparedness for future outbreaks, emphasizing a collective global response to combat infectious diseases (Jackson et al., 2016).

9.5 PUBLIC HEALTH AGENCIES AND THEIR ROLES

9.5.1 CENTERS FOR DISEASE CONTROL AND PREVENTION

The Centers for Disease Control and Prevention (CDC) is a leading public health agency headquartered in Atlanta, USA. Established in 1946, the CDC focuses on disease prevention, health promotion, and outbreak control (Gould et al., 2013). It conducts disease surveillance, investigates outbreaks, and disseminates evidence-based information to the public and healthcare providers. Engaging in research and collaboration globally, the CDC is pivotal in shaping public health policies, addressing emerging health threats, and promoting overall health and well-being at both national and international levels (Benedict et al., 2017).

9.5.2 WHO

The WHO is a specialized agency of the United Nations, established in 1948, and headquartered in Geneva, Switzerland (Chisholm, 1950). It is responsible for international public health and leads global efforts to combat diseases, set health standards, and provide technical assistance and guidance to countries. The WHO plays a central role in coordinating responses to health emergencies, conducting research, establishing health policies, and advocating for universal healthcare access. With a focus on disease prevention, health promotion, and equitable healthcare systems, the WHO remains a critical authority in shaping global health agendas and ensuring health security worldwide (Howard-Jones, 1981).

9.5.3 NATIONAL HEALTH SERVICE (NHS)

The NHS in the United Kingdom is a cornerstone of public healthcare. It provides comprehensive medical services, from primary care to specialized treatments, to all UK residents based on need rather than the ability to pay. With its vast network of hospitals, clinics, general practitioners, and healthcare professionals, the NHS aims to ensure everyone receives timely, high-quality care. In the context of microbial outbreak investigations, the NHS is crucial in detecting and managing outbreaks, conducting diagnostic tests, treating infected individuals, and implementing preventive measures. Its expertise and integrated healthcare system play a vital role in controlling and mitigating the impact of infectious disease outbreaks within the UK population (Waterson, 2014).

9.5.4 PUBLIC HEALTH AGENCY OF CANADA (PHAC)

The PHAC is a federal agency dedicated to safeguarding the health of Canadians. It focuses on disease prevention, health promotion, and responding to public health emergencies, including infectious disease outbreaks. PHAC conducts surveillance, research, and risk assessments to identify health threats, including microbial outbreaks, and provides guidance for their control and management. Through collaboration with various partners, including provincial and territorial health authorities, PHAC works to limit the spread of infectious diseases, ensures effective communication to the public during outbreaks, and implements strategies to protect health and safety of people (Bielska et al., 2015).

9.6 STEPS IN OUTBREAK INVESTIGATION

9.6.1 RECOGNITION OF A POTENTIAL OUTBREAK

The term "outbreak detection" refers to bio-surveillance methods used to identify the presence of outbreaks. Clinicians might detect an outbreak by diagnosing a highly contagious disease like measles or a rare ailment such as anthrax. They treat a single case of such a disease as potential evidence of an outbreak until proven otherwise. For instance, the 2003 hepatitis A outbreak was spotted by vigilant clinicians, while bio-surveillance organizations might detect outbreaks by analyzing surveillance data. These organizations are increasingly automating the collection and analysis of surveillance data, allowing computers to potentially identify outbreaks (Friis and Sellers, 2020). Outbreak detection often stems from individual cases of highly contagious or unusual diseases. The 2004 SARS outbreak and the foot-and-mouth disease outbreak in the UK illustrate instances where clinicians, veterinarians, or pathologists encountered individuals with rare diseases. Measles, botulism, and tuberculosis outbreaks have been identified in similar ways. Another means of detection is through astute observation. Diseases like Lyme disease, hepatitis A, AIDS, cryptosporidium, SARS (2003), and Legionnaire's disease were discovered when an observant individual noticed clusters of illness and reported them to health departments. Bio-surveillance organizations use surveillance data analysis to detect outbreaks. Diseases like certain diarrheal illnesses occur sporadically, so a single case report might not be considered evidence of an outbreak. Examples include the New York State Department of Health detecting an *E. coli* outbreak after hospitalizations and the Volusia County Health Department discovering a *Shigella sonnei* outbreak due to common exposure at a park. Hospital infection control units also conduct surveillance of various infections, such as antibiotic-resistant organisms and *C. difficile*. Computers play an increasingly vital role in outbreak detection by analyzing different data sources to identify clusters of cases. These data sources can include cases reported by clinicians, aggregate health population data (like thermometer or diarrhea remedy sales), or clinical data repositories in hospitals for nosocomial infection surveillance. However, the precision of diagnostic data used by detection algorithms can vary significantly, ranging from precise data on notifiable diseases to broader indicators like the number of absentees from work or sales of diarrhea remedies (Raslan, 2011).

9.6.2 CASE DEFINITION AND IDENTIFICATION

A case definition is essential, outlining specific criteria based on time, place, biological, and clinical aspects. It should precisely detail inclusion and exclusion criteria and may categorize cases as definite, probable, or possible, also distinguishing between infection and colonization (Anderson, 2020). There are four common factors listed below:

1. Introduction of susceptible individuals to areas where the disease is prevalent.

2. Movement of susceptible humans or animals from endemic areas into populations where the disease is not common, or contamination of food, water, or other vehicles by uncommon infectious agents (e.g., anthrax spores in mailed letters as a deliberate act).
3. Emergence of pre-existing infections in low-endemic areas due to new social, behavioral, sexual, or cultural practices, like migration during conflicts or pilgrimages.
4. Alteration in host susceptibility or response due to natural or drug-induced immunosuppression (e.g., cancer treatment, malnutrition, or conditions like AIDS).

The investigation of outbreaks aims to curb further disease spread by fulfilling three primary objectives mentioned below (Williams, 1954):

1. Identification of the causative agent.
2. Determination of the infection source by assessing disease occurrence concerning people, place, and time, as well as computing specific attack rates.
3. Development of recommendations to prevent future transmissions.

The Infection Control Committee carries out several steps to investigate a suspected communicable disease outbreak. Steps are discussed in the following section:

1. Confirmation of the outbreak's existence by comparing current cases with baseline incidences, either local or from national surveillance systems.
2. Assessment for changes in case identification or diagnostics that might influence the reported outbreak.
3. Establishment of diagnoses for reported cases based on population risk factors, clinical data, and laboratory results.
4. Identification of additional cases retrospectively or concurrently through data collection from various sources like laboratory reports, medical records, and patient charts.
5. Characterization of cases involves assembling and organizing information based on time, place, and person. This includes calculating incidence and attack rates, stratifying these rates by different characteristics, and describing the population at risk accurately.
6. Formulation of a hypothesis regarding the outbreak's cause based on epidemiological and clinical data.

7. Testing the hypothesis, which may require a special study, typically conducted when facing severe problems or high morbidity/mortality issues.
8. Analyzing case investigation data to determine transmission sources and associated risk factors.
9. Refinement of the hypothesis based on the investigation's findings and conducting additional studies if necessary to further validate the findings.

9.6.2.1 EPIDEMIOLOGICAL STUDIES AND DATA COLLECTION

Identifying the origin of infection can be done in several ways:

1. Common source (single-point source): Arises from a singular origin, where a single person or vehicle serves as the primary reservoir or transmission route.
2. Propagated or ongoing source: Infections are transmitted between individuals, making it challenging to attribute cases to a single source.

Both common and propagated source (intermittent source): Occasional exposure to a common source lead to an epidemic curve marked by irregularly spaced peaks (Dicker et al., 2006).

When a health department suspects an outbreak, its staff initiates a preliminary inquiry to verify available information and assess the severity and scope of the event. By reviewing medical records, conducting interviews, and considering factors like illness severity, potential spread, and available resources, they decide if a field investigation is necessary. Once the investigation starts, a team or individual investigator interviews affected individuals, examines various data sources, and may issue alerts to healthcare providers or the public. They collect specimens, aiming to identify the outbreak's cause, sources, and affected individuals. While initial investigations may reveal some details, ongoing efforts involve analytical techniques to uncover more information. Investigators continuously refine hypotheses, gather additional data, and apply control measures based on likely causes. Outbreak investigations are intensive, involving visits to multiple locations, and technology aids in managing and organizing the amassed data, supporting efforts of investigators (Dato et al., 2004).

9.7 LABORATORY TECHNIQUES IN OUTBREAK INVESTIGATION

9.7.1 ISOLATION AND IDENTIFICATION OF PATHOGENS

Sample collection serves as the cornerstone in diagnosing infections and uncovering the root causes of diseases. It involves procuring diverse biological specimens from individuals or environments to pinpoint potential pathogens responsible for illnesses or contaminations. These samples fall into two broad categories: clinical and environmental. Clinical samples encompass blood, urine, sputum, stool, and tissue, obtained directly from patients suspected of harboring infections. They provide crucial insights into various infections affecting different bodily systems. On the other hand, environmental samples, sourced from surfaces, water, air, or food, help assess potential contamination sources or outbreak origins. Collecting these samples demands aseptic techniques, proper containers, and sometimes preservation methods to maintain sample integrity. Timing, site selection, and adherence to ethical guidelines pose challenges. Yet, the collected samples serve a pivotal role in accurate diagnosis, understanding disease patterns, and guiding effective treatment strategies, forming the bedrock of informed healthcare decisions and public health measures (Harris et al., 2003).

9.7.2 ANTIMICROBIAL SUSCEPTIBILITY TESTING (AST)

AST serves as a crucial tool in clinical microbiology labs, aiding in the selection of appropriate antibiotics for bacterial infections. This testing provides essential insights into the general antimicrobial susceptibility patterns, which aids medical practitioners in determining effective therapy of antimicrobials (Holmes et al., 2016). For example, if a particular pathogen exhibits a resistance rate above 20%, caution is warranted against employing that antibiotic as the primary treatment. Additionally, AST assists in monitoring resistant pathogens like Methicillin-resistant *S. aureus* (MRSA), Vancomycin-resistant *Enterococci* (VRE), and Extended-Spectrum Beta-Lactamase (ESBL), among others, contributing to infection prevention measures. The monitoring of resistance to antimicrobials relies on continuous data of susceptibility, contributing to systems like the Global Antimicrobial Resistance and Use Surveillance System and the European Antimicrobial Resistance Surveillance Network (Holmes et al., 2016). The currently used methods for AST are discussed in the following section.

9.7.2.1 BROTH AND AGAR DILUTION METHODS

In spite of novel techniques that have emerged for assessing bacterial susceptibility to antimicrobial agents, traditional methods remain widely utilized. Broth and agar dilution techniques, along with disc diffusion tests, persist as prevalent approaches. Among these, broth macro- and micro-dilution, and agar dilution methods, are regarded as primary reference methods. These techniques help determine the minimum inhibitory concentrations (MICs) of antibiotics that halts microorganism growth (Mirzaei et al., 2020). MIC values ascertain the pathogen's susceptibility category to a specific antibiotic and aid in ambiguous result cases or when clinical breakpoints for disc diffusion are absent. Unlike qualitative methods, MIC values gauge the degree of susceptibility or resistance to antibiotics. Broth dilution methods additionally provide the MBC also known as Minimum bacterial concentration, which is responsible for killing 99.9% bacteria (Vasilijević et al., 2019). The macro dilution method involves serial dilution of antimicrobials in test tubes with bacterial suspension, while the time-kill methodology tracks the effect of varied antimicrobial concentrations on bacterial death rate. The broth microdilution (BMD) method, performed in microtiter plates, allows multiple antimicrobial tests concurrently and uses a color indicator to monitor bacterial activity. There are commercially available systems like MBD Sensititre and ComASP Colistin, offering ease and efficiency in BMD testing. In contrast, the agar dilution method applies different antibiotic concentrations to a nonselective medium before bacterial inoculation, to determine MIC by observing growth. This method enables concurrent analysis of a variety of strains and species of bacteria (Tebano et al., 2020).

9.7.2.2 ANTIMICROBIAL GRADIENT METHOD

The antimicrobial gradient method, blending features of disk diffusion (DD) and dilution techniques, efficiently determines MICs, while maintaining simplicity. This approach relies on an antibiotic's diffusion through agar with a continuous gradient, allowing for MIC determination in a user-friendly manner. Studies show high agreement between gradient tests and the gold standard BMD method for some antibiotics, like ceftazidime–avibactam and ceftolozane–tazobactam (Ferro et al., 2015). However, certain antibiotics, notably colistin and tigecycline, exhibit controversial outcomes due to agar-related factors affecting diffusion, making BMD the preferable method for their MIC determination. Commercially strip tests such as MIC Test Strip, Etest, M.I.C. Evaluator, and Ezy MIC Strip are available for analyzing the microbial susceptibility of microbes against chemotherapeutic agents. These strips, impregnated with antibiotics, are placed on inoculated agar to determine MIC by measuring the intersection of inhibition zones with the strip (Mirajkar and Gebhart, 2016). Automated systems like the ADAGIO Automated System can read the results. Variants of gradient tests exist for detecting various antimicrobial resistance (AMR) phenotypes, like ESBL production in enterobacteria and metallo-beta-lactamase-producing bacteria. These tests offer simplicity, flexibility, and ease of use, making them suitable for screening emerging resistance patterns in clinically relevant bacteria, despite their relatively higher cost per strip compared to disks. However, the incubation period required (16–24 hours) may be a drawback compared to more rapid automated systems for MIC determination (Matuschek et al., 2023).

9.7.2.3 DD TEST

The DD test, conceived in the 1940s, stands as the most commonly employed routine method for AST in clinical microbiological laboratories. This technique, continually standardized and adapted to diverse bacteria and antibiotics, involves placing disks loaded with antibiotic on agar which has been injected previously with the suspension of bacteria. As the outward diffusion of antibiotic is observed, they form inhibition zones, which are measured after incubation for 24 h at 35±1°C (Humphries et al., 2018). The interpretation of results follows clinical breakpoints, aiding in susceptibility categorization. Although widely used due to its affordability, flexibility in antibiotic selection, and applicability across various bacterial species, the DD method has limitations. It cannot determine the MIC and might lead to delayed results. This delay can impact critical patient care, emphasizing the need for faster methods. Attempts to expedite this method have led to automation, like the WASPLab and BD Kiestra systems, reducing turnaround times significantly. Additionally, the introduction of Rapid AST (RAST) from positive blood culture bottles, following EUCAST guidelines, provides a faster alternative.

Combining MALDI–TOF MS for bacterial identification and RAST expedites reporting AST results within 24 h, improving turnaround time compared to conventional culturing. Quality control measures are crucial to ensure the accuracy of DD, as it remain valuable for detecting specific resistance phenotypes and screening susceptibility to various antibiotics or resistance patterns. Overall, despite its limitations, the DD method is expected to persist as a primary AST technique due to its versatility and applicability in diverse scenarios (Gajic et al., 2022).

9.7.2.4 IDENTIFICATION OF ANTIBIOTIC-RESISTANT BACTERIA WITH CHROMOGENIC AGAR MEDIA

Numerous chromogenic media have emerged to identify clinically significant resistant pathogens like MRSA, VRE, ESBL, and colistin-resistant Gram-negative bacteria. These specialized media aim to expedite the identification of resistant microorganisms by leveraging specific enzyme systems that metabolize substrates, triggering a distinct color change in the medium known as a chromogen (Yusof et al., 2008). The resultant-colored colonies allow for visual identification of targeted pathogens. The utilization of these chromogenic agar is economic and less time consuming. Primarily used for screening patients harboring various pathogens, these media play a crucial role in infection prevention and control within healthcare settings (Le Page et al., 2016). However, the major concern regarding the use of these media is the variation in their sensitivity and specificity which has been found to be varied depending upon the manufacturer and the detected microorganism, which often necessitates the confirmation of identification of resistant bacteria. Given their broad applicability, ongoing efforts persist in developing new chromogenic media for enhanced detection capabilities (Idelevich et al., 2017).

9.7.2.5 DETECTING ANTIMICROBIAL-RESISTANT BACTERIA USING COLORIMETRIC TESTS

Colorimetric tests are phenotypic methods designed for detecting AMR. They rely on bacterial enzymes that alter test components, leading to pH changes and the appearance of chromogenic substances (Åhman et al., 2019). In these tests, bacterial or lysed bacterial suspensions are combined with a detection solution containing antibiotics and pH-sensitive dyes. Over a short incubation, typically a few hours, bacterial growth or enzyme activity alters the solution's pH and color. This color change is indicative of antibiotic-resistant bacteria and can be visually observed. These tests are known for their speed, simplicity, and high sensitivity. One prominent example is the Carba NP test by bioMérieux, which swiftly identifies carbapenemase-producing bacteria within 30 minutes to 2 hours, providing efficient control over these resistant strains (Ledeboer et al., 2007).

9.7.3 MOLECULAR TYPING AND FINGERPRINTING METHODS

Typing is the process of identifying various organisms within a species. Traditional methods like serotype, biotype, and antibiogram based on phenotype have been the norm for years. However, molecular techniques examining isolates at a molecular level have transformed our ability to distinguish bacterial types. Selecting the right molecular typing method depends on the specific problem to solve, epidemiological context, time, and geographical scale of use. Pathogens within a species can be diverse, demanding excellent typeability from typing techniques to cover all studied isolates (Van Belkum et al., 2007). During outbreaks, the typing method needs to differentiate all unrelated isolates and even closely related ones to track person-to-person strain transmission, facilitating preventive strategies. It should be rapid, cost-effective, reproducible, easily interpretable, and implementable for continuous surveillance, ensuring stable results over time for efficient infection control measures (Arbeit et al., 1990). An ideal typing method for international use should generate portable data, accessible through open-source databases, using standardized nomenclature and applicable across various bacterial species. Robust quality checks are crucial to ensure high-quality typing data, and the availability of software aids in automated quality control, pattern assignment, clustering of isolates, outbreak detection, and data management. Although numerous molecular methods exist for bacterial isolate characterization, no single method suits all investigations. Typing methods predominantly impacts public health or gains increasing interest in clinical usage, delineating their advantages and disadvantages in bacterial disease outbreak investigations and active surveillance networks (Arbeit et al., 1990).

9.7.3.1 PFGE

PFGE has long been regarded as a leading molecular typing technique for various clinically significant bacteria. Its significant influence in the field is evident from over 2700 PubMed publications retrieved using "PFGE and typing" as search terms (Gordillo et al., 1993). Adopted as an epidemiological tool for most bacterial species in the 1990s, PFGE remains a primary approach for characterizing bacterial isolates during outbreaks. A focused search on PubMed between January 2011 and the present day revealed 183 hits for "PFGE and outbreak," surpassing other typing methods in combination with the term "outbreak" (Prevost et al., 1991). PFGE has been pivotal in analyzing center-to-center transmission events and has shown success in large-scale epidemiological investigations due to its exceptional discriminatory power and high epidemiological concordance. It is a relatively cost-effective method with excellent typeability and reproducibility within laboratories. Over the past decade, standardized protocols and inter-laboratory comparisons through initiatives like PulseNet and Harmony have further bolstered its reliability. International fingerprinting databases have facilitated rapid identification of emerging clones and monitoring of pathogenic bacterial strains across regions. The PFGE technique involves cleaving highly purified genomic DNA with a restriction endonuclease, separating resulting large restriction fragments through "pulsed-field" electrophoresis on an agarose gel, forming a distinct PFGE pattern (Tenover et al., 1995). It typically resolves DNA fragments ranging from approximately 30 kb to over 1 Mb for most bacteria, simplifying result analysis due to the limited number of bands produced. PFGE largely addresses a significant portion (>90%) of the investigated genome, detecting changes resulting from insertions, deletions, or large recombination events within genomic DNA (Tosh et al., 2011). However, despite its widespread use and advantages, PFGE has drawbacks. It demands technical expertise, is time-consuming, and labor-intensive. Additionally, it may struggle to differentiate bands of nearly identical size and lacks the objectivity, continuous quality control, and data portability offered by sequence-based methods (Yu et al., 2012).

9.7.3.2 AMPLIFIED FRAGMENT LENGTH POLYMORPHISM (AFLP)

The AFLP technique involves cutting genomic DNA using two restriction enzymes and attaching double-stranded adaptors to one end of the resulting restriction fragments. Through PCR using specific primers, the fragments joined with the adaptor are selectively amplified under stringent conditions (Lanini et al., 2011). Typically, AFLP allows the simultaneous amplification of a large number of restriction fragments, usually between 50 and 100, and often employs fluorescent dye-labeled PCR primers to enable fragment detection post-separation by size on an automated DNA sequences. A computer-assisted analysis of these banding patterns derived from AFLP facilitates the determination of genetic relatedness among analyzed bacterial isolates. Studies have indicated that AFLP exhibits discriminatory power comparable to PFGE. Additionally, AFLP is reproducible, automatable, and yields portable results. However, its drawbacks include being labor-intensive, requiring approximately 3 days for analysis, and the associated costs with DNA extraction kits, enzymes, fluorescence detection systems, and adaptors (Cavanagh et al., 2012).

9.7.3.3 RANDOM AMPLIFICATION OF POLYMORPHIC DNA

Random Amplification of Polymorphic DNA (RAPD) and Arbitrarily Primed PCR (AP-PCR) are techniques used in molecular biology for the identification and typing of bacterial strains. RAPD works by amplifying various DNA fragments simultaneously using short, arbitrary sequences as primers, targeting unspecified genomic sequences (Li et al., 2009). The amplification occurs at a lower annealing temperature, allowing the hybridization of multiple mismatched sequences. Generated amplicons cover the sequence between primer binding sites, unique to each bacterial strain. Despite being less discriminatory than PFGE, RAPD is commonly employed for outbreak typing due to its simplicity, low cost, and rapidity. However, its drawbacks include low intra-laboratory reproducibility due to the usage of very low annealing temperatures, and the lack of inter-laboratory reproducibility sensitive to differences in reagents, protocols, and machinery (Sabat et al., 2006). AP-PCR, often referred to as RAPD, is a variant of RAPD methodology involving certain technical differences. In AP-PCR, the amplification is divided into three parts, each with different stringencies and concentrations of components. Higher primer concentrations are used in initial PCR cycles, and primers of variable length designed for different purposes are utilized. AP-PCR shares both advantages and limitations with RAPD as it faces similar issues with reproducibility and sensitivity to protocol and equipment variations (Healy et al., 2005).

9.7.3.4 REPETITIVE-ELEMENT PCR (REP-PCR)

The rep-PCR technique utilizes genomic fingerprint patterns to classify bacterial isolates. It employs primers targeting noncoding intergenic repetitive sequences in the genome, amplifying the DNA between these elements. The resulting amplicons, analyzed via electrophoresis, provide banding patterns for comparison, determining genetic relatedness among bacterial strains (Babouee et al., 2011). Various repeat sequences like ERIC, REP, and BOX have been utilized successfully in rep-PCR typing, offering a relatively quick and cost-effective approach for bacterial differentiation. However, traditional rep-PCR combined with gel electrophoresis often lacks reproducibility due to reagent and system variability (Overdevest et al., 2011). The DiversiLab system, a semiautomated method based on rep-PCR, enhances resolution and reproducibility using microfluidic capillary electrophoresis. This system offers rapid and reproducible typing results for a wide range of microorganisms, particularly useful for outbreak detection in hospital settings. However, studies have shown limitations in typing certain bacterial species, such as *Pseudomonas aeruginosa*, *Enterococcus faecium*, and MRSA. Despite its utility, concerns remain about its limitations in interlaboratory reproducibility and data security, housed on a manufacturer server. Further evaluations are necessary to assess its broader usefulness in regional and national bacterial genotype surveillance (Köser et al., 2012).

9.7.3.5 VARIABLE-NUMBER TANDEM REPEAT (VNTR)

VNTR typing method utilizes repeated DNA sequences in bacterial genomes to classify isolates. VNTR loci are regions where the number of repeats varies among isolates. Multilocus VNTR Analysis (MLVA) examines these repeats at different loci, employing PCR to amplify specific VNTR regions. While traditional agarose gel electrophoresis can be used, microfluidic chip-based analysis offers enhanced resolution and reproducibility. Capillary electrophoresis on DNA sequencers further refines the typing, accurately determining repeat numbers per locus and generating an allelic profile. However, VNTR typing requires specific primers for each targeted species and may lack complete reproducibility without sequencing the amplicons. Despite its potential, MLVA methods need further validation for use in clinical surveillance networks (Francois et al., 2005).

9.7.3.6 SINGLE LOCUS SEQUENCE TYPING (SLST)

SLST examines sequence variations in a single target gene to establish relationships among bacterial isolates. This method, akin to multilocus sequence typing (MLST), focuses on one specific gene for analysis. For instance, in group A *Streptococcus* (GAS), the emm gene, responsible for the M-protein on the bacterial surface, is commonly sequenced to distinguish isolates. The emm-typing technique has replaced traditional serological methods, providing a gold standard for GAS molecular typing, revealing over 200 emm types (Grundmann et al., 2010). However, to achieve complete discrimination among GAS clones, emm-typing is often used alongside other methods like PFGE or MLST. Similarly, in *Campylobacter*, sequencing the short variable region of the flaB gene offers rapid, reproducible, and discriminatory insights into the bacteria's epidemiology. While PFGE remains highly discriminating, flaB sequence-typing, especially when combined with MLST, effectively differentiates closely related or outbreak-related isolates. The prevalence of publications on "emm" or "flaB" typing in PubMed, totaling 238 hits, underlines the significance of these methods for GAS and *Campylobacter* typing (Dingle et al., 2001).

9.7.3.7 MULTILOCUS SEQUENCE TYPING

Multilocus Sequence Typing (MLST), a method based on phenotypic multilocus enzyme electrophoresis principles, was developed to overcome the limitations of traditional typing approaches. This technique sequences internal segments of seven housekeeping genes, assigning unique numbers (alleles) to their sequences and determining a sequence type (ST) based on the combination of these alleles. MLST gained popularity for global epidemiological studies and pathogen evolution analysis, producing unambiguous and reproducible data (Enright and Spratt, 1999). Central databases like PubMLST and MLST.net store allele sequences and ST profiles, offering tools to assess genetic relatedness between bacterial strains within a species. Despite its standardized nomenclature, easy accessibility via the Internet, and reliable results, MLST is costly, labor-intensive, and may lack discrimination for some outbreaks. To enhance discrimination, variants like NG-MAST (*Neisseria gonorrhoeae* multiantigen sequence typing) for gonorrhoeae or MLST schemes incorporating virulence genes (MVLST) have been developed. MVLST might offer higher discrimination, but more research and validation are necessary for its widespread application in epidemiological typing (Larsen et al., 2012).

9.7.3.8 WHOLE GENOME SEQUENCING (WGS)

NGS revolutionized genetic investigations by offering a cost-effective method to detect genome-wide variations. It is distinguished from first-generation sequencing (like the Sanger method) by its ability to produce millions of short reads at a lower cost (Men et al., 2008). NGS technology generates sequence data that can be assembled either by overlapping regions or compared to existing reference genomes. WGS holds promise for epidemiological studies and clinical use, enabling accurate identification of bacterial isolates. However, challenges persist in swiftly processing and interpreting the vast data produced by NGS, particularly due to short read lengths leading to gaps in genome assembly, mainly caused by repeated sequences (Balloux et al., 2018).

9.8 RISK ASSESSMENT AND CONTROL MEASURES

9.8.1 ASSESSING THE SCOPE AND SEVERITY OF AN OUTBREAK

During microbial outbreak investigations, risk assessment plays a pivotal role. Initially, hazard identification involves pinpointing the pathogen responsible and understanding its transmission dynamics. This leads to an evaluation of the risks, considering the severity of the outbreak, its spread, and the potential impact on the population. Subsequently, control measures are determined based on this assessment. Strategies such as isolating infected individuals, improving hygiene, vaccination, and treatment are formulated (Havelaar et al., 2008). Continuous monitoring and review of these measures occur throughout the investigation to adapt to the evolving situation effectively. Control measures in outbreak management encompass a multifaceted approach. Isolation and quarantine measures aim to prevent further transmission by separating infected individuals and restricting the movement of exposed individuals. Emphasis on hygiene practices, sanitation, and disinfection helps curb the spread of the pathogen. Vaccination and medical care are crucial to minimize the severity and impact of the outbreak. Public education about the outbreak and necessary preventive measures enhances community cooperation. Environmental control to eliminate contamination sources, surveillance, contact tracing, and effective communication among health authorities and the public are pivotal in containing the outbreak swiftly and effectively (Aljeldah, 2022). Each measure contributes as a piece of a comprehensive strategy, aimed at mitigating risks and controlling the outbreak's impact on public health.

9.8.2 IMPLEMENTING CONTAINMENT STRATEGIES

During a microbial outbreak, implementing effective containment strategies is pivotal to curtail further spread and safeguard public health. These strategies encompass a multifaceted approach, starting with rapid isolation and quarantine measures for confirmed cases and individuals in close contact. Rigorous contact tracing aids in identifying potential spreaders, allowing for their isolation or quarantine to prevent transmission. Reinforcing stringent hygiene practices, promoting public health communication, and enforcing healthcare protocols with proper personal protective equipment usage and infection control measures in medical facilities are critical elements (Khandia et al., 2022). Additionally, travel restrictions, vaccination campaigns, community engagement, continuous surveillance, and adaptive response mechanisms form integral parts of containment. Successful execution of these measures requires collaboration among diverse stakeholders and adaptive strategies tailored to the evolving nature of the outbreak. Such a comprehensive and coordinated approach is essential to effectively contain and manage microbial outbreaks while minimizing their impact on public health (Tambolkar et al., 2022).

9.8.3 PUBLIC COMMUNICATION AND EDUCATION

Public communication and education during a microbial outbreak play a pivotal role in disseminating accurate information, mitigating panic, and fostering cooperation among the populace. Clear, transparent, and timely communication through various channels is vital to keep the public informed about the outbreak's nature, risks, preventive measures, and government interventions (Anwar et al., 2020). Educating the community about proper hygiene practices, symptom recognition, and the importance of seeking medical attention, when necessary, helps in early detection and containment. Providing reliable information through press releases, social media, dedicated hotlines, and public health campaigns aids in dispelling myths, reducing misinformation, and instilling confidence in public health measures. Moreover, engaging community leaders, healthcare professionals, and influencers to endorse and disseminate accurate information fosters trust and compliance with recommended protocols. Ultimately, effective public communication and education are instrumental in garnering public support, encouraging cooperation, and ensuring community adherence to containment measures, thus contributing significantly to managing and controlling microbial outbreaks (Dry and Leach, 2010).

9.9 CASE STUDIES IN MICROBIAL OUTBREAKS

Investigation of microbial outbreaks can help in preventing their recurrence in the future. This helps in monitoring and taking preventive measures to control the outbreak thereby minimizing its spread across the globe. Table 9.1 highlights the recent outbreaks, its impact globally and the causative agent.

TABLE 9.1 Case Studies in Microbial Outbreaks

Outbreak	Year	Country	Pathogen	Findings	References
Ebola Virus Outbreak	2014–2016	Multiple	Ebola virus	Swift global response and cooperation are vital, emphasizing the need for robust healthcare systems in affected areas.	Magassouba et al. (2020)
Salmonella Outbreak in the US	2008	United States	Salmonella	Food supply chain vulnerabilities require stringent regulations for safer food handling and distribution.	Barton Behravesh et al. (2011)
SARS Outbreak	2002–2003	Multiple	SARS-CoV	Rapid transmission highlights the necessity for early detection and global cooperation in implementing quarantine measures.	Cherry (2004)
Legionnaires' Disease Outbreak (Philadelphia)	1976	United States	*Legionella pneumophila*	Monitoring water systems in public buildings is crucial to prevent similar disease outbreaks, following the discovery of Legionella bacteria.	Tsai et al. (1979)

9.10 SURVEILLANCE AND MONITORING SYSTEMS

Surveillance and monitoring systems serve as essential pillars in managing microbial outbreaks by systematically collecting, analyzing, and interpreting health-related data. These systems encompass various facets, including the comprehensive collection of information from healthcare facilities, laboratories, and public health agencies. Through sophisticated analysis techniques, they evaluate this data to detect patterns, unusual trends, or clusters of cases that might signify an outbreak. Rapid reporting and effective communication of findings to relevant authorities, healthcare professionals, and the public are crucial in triggering necessary responses and preventive measures (Agustin et al., 2022). Utilizing early warning systems and statistical models, these systems aim to promptly identify potential outbreaks, facilitating timely intervention measures such as quarantine or vaccination campaigns. International collaboration and coordination are also pivotal, enabling the exchange of information across borders and fostering a unified response to global health threats. Overall, surveillance and monitoring systems play a pivotal role in early detection, prompt response, and effective management of microbial outbreaks (Choi, 2012).

9.11 CHALLENGES AND FUTURE DIRECTIONS

Addressing the challenges and charting future directions in managing microbial outbreaks is pivotal for global health security. The challenges encompass rapid pathogen evolution, global dissemination, AMR, data standardization, resource allocation, and effective public communication. Looking ahead, advancements in surveillance technologies, vaccine development, international collaboration, One Health strategies, policy reforms, and capacity building stand as pivotal future directions. Embracing artificial intelligence, genomics, and big data analytics, prioritizing research for vaccines, fostering global partnerships, integrating One Health approaches, implementing agile policies, and fortifying healthcare infrastructure are paramount. By navigating these challenges and committing to these directions, the global community can bolster preparedness and response capacities to effectively confront and contain microbial outbreaks. Microbial surveillance and outbreak investigation are critical pillars in safeguarding public health. They empower us to detect, contain, and mitigate the impact of infectious diseases on communities. Through robust surveillance systems, early detection becomes possible, allowing for prompt response measures. Utilizing diverse molecular typing techniques enhances our understanding of pathogen transmission, aiding in effective outbreak control. Challenges persist, from the rapid spread of emerging diseases to technological limitations in data analysis. However, ongoing advancements in technology, coupled with global collaboration and continuous improvement in healthcare systems, offer hope for better preparedness and response in the face of future microbial threats. Emphasizing education, preparedness, and international cooperation will be pivotal in enhancing our ability to combat infectious diseases, ensuring a safer and healthier world.

KEYWORDS

- **epidemiology**
- **pathogen identification**
- **genomic sequencing**
- **public health agencies**
- **zoonotic diseases**
- **containment strategies**
- **surveillance networks**
- **outbreak management**
- **antimicrobial resistance**
- **risk assessment**

REFERENCES

Abiddin, N. Z., Ibrahim, I., Abdul Aziz, S. A. (2022). Non-governmental organisations (NGOs) and their part towards sustainable community development. *Sustainability*, *14*(8), 4386.

Agustin, N. D., Aritonang, S., Pane, M. (2022). Analysis of the early warning alert and response system to anticipate an outbreak in Indonesia. *Journal of Advanced Research in Defense and Security Studies*, *1*(1), 53–64.

Åhman, J., Matuschek, E., Kahlmeter, G. (2019). The quality of antimicrobial discs from nine manufacturers—EUCAST evaluations in 2014 and 2017. *Clinical Microbiology and Infection*, *25*(3), 346–352.

Aljeldah, M. M. (2022). Antimicrobial resistance and its spread is a global threat. *Antibiotics*, *11*(8), 1082.

Anderson, R. P. (2020). *Outbreak: Cases in Real-world Microbiology*. John Wiley & Sons.

Anwar, A., Malik, M., Raees, V., Anwar, A. (2020). Role of mass media and public health communications in the COVID-19 pandemic. *Cureus*, *12*(9), e10453.

Arbeit, R. D., Arthur, M., Dunn, R., Kim, C., Selander, R. K., Goldstein, R. (1990). Resolution of recent evolutionary divergence among *Escherichia coli* from related lineages: The application of pulsed field electrophoresis to molecular epidemiology. *Journal of Infectious Diseases*, *161*(2), 230–235.

Arias, K. M. (2000). *Quick Reference to Outbreak Investigation and Control in Health Care Facilities*. Jones & Bartlett Learning.

Babouee, B., Frei, R., Schultheiss, E., Widmer, A. F., Goldenberger, D. (2011). Comparison of the DiversiLab repetitive element PCR system with spa typing and pulsed-field gel

electrophoresis for clonal characterization of methicillin-resistant *Staphylococcus aureus*. *Journal of Clinical Microbiology*, *49*(4), 1549–1555.
Baker, B., Wisely, S. (2023). Facts about wildlife diseases: Highly pathogenic avian influenza (HPAI): WEC457/UW502, 2/2023. *EDIS*, *2023*(1).
Baker, M. G., Fidler, D. P. (2006). Global public health surveillance under new international health regulations. *Emerging Infectious Diseases*, *12*(7), 1058.
Balloux, F., Brynildsrud, O. B., Van Dorp, L., Shaw, L. P., Chen, H., Harris, K. A., Wang, H., Eldholm, V. (2018). From theory to practice: Translating whole-genome sequencing (WGS) into the clinic. *Trends in Microbiology*, *26*(12), 1035–1048.
Barton Behravesh, C., Mody, R. K., Jungk, J., Gaul, L., Redd, J. T., Chen, S., et al. (2011). 2008 Outbreak of Salmonella Saintpaul infections associated with raw produce. *New England Journal of Medicine*, *364*(10), 918–927.
Bell, B. P. (2016). Overview, control strategies, and lessons learned in the CDC response to the 2014–2016 Ebola epidemic. *MMWR Supplements*, *65*.
Benedict, K. M., Reses, H., Vigar, M., Roth, D. M., Roberts, V. A., Mattioli, M., et al. (2017). Surveillance for waterborne disease outbreaks associated with drinking water—United States, 2013–2014. *Morbidity and Mortality Weekly Report*, *66*(44), 1216.
Bielska, I. A., Drobot, A. C., Moir, M., Nartowski, R. O., Lee, R., Lukewich, J., Lukewich, M. K. (2015). Public health in Canada: An overview. Zeszyty Naukowe Ochrony Zdrowia. *Zdrowie Publiczne i Zarzadzanie*, *13*(2), 165.
Brownson, R. C., Petitti, D. B. (1998). *Applied Epidemiology: Theory to Practice*. Oxford University Press: USA.
Buttner, M. P., Cruz, P., Stetzenbach, L. D., Cronin, T. (2007). Evaluation of two surface sampling methods for detection of *Erwinia herbicola* on a variety of materials by culture and quantitative PCR. *Applied and Environmental Microbiology*, *73*(11), 3505–3510.
Cassola, A., Fafard, P., Nagi, R., Hoffman, S. J. (2022). Tensions and opportunities in the roles of senior public health officials in Canada: A qualitative study. *Health Policy*, *126*(10), 988–995.
Cavanagh, J. P., Klingenberg, C., Hanssen, A.-M., Fredheim, E. A., Francois, P., Schrenzel, J., et al. (2012). Core genome conservation of *Staphylococcus haemolyticus* limits sequence based population structure analysis. *Journal of Microbiological Methods*, *89*(3), 159–166.
Charalambous, M., Mitosis, K., Talias, M. A. (2018). Strategic application of the hazard analysis and critical control point system for new export markets for Cyprus' small and medium food enterprises during the 2012 economic crisis. *International Journal of Export Marketing*, *2*(1), 47–62.
Cherry, J. D. (2004). The chronology of the 2002–2003 SARS mini pandemic. *Paediatric Respiratory Reviews*, *5*(4), 262–269.
Chinn, R. Y. W., Sehulster, L. (2003). *Guidelines for Environmental Infection Control in Health-care Facilities*. Recommendations of CDC and Healthcare Infection Control Practices Advisory Committee (HICPAC).
Chisholm, B. (1950). The World Health Organization. *British Medical Journal*, *1*(4661), 1021.
Choi, B. C. K. (2012). The past, present, and future of public health surveillance. *Scientifica*, *2012*.

Craun, G. F. (1990). *Methods for the Investigation and Prevention of Waterborne Disease Outbreaks*: Health Effects Research Laboratory, US Environmental Protection Agency.

Dancer, S. J. (2004). How do we assess hospital cleaning? A proposal for microbiological standards for surface hygiene in hospitals. *Journal of Hospital Infection, 56*(1), 10–15.

Dancer, S. J. (2014). Controlling hospital-acquired infection: Focus on the role of the environment and new technologies for decontamination. *Clinical Microbiology Reviews, 27*(4), 665–690.

Dato, V., Wagner, M. M., Fapohunda, A. (2004). How outbreaks of infectious disease are detected: A review of surveillance systems and outbreaks. *Public Health Reports, 119*(5), 464–471.

Di Bari, C., Venkateswaran, N., Fastl, C., Gabriël, S., Grace, D., Havelaar, A. H., et al. (2023). The global burden of neglected zoonotic diseases: Current state of evidence. *One Health, 17*, 100595.

Dicker, R. C., Coronado, F., Koo, D., Parrish, R. G. (2006). Principles of epidemiology in public health practice; an introduction to applied epidemiology and biostatistics.

Dingle, K. E., Colles, F. M., Wareing, D. R. A., Ure, R., Fox, A. J., Bolton, F. E., et al. (2001). Multilocus sequence typing system for *Campylobacter jejuni*. *Journal of Clinical Microbiology, 39*(1), 14–23.

Downey, A. S., Da Silva, S. M., Olson, N. D., Filliben, J. J., Morrow, J. B. (2012). Impact of processing method on recovery of bacteria from wipes used in biological surface sampling. *Applied and Environmental Microbiology, 78*(16), 5872–5881.

Dry, S., Leach, M. (2010). *Epidemics: Science, Governance and Social Justice*. Routledge.

Enright, M. C., Spratt, B. G. (1999). Multilocus sequence typing. *Trends in Microbiology, 7*(12), 482–487.

Fenton, A., Pedersen, A. B. (2005). Community epidemiology framework for classifying disease threats. *Emerging Infectious Diseases, 11*(12), 1815.

Ferro, B. E., van Ingen, J., Wattenberg, M., van Soolingen, D., Mouton, J. W. (2015). Time–kill kinetics of antibiotics active against rapidly growing mycobacteria. *Journal of Antimicrobial Chemotherapy, 70*(3), 811–817.

Francois, P., Huyghe, A., Charbonnier, Y., Bento, M., Herzig, S., Topolski, I., et al. (2005). Use of an automated multiple-locus, variable-number tandem repeat-based method for rapid and high-throughput genotyping of *Staphylococcus aureus* isolates. *Journal of Clinical Microbiology, 43*(7), 3346–3355.

Friis, R. H., Sellers, T. (2020). *Epidemiology for Public Health Practice*. Jones & Bartlett Learning.

Frumkin, H. (2016). *Environmental Health: From Global to Local*. John Wiley & Sons.

Gajic, I., Kabic, J., Kekic, D., Jovicevic, M., Milenkovic, M., Mitic Culafic, D., Opavski, N. (2022). Antimicrobial susceptibility testing: A comprehensive review of currently used methods. *Antibiotics, 11*(4), 427.

Getchell-White, S. I., Donowitz, L. G., Groschel, D. H. M. (1989). The inanimate environment of an intensive care unit as a potential source of nosocomial bacteria: Evidence for long survival of *Acinetobacter calcoaceticus*. *Infection Control and Hospital Epidemiology, 10*(9), 402–407.

Gordillo, M. E., Singh, K. V., Baker, C. J., Murray, B. E. (1993). Typing of group B streptococci: Comparison of pulsed-field gel electrophoresis and conventional electrophoresis. *Journal of Clinical Microbiology, 31*(6), 1430–1434.

Gould, L. H., Walsh, K. A., Vieira, A. R., Herman, K., Williams, I. T., Hall, A. J., Cole, D. (2013). Surveillance for foodborne disease outbreaks—United States, 1998–2008. Morbidity and Mortality Weekly Report: Surveillance *Summaries*, *62*(2), 1–34.

Green, M. S., Kaufman, Z. (2002). Surveillance for early detection and monitoring of infectious disease outbreaks associated with bioterrorism. *The Israel Medical Association Journal*, *4*(7), 503–506.

Grundmann, H., Aanensen, D. M., Van Den Wijngaard, C. C., Spratt, B. G., Harmsen, D., Friedrich, A. W., European Staphylococcal Reference Laboratory Working, G. (2010). Geographic distribution of *Staphylococcus aureus* causing invasive infections in Europe: A molecular-epidemiological analysis. *PLoS Medicine*, *7*(1), e1000215.

Haining, R. P. (2003). *Spatial Data Analysis: Theory and Practice*. Cambridge University Press.

Haque, M., Sartelli, M., McKimm, J., Bakar, M. A. (2018). Health care-associated infections–an overview. *Infection and Drug Resistance*, *11*, 2321–2333.

Harris, L. J., Farber, J. N., Beuchat, L. R., Parish, M. E., Suslow, T. V., Garrett, E. H., Busta, F. F. (2003). Outbreaks associated with fresh produce: Incidence, growth, and survival of pathogens in fresh and fresh-cut produce. *Comprehensive Reviews in Food Science and Food Safety*, *2*, 78–141.

Havelaar, A. H., Evers, E. G., Nauta, M. J. (2008). Challenges of quantitative microbial risk assessment at EU level. *Trends in Food Science and Technology*, *19*, S26–S33.

Healy, M., Huong, J., Bittner, T., Lising, M., Frye, S., Raza, S., et al. (2005). Microbial DNA typing by automated repetitive-sequence-based PCR. *Journal of Clinical Microbiology*, *43*(1), 199–207.

Hebebci, M. T., Bertiz, Y., Alan, S. (2020). Investigation of views of students and teachers on distance education practices during the Coronavirus (COVID-19) Pandemic. International *Journal of Technology in Education and Science*, *4*(4), 267–282.

Hertzman, P. A., Blevins, W. L., Mayer, J., Greenfield, B., Ting, M., Gleich, G. J. (1990). Association of the eosinophilia–myalgia syndrome with the ingestion of tryptophan. *New England Journal of Medicine*, 322(13), 869–873.

Heymann, D. L., Rodier, G. (2004). Global surveillance, national surveillance, and SARS. *Emerging Infectious Diseases*, *10*(2), 173.

Hitchcock, P., Chamberlain, A., Van Wagoner, M., Inglesby, T. V., O'Toole, T. (2007). Challenges to global surveillance and response to infectious disease outbreaks of international importance. *Biosecurity and Bioterrorism: Biodefense Strategy, Practice, and Science*, *5*(3), 206–227.

Holmes, A. H., Moore, L. S. P., Sundsfjord, A., Steinbakk, M., Regmi, S., Karkey, A., et al. (2016). Understanding the mechanisms and drivers of antimicrobial resistance. *The Lancet*, *387*(10014), 176–187.

Holmes, E. C. (2022). COVID-19—lessons for zoonotic disease. In: *American Association for the Advancement of Science*.

Hopkins, R. S., Shillam, P., Gaspard, B., Eisnach, L., Karlin, R. J. (1985). Waterborne disease in Colorado: Three years' surveillance and 18 outbreaks. *American Journal of Public Health*, *75*(3), 254–257.

Horan, T. C., Andrus, M., Dudeck, M. A. (2008). CDC/NHSN surveillance definition of health care–associated infection and criteria for specific types of infections in the acute care setting. *American Journal of Infection Control*, *36*(5), 309–332.

Howard-Jones, N. (1981). The world Health organization in historical perspective. *Perspectives in Biology and Medicine*, *24*(3), 467–482.

Humphries, R. M., Hindler, J. A., Magnano, P., Wong-Beringer, A., Tibbetts, R., Miller, S. A. (2018). Performance of ceftolozane-tazobactam Etest, MIC test strips, and disk diffusion compared to reference broth microdilution for β-lactam-resistant *Pseudomonas aeruginosa* isolates. *Journal of Clinical Microbiology*, *56*(3), 10–1128.

Hutwagner, L., Thompson, W., Seeman, G. M., Treadwell, T. (2003). The bioterrorism preparedness and response early aberration reporting system (EARS). *Journal of Urban Health*, *80*, i89–i96.

Idelevich, E. A., Hoy, M., Görlich, D., Knaack, D., Grünastel, B., Peters, G., et al. (2017). Rapid phenotypic detection of microbial resistance in gram-positive bacteria by a real-time laser scattering method. *Frontiers in Microbiology*, *8*, 1064.

Jackson, B. R., Tarr, C., Strain, E., Jackson, K. A., Conrad, A., Carleton, H., et al. (2016). Implementation of nationwide real-time whole-genome sequencing to enhance listeriosis outbreak detection and investigation. *Reviews of Infectious Diseases*, *63*(3), 380–386.

Kaiser, F. M. (2008). *GAO: Government Accountability Office and General Accounting Office*. Congressional Research Service.

Khandia, R., Singhal, S., Alqahtani, T., Kamal, M. A., Nahed, A., Nainu, F., et al. (2022). Emergence of SARS-CoV-2 Omicron (B. 1.1. 529) variant, salient features, high global health concerns and strategies to counter it amid ongoing COVID-19 pandemic. *Environmental Research*, *209*, 112816.

Knobler, S., Mahmoud, A., Lemon, S., Pray, L. (2006). *The Impact of Globalization on Infectious Disease Emergence and Control: Exploring the Consequences and Opportunities*. Workshop Summary. Washington (DC): National Academies Press, USA.

Köser, C. U., Holden, M. T. G., Ellington, M. J., Cartwright, E. J. P., Brown, N. M., Ogilvy-Stuart, A. L., et al. (2012). Rapid whole-genome sequencing for investigation of a neonatal MRSA outbreak. *New England Journal of Medicine*, *366*(24), 2267–2275.

Kulldorff, M., Heffernan, R., Hartman, J., Assunçao, R., Mostashari, F. (2005). A space–time permutation scan statistic for disease outbreak detection. *PLoS Medicine*, *2*(3), e59.

Kulski, J. K. (2016). Next-generation sequencing—an overview of the history, tools, and "Omic" applications. *Next Generation Sequencing—Advances, Applications and Challenges*, *10*, 61964.

Lagier, J.-C., Edouard, S., Pagnier, I., Mediannikov, O., Drancourt, M., Raoult, D. (2015). Current and past strategies for bacterial culture in clinical microbiology. *Clinical Microbiology Reviews*, *28*(1), 208–236.

Lanini, S., D'Arezzo, S., Puro, V., Martini, L., Imperi, F., Piselli, P., et al. (2011). Molecular epidemiology of a Pseudomonas aeruginosa hospital outbreak driven by a contaminated disinfectant-soap dispenser. *PLoS One*, *6*(2), e17064.

Larsen, M. V., Cosentino, S., Rasmussen, S., Friis, C., Hasman, H., Marvig, R. L., et al. (2012). Multilocus sequence typing of total-genome-sequenced bacteria. *Journal of Clinical Microbiology*, *50*(4), 1355–1361.

Le Page, S., Dubourg, G., Rolain, J.-M. (2016). Evaluation of the Scan® 1200 as a rapid tool for reading antibiotic susceptibility testing by the disc diffusion technique. *Journal of Antimicrobial Chemotherapy*, *71*(12), 3424–3431.

Leclerc, H., Schwartzbrod, L., Dei-Cas, E. (2002). Microbial agents associated with waterborne diseases. *Critical Reviews in Microbiology*, *28*(4), 371–409.

Ledeboer, N. A., Das, K., Eveland, M., Roger-Dalbert, C., Mailler, S., Chatellier, S., Dunne, W. M. (2007). Evaluation of a novel chromogenic agar medium for isolation and differentiation of vancomycin-resistant *Enterococcus faecium* and *Enterococcus faecalis* isolates. *Journal of Clinical Microbiology*, *45*(5), 1556–1560.

Li, W., Raoult, D., Fournier, P.-E. (2009). Bacterial strain typing in the genomic era. *FEMS Microbiology Reviews*, *33*(5), 892–916.

Lober, W. B., Karras, B. T., Wagner, M. M., Overhage, J. M., Davidson, A. J., Fraser, H., et al. (2002). Roundtable on bioterrorism detection: Information system–based surveillance. *Journal of the American Medical Informatics Association*, *9*(2), 105–115.

Longfield, J. N. Outbreak investigation.

Lutz, J. K., Crawford, J., Hoet, A. E., Wilkins Iii, J. R., Lee, J. (2013). Comparative performance of contact plates, electrostatic wipes, swabs and a novel sampling device for the detection of Staphylococcus aureus on environmental surfaces. *Journal of Applied Microbiology*, *115*(1), 171–178.

Magassouba, A. S., Diallo, B. D., Camara, L. M., Sow, K., Camara, S., Bah, B., et al. (2020). Impact of the Ebola virus disease outbreak (2014–2016) on tuberculosis surveillance activities by Guinea's National Tuberculosis Control Program: A time series analysis. *BMC Public Health*, *20*, 1–9.

Matuschek, E., Copsey-Mawer, S., Petersson, S., Åhman, J., Morris, T. E., Kahlmeter, G. (2023). The European committee on antimicrobial susceptibility testing disc diffusion susceptibility testing method for frequently isolated anaerobic bacteria. *Clinical Microbiology and Infection*, *29*(6), 795–e791.

Men, A. E., Wilson, P., Siemering, K., Forrest, S. (2008). Sanger DNA sequencing. *Next Generation Genome Sequencing: Towards Personalized Medicine*, 1–11.

Mirajkar, N. S., Gebhart, C. J. (2016). Comparison of agar dilution and antibiotic gradient strip test with broth microdilution for susceptibility testing of swine Brachyspira species. *Journal of Veterinary Diagnostic Investigation*, *28*(2), 133–143.

Mirzaei, R., Goodarzi, P., Asadi, M., Soltani, A., Aljanabi, H. A. A., Jeda, A. S., et al. (2020). Bacterial co-infections with SARS-CoV-2. *IUBMB Life*, *72*(10), 2097–2111.

Moe, C. L. (2007). Waterborne transmission of infectious agents. In: *Manual of Environmental Microbiology* (pp. 222–248).

Morgantini, L. A., Naha, U., Wang, H., Francavilla, S., Acar, Ö., Flores, J. M., et al. (2020). Factors contributing to healthcare professional burnout during the COVID-19 pandemic: A rapid turnaround global survey. *PLoS ONE*, *15*(9), e0238217.

Mostashari, F., Hartman, J. (2003). *Syndromic Surveillance: A Local Perspective* (Vol. 80, pp. i1–i7), Springer.

Nakase, J. Y. (2000). Update on emerging infections from the Centers for Disease Control and Prevention. *Annals of Emergency Medicine*, *36*(3), 268–270.

Nelson, K. E., Williams, C. M. (2014). *Infectious Disease Epidemiology: Theory and Practice*. Jones & Bartlett Publishers.

Neves, E., Lourenço, A., Silva, A. C., Coutinho, R., Brito, L. (2008). Pulsed-field gel electrophoresis (PFGE) analysis of *Listeria monocytogenes* isolates from different sources and geographical origins and representative of the twelve serovars. *Systematic and Applied Microbiology*, *31*(5), 387–392.

Ortiz, E., Clancy, C. M. (2003). Use of information technology to improve the quality of health care in the United States. *Health Services Research*, *38*(2), 10.

Otten, E. J. (2000). Chemical and Biological terrorism: Research and development to improve civilian medical response; National Academy Press, 1999. *Journal of Emergency Medicine*, *18*(1), 138.

Overdevest, I., Willemsen, I., Elberts, S., Verhulst, C., Rijnsburger, M., Savelkoul, P., Kluytmans, J. (2011). Evaluation of the DiversiLab typing method in a multicenter study assessing horizontal spread of highly resistant gram-negative rods. *Journal of Clinical Microbiology*, *49*(10), 3551–3554.

Pinto, F., Hiom, S., Girdlestone, S., Maillard, J. Y. (2009). Evaluation of the effectiveness of commercially available contact plates for monitoring microbial environments. *Letters in Applied Microbiology*, *48*(3), 379–382.

Pitchai, K., Chen, J., Birla, S., Gonzalez, R., Jones, D., Subbiah, J. (2014). A microwave heat transfer model for a rotating multi-component meal in a domestic oven: Development and validation. *Journal of Food Engineering*, *128*, 60–71.

Polonsky, J. A., Baidjoe, A., Kamvar, Z. N., Cori, A., Durski, K., Edmunds, W. J., et al. (2019). Outbreak analytics: A developing data science for informing the response to emerging pathogens. *Philosophical Transactions of the Royal Society B*, *374*(1776), 20180276.

Prevost, G., Pottecher, B., Dahlet, M., Bientz, M., Mantz, J. M., Piemont, Y. (1991). Pulsed field gel electrophoresis as a new epidemiological tool for monitoring methicillin-resistant *Staphylococcus aureus* in an intensive care unit. *Journal of Hospital Infection*, *17*(4), 255–269.

Pulvirenti, J. J., Mehra, T., Hafiz, I., DeMarais, P., Marsh, D., Kocka, F., et al. (2002). Epidemiology and outcome of *Clostridium difficile* infection and diarrhea in HIV infected inpatients. *Diagnostic Microbiology and Infectious Disease*, *44*(4), 325–330.

Rabuza, U., Šostar-Turk, S., Fijan, S. (2012). Efficiency of four sampling methods used to detect two common nosocomial pathogens on textiles. *Textile Research Journal*, *82*(20), 2099–2105.

Racaniello, V. R. (2004). Emerging infectious diseases. *Journal of Clinical Investigation*, *113*(6), 796–798.

Raslan, O. (2011). Outbreak management. *IFIC Basic Concepts of Infection Control*, *57*.

Rasmussen, S. A., Goodman, R. A. (2018). *The CDC Field Epidemiology Manual*. Oxford University Press.

Robertson, L. J., Sprong, H., Ortega, Y. R., van der Giessen, J. W. B., Fayer, R. (2014). Impacts of globalisation on foodborne parasites. *Trends in Parasitology*, *30*(1), 37–52.

Roelofsen, E., Van Leeuwen, M., Meijer-Severs, G. J., Wilkinson, M. H. F., Degener, J. E. (1999). Evaluation of the effects of storage in two different swab fabrics and under three different transport conditions on recovery of aerobic and anaerobic bacteria. *Journal of Clinical Microbiology*, *37*(9), 3041–3043.

Rose, L., Jensen, B., Peterson, A., Banerjee, S. N., Arduino, M. J. (2004). Swab materials and *Bacillus anthracis* spore recovery from nonporous surfaces. *Emerging Infectious Diseases*, *10*(6), 1023.

Sabat, A., Malachowa, N., Miedzobrodzki, J., Hryniewicz, W. (2006). Comparison of PCR-based methods for typing *Staphylococcus aureus* isolates. *Journal of Clinical Microbiology*, *44*(10), 3804–3807.

Siegel, J. D., Rhinehart, E., Jackson, M., Chiarello, L. (2007). Management of multidrug-resistant organisms in health care settings, 2006. *American Journal of Infection Control*, *35*(10), S165–S193.

Stephens, P. R., Gottdenker, N., Schatz, A. M., Schmidt, J. P., Drake, J. M. (2021). Characteristics of the 100 largest modern zoonotic disease outbreaks. *Philosophical Transactions of the Royal Society B, 376*(1837), 20200535.

Stephens, P. R., Sundaram, M., Ferreira, S., Gottdenker, N., Nipa, K. F., Schatz, A. M., et al. M. (2022). Drivers of African filovirus (ebola and marburg) outbreaks. *Vector-Borne and Zoonotic Diseases, 22*(9), 478–490.

Tambolkar, S., Pustake, M., Giri, P., Tambolkar, I. (2022). Comparison of public health measures taken during Spanish flu and COVID-19 pandemics: A narrative review. *Journal of Family Medicine and Primary Care, 11*(5), 1642.

Tebano, G., Mouelhi, Y., Zanichelli, V., Charmillon, A., Fougnot, S., Lozniewski, A., et al. (2020). Selective reporting of antibiotic susceptibility testing results: A promising antibiotic stewardship tool. *Expert Review of Anti-infective Therapy, 18*(3), 251–262.

Teljeur, E. (2002). Response of non-governmental organisations, community-based organisations and communities. *HIV/AIDS, Economics and Governance in South Africa: Key Issues in Understanding Response*, 57.

Tenover, F. C., Arbeit, R. D., Goering, R. V., Mickelsen, P. A., Murray, B. E., Persing, D. H., Swaminathan, B. (1995). Interpreting chromosomal DNA restriction patterns produced by pulsed-field gel electrophoresis: Criteria for bacterial strain typing. *Journal of Clinical Microbiology, 33*(9), 2233–2239.

Tosh, P. K., Disbot, M., Duffy, J. M., Boom, M. L., Heseltine, G., Srinivasan, A., Berríos-Torres, S. I. (2011). Outbreak of *Pseudomonas aeruginosa* surgical site infections after arthroscopic procedures: Texas, 2009. *Infection Control and Hospital Epidemiology, 32*(12), 1179–1186.

Tsai, T. F., Finn, D. R., Plikaytis, B. D., McCauley, W., Martin, S. M., Fraser, D. W. (1979). Legionnaires' disease: Clinical features of the epidemic in Philadelphia. *Annals of Internal Medicine*, 90(4), 509–517.

Tumpey, A. J., Daigle, D., Nowak, G. (2018). Communicating during an outbreak or public health investigation. In: *The CDC Field Epidemiology Manual* (pp. 243–259).

Van Belkum, A., Tassios, P. T., Dijkshoorn, L., Haeggman, S., Cookson, B., Fry, N. K., Gerner-Smidt, P. (2007). Guidelines for the validation and application of typing methods for use in bacterial epidemiology. *Clinical Microbiology and Infection, 13*, 1–46.

Vasilijević, B., Mitić-Ćulafić, D., Djekic, I., Marković, T., Knežević-Vukčević, J., Tomasevic, I., Nikolić, B. (2019). Antibacterial effect of Juniperus communis and Satureja montana essential oils against *Listeria monocytogenes* in vitro and in wine marinated beef. *Food Control, 100*, 247–256.

Wang, G., Doyle, M. P. (1998). Survival of enterohemorrhagic *Escherichia coli* O157: H7 in water. *Journal of food Protection, 61*(6), 662–667.

Waterson, P. (2014). Health information technology and sociotechnical systems: A progress report on recent developments within the UK National Health Service (NHS). *Applied Ergonomics, 45*(2), 150–161.

Williams, R. E. O. (1954). Investigation of outbreaks of infection. *British Medical Journal, 1*(4853), 91.

World Health, O. (2004). International Health Regulations—update on the revised version.

World Health, O. (2008). *International Health Regulations (2005)*. World Health Organization.

World Health, O. (2018). Identifying and responding to serious adverse events following immunization, following use of smallpox vaccine during a public health emergency: A guidance document for smallpox vaccine safety surveillance.

World Health, O. (2021). Pandemic influenza preparedness (PIP) framework: Partnership contribution (PC) preparedness high-level implementation plan II 2018–2023.

Yu, F., Ying, Q., Chen, C., Li, T., Ding, B., Liu, Y., Salgado, C. (2012). Outbreak of pulmonary infection caused by *Klebsiella pneumoniae* isolates harbouring bla IMP-4 and bla DHA-1 in a neonatal intensive care unit in China. *Journal of Medical Microbiology, 61*(7), 984–989.

Yusof, A., Engelhardt, A., Karlsson, A. S., Bylund, L., Vidh, P., Mills, K., Walsh, T. R. (2008). Evaluation of a new Etest vancomycin-teicoplanin strip for detection of glycopeptide-intermediate *Staphylococcus aureus* (GISA), in particular, heterogeneous GISA. *Journal of Clinical Microbiology, 46*(9), 3042–3047.

Zhan, H., Li, R., Liu, X. (2014). Foodborne illness. http://hdl. handle. net/1800/3166.

CHAPTER 10

Nanotechnology and Its Role in Pharmaceutical Microbiology

ZAINAB IRFAN,[1] SUMON GIRI,[1] and SOFIA KHANAM[2*]

[1]*Department of Pharmaceutical Technology, Brainware University, Kolkata, West Bengal, India*

[2]*Department of Drug Design and Pharmacology, University of Copenhagen, Denmark*

*Corresponding author

ABSTRACT

The domains of microbiology and nanotechnology have been instrumental in the evolution of science and technology by bringing forth novel approaches for promoting human well-being as well as preserving ecological and environmental harmony. The recurrent use of drugs causing antibiotic resistance, as well as the distribution of metal nanoparticles (NPs), is having an effect on the trophic levels. To combat human health problems, it is essential to produce multifaceted techniques amalgamating the aspects of both microbiology and nanotechnology. With reference to NP synthesis processes, their mechanism of action, characterization methods, and utilization, there has been a notable elevation in the field of nanotechnology. The synthesis of metal NPs and oxides through chemical and physical processes is growing, but their discharge into the environment is having ecotoxicological impacts. In light of this, "biosynthesis" of NPs using microbes is receiving an array of attention. To overcome microbiological constraints, both domains have been successfully merged in fields like pharmaceuticals. This chapter emphasizes the relationship between

Advances in Pharmaceutical Microbiology: From Bench to Bedside. Harpreet Singh, Arun Kumar Mishra, Jeyabalan Sangeetha, and Devarajan Thangadurai (Eds.)

DOI: 10.1201/9781779640918-14

pharmaceutical microbiology and nanotechnology and the vast opportunities provided by the interdisciplinary study. Additionally, it addresses how nanotechnology is being used in numerous areas of pharmaceutical microbiology, including the manufacture of nanomaterials from microbes and microbial nanoformulations.

10.1 INTRODUCTION

Nanotechnology revolves around the investigation and manipulation of materials at the nanoscale, that is, in the size range of 1–100 nanometers (nm). This new field encompasses novel phenomena occurring specifically at this scale, leading toward innovative applications (Nasrollahzadeh et al., 2019). Involving a broadscale of scientific knowledge that ranges from microbiology, chemistry, physics, material science, engineering and manufacturing, nanotechnology can be termed as a 21st century technology involving the effect on society and economy similar to that of semiconductor technology, information technology, and cellular and molecular biology associated with various technologies in the 20th century (Bhushan, 2017). As we explore the complexities of nanotechnology, we uncover the possibility of revolutionary breakthroughs that might fundamentally alter a number of facets of our existence. Nanotechnology, which offers previously unheard-of chances for creativity and discovery, is at the vanguard of scientific and technological evolution, from the microscopic manipulation of materials to the macroscopic impact on society (Ball et al., 2019).

Microbiology, a field that delves into the study of microscopic organisms, marks a pivotal intersection of biology and the unseen world. At its core, microbiology explores the intricacies of microbes, including bacteria, fungi, viruses, and protozoa, whose existence often eludes the naked eye. The significance of microbiology extends far beyond the realm of invisibility, as these microorganisms play fundamental roles in shaping life on earth (Gilmore and Denyer, 2023). The implementation of microbiology in pharmaceutical and healthcare settings is known as pharmaceutical microbiology. Pharmaceutical microbiology has a wide range of applications. The safe production of medical equipment and pharmaceutical and healthcare products is, nevertheless, its primary duty. Testing and validating pharmaceutical products, in-process samples, and raw materials are all included in the field of pharmaceutical microbiology. This comprises microbiological limits assessment, sterility evaluation, and microorganism identification. Pharmaceutical microbiologists also work on aseptic production process development and monitoring, cleanroom environmental monitoring, and sterilization technique validation (Sandle, 2016; Jeevanandam et al., 2022). This emerging discipline of pharmaceutical microbiology is crucial to the industry because it uses special nanoscale phenomena to transform drug delivery, development, and diagnostics. In pharmaceutical microbiology, nanotechnology is important because it can bring forth novel approaches that lead to improved medication formulations, targeted delivery systems, and diagnostic instruments. The future of medicine may be shaped by this synergy between nanotechnology and pharmaceutical microbiology, which has the potential to advance therapeutic methods and solve difficulties in the microbiological elements of drug development (Jeevanandam et al., 2022). This chapter highlights the confluence of nanotechnology and pharmaceutical microbiology focusing on the development of nanoformulations from microbes synthesized nanomaterials (NMs) and its application to various diseases.

10.2 PHARMACEUTICAL MICROBIOLOGY AND ITS IMPORTANCE

Pharmaceutical microbiology entails researching the microorganisms involved in the manufacturing of pharmaceuticals, like reducing the number of microbes in a process environment, eliminating microbes and microbial byproducts from water and other raw materials, and assuring the sterility of the pharmaceutical product when it is finished (Denyer et al., 2004). The investigation and synthesis of anti-infective agents, the use of microbes to identify potential drug mutagenic and carcinogenic activity, and the application of microorganisms in the manufacture of pharmaceuticals like insulin and human growth hormone are additional facets of pharmaceutical microbiology. In order to guarantee the effectiveness and safety of pharmaceutical goods, pharmaceutical microbiology is essential. This particular area of microbiology is concerned with the study of microorganisms, such as bacteria, viruses, fungi, and other microbes, that are important to the pharmaceutical sector (Sandle, 2016). In recent decades, the pharmaceutical sector has grown in tandem with the rise in product quality requirements and the tightening of regulations around production processes. An effective, safe, and high-quality modern medicine must be demonstrated in order to obtain a production license (Kapoor et al., 2020). The majority of medications are made up of an active component plus a number of other ingredients, or excipients, which are added to the medication to make it safe, pleasant, and effective throughout usage and storage. Numerous other areas contribute to the overall effectiveness, safety, and quality of the manufactured product, even though pharmacologists and toxicologists are responsible for the effectiveness and safety aspects of the active ingredient, respectively (Demain, 2002). The primary responsibility for guaranteeing that the medicinal ingredients are present in the appropriate physical form and concentration lies with analytical chemists. However, the quality of a product is not only determined by its physicochemical characteristics; microorganisms can also impact its safety and efficacy (Waters et al., 2010).

For pharmaceutical products to be safe and of high quality, pharmaceutical microbiology is essential. To reduce the possibility of microbial contamination compromising pharmaceutical product safety, stringent testing and control procedures are necessary (Magdy, 2014). Pharmaceutical microbiologists use strict procedures to validate and maintain the sterility of sterile goods, such as injectables and implants, and they play a vital role in preventing contamination during the drug-production process (von Woedtke and Kramer, 2008). In the pharmaceutical sector, microbiological testing, which includes evaluating raw materials, in-process samples, and final products, is essential to quality assurance. Furthermore, microbiologists keep an eye on production areas and clean rooms to identify and stop the entrance of contaminants that can lower the quality of the final product. Global regulatory organizations require stringent microbiological testing and adherence to set standards; fulfilling these obligations is crucial for gaining market acceptance and preserving public confidence (Demain and Adrio, 2008). Pharmaceutical microbiology assists in the discovery and characterization of microbial agents pertinent to drug development during the research and development stage. With the development of biopharmaceuticals, microbiology now plays a bigger part in maintaining cell cultures under control and making sure impurities do not affect the quality of pharmaceuticals obtained from biological sources. Pharmaceutical microbiology testing services, including environmental monitoring, microbial contamination testing, and sterility testing, are provided by a number of companies (Lambert et al., 2006). In summary, by ensuring the microbiological purity of pharmaceutical goods, pharmaceutical microbiology plays a critical role in protecting public health. Extensive microbiological practices are crucial in the pharmaceutical sector, and its impact extends across the entire pharmaceutical life cycle, from research and development to manufacturing and quality control.

10.3 THE BOOM OF NANOTECHNOLOGY

A disruptive period marked by the manipulation and application of materials at the nanoscale, usually ranging from 1 to 100 nm, is reflected in the growth of nanotechnology. Nanotechnology is the survey and development of structures and systems at the atomic or molecular level for various applications, according to the US National Nanotechnology Initiative (Balzani, 2005; Ball et al., 2019). This rapidly developing field has experienced exponential expansion, penetrated numerous industries, and resulted in ground-breaking discoveries with far-reaching effects. Nanotechnology takes advantage of the distinct physical and chemical features that arise at the nanoscale to achieve miniaturization and enhanced properties. Materials' characteristics frequently diverge significantly from those at larger scales as they are shrunk down. Unprecedented control over substances is made possible by this miniaturization, which results in the production of innovative materials with improved strength, conductivity, and reactivity (Rambaran and Schirhagl, 2020). It has a wide range of applications in a number of industries, including electronics, medical, energy, and materials science. For example, nanoscale electronics components allow for the development of more compact and potent devices. Nanoparticles (NPs) are transforming drug delivery and diagnostics in medicine, enabling more precise and effective treatment plans. The innovation of nanomedicine has been made possible by nanotechnology, which has ushered in a new era in healthcare. Engineers are developing nanostructures and particles for precise medicine delivery, imaging, and diagnostics (Malik et al., 2023). This focused strategy improves therapeutic efficacy while reducing adverse effects, which represents a major improvement in patient care. Applications of nanotechnology have also been advantageous for the environmental field. Sustainable solutions are produced by innovations in water treatment, environmental remediation, and renewable energy that take advantage of the special qualities of NMs (Navya and Daima 2016). The development of eco-friendly technologies with less ecological footprints is greatly aided by nanotechnology. Nanotechnology functions at the nexus of several scientific fields, encouraging cooperation and convergence. In order to investigate the many uses of NMs, scientists from the fields of physics, chemistry, biology, and engineering come together and produce ground-breaking findings and solutions (Ball et al., 2019). The boom of nanotechnology has had a major impact on the economy in addition to advancing science. Increased funding and investment in nanotechnology research and development is a result of governments, industry, and investors refer to the potential for innovation and economic prosperity. As nanotechnology develops further, it is becoming more crucial to take ethical and regulatory issues into account. To ensure responsible and sustainable development, questions regarding the safety of NMs, their possible impact on the environment, and their ethical usage in medicine need to be carefully examined (Dykman and Khlebtsov, 2012). In summary, the development of nanotechnology is a revolutionary force that is reshaping our understanding of and ability to work with matter. Its relevance in the current technology landscape is highlighted by its broad impact on a variety of industries and its capacity to address complicated challenges. This points to a future filled with never-before-seen developments and opportunities.

10.4 RELATION BETWEEN PHARMACEUTICAL MICROBIOLOGY AND NANOTECHNOLOGY

Microorganisms involved in the synthesis of therapeutic compounds are the focus of the discipline of pharmaceutical microbiology. In the early days of pharmaceutical microbiology, antibiotics were utilized to treat illnesses that were infectious by eliminating the microorganisms triggering the disease. Owing to their multitude of applications, antibiotics continue to be considered by the pharmaceutical industry as an essential drug for life (Uddin et al., 2021). Because of their unique physiological and biochemical characteristics, microorganisms have been used for food preservation, baking, and brewing since ancient times (Lorenzo et al., 2018). More recently, these features have been used to produce antibiotics, solvents, amino acids, feed additives, and chemical feedstuffs. However, because of their symbiotic properties, many microbes are also frequently exploited nowadays for the production of pharmaceutical products. Microbes play a role, for instance, in the manufacture of pharmaceutical articles like human growth hormones and insulin, as well as in the identification of mutagenic and carcinogenic activity (Maurya et al., 2021).

Using materials at the nanoscale, the multidisciplinary area of nanotechnology combines science and technology. It concentrated on the production of materials with applications in agriculture, medicine, pharmacology, the environment, and other diverse sectors at the 1–100 nm scale (Lateef et al., 2018; Elegbede and Lateef 2020). Merging pharmaceutical microbiology and nanotechnology allows for the achievable and innovative methods to address environmental and ecological challenges, as well as subsequent human health issues such as antibiotic or multidrug resistance (Ball et al., 2019). Notably designed NMs are synthesized to deliver drugs, proteins, plasmids, antibodies, oligonucleotides, fluorophores, ligands, polymers, radioisotopes, tissue-engineered products, etc., to the human body and influence target cells. Many different types of microbes have demonstrated the capacity to synthesize unique nanostructured materials. Examples of these include silicified frustules (Kröger and Poulsen, 2008), calcified coccoliths, magnetosomes (Yan et al., 2017), and organic NMs such as bacterial nanowires (Malvankar and Lovley, 2012), microbial nanocellulose (Hasanin et al., 2018), and exopolysaccharide NPs. Microbiologically mediated NM biosynthesis is a potentially greener alternative to physical and chemical approaches to nanosynthesis, and it is a biotechnologically based nanomanufacturing method. Consequently, the field of nanotechnology has acquired symbolic consideration recently in the interest of its novel utilization in pharmaceutical research utilizing microbes (Grasso et al., 2019).

10.5 RELEVANCE OF NANOTECHNOLOGY IN VARIOUS AREAS OF PHARMACEUTICAL MICROBIOLOGY

In the last several decades, multidisciplinary nanotechnology has developed and is now heavily involved in industry, pharmaceuticals, agriculture, and the environment (Fariq et al., 2017). The global market for NMs is foreseen to grow at a compound annual growth rate of 20% or more between 2016 and 2022 (Inshakova and Inshakov, 2017). An important obstacle to the worldwide production of the NMs industry is the environmental sustainability of the technologies used in nanomanufacturing. These materials provide unique features for biomedical applications due to their nanoscale diameters, which also give them a significant surface/volume ratio, distinctive shapes, and comparable dimensions to biomolecules (Ghosh et al., 2021). Considering their equivalent sizes to biomolecules and ease of penetration, particles less than 100 nm are generally considered effective for most purposes. Biologists may conduct a wide range of research projects with NMs because of their smaller size. NMs can connect with intricate biological systems in novel ways due to their size, which is analogous to that of biomolecules. Multifunctional NMs that can be used to target, diagnose, and cure critical illnesses like cancer have been designed and developed thanks to this quickly developing sector (Sardar et al., 2014; Pastorino et al., 2019). Because they are nearly the same size as biological things, nanoscale chemicals, parts, and gadgets are able to pass across blood-tissue barriers with ease. For precise and regulated medication delivery to a particular location, novel techniques, including drug delivery using nanocarriers, are being employed. They support the reduction of drug toxicity and enhancement of pharmacological effectiveness in illness therapy (Blanco et al., 2015; Ahmad et al., 2021). Furthermore, the interactions that nanocarriers have with the biomolecules within and on the surface of cells do not change the biochemical characteristics and behavior of these molecules (Abdulla et al., 2021). Biological synthesis techniques can get beyond the drawbacks of the chemical and physical approaches to creating NMs. It is now well acknowledged that a broad range of organisms are capable of producing inorganic compounds extracellularly or intracellularly (Jeevanandam et al., 2016). Since the majority of nutraceuticals come from plants, they are more likely to degrade and experience chemical instability, poor solubility, bad taste, and loss of bioactivity before being absorbed at the intended location (Shende and Mallick 2020). An ample amount of effort has been paid to encapsulation methods that use food-grade substances such as proteins, lipids, polysaccharides, liposomes, etc. In particular, polysaccharides have become more well-known because of their molecular similarities to human extracellular matrices, which allow the body to recognize them with ease (Miao et al., 2018). Their involvement extends to several biological processes, such as immune recognition and cell signaling, which trigger the body's antimicrobial and anti-inflammatory responses. Plants, mammals, fungi, bacteria, and algae all contain polysaccharides, which are long chains of branched or unbranched sugar monomeric units connected by glycosidic bonds (Casillo et al., 2018). Microbially obtained polysaccharides have gained popularity among them because of a number of benefits, including a fast fermentation process, economical large-scale production, biocompatibility, nonimmunogenicity, and biodegradability. Additionally, the majority of these polysaccharides have US-FDA approval, indicating that they are safe for human consumption (Srivastava and Choudhury, 2021).

Individually, the fields of microbiology and nanotechnology have advanced science and technology by providing cutting-edge remedies for human health and preserving ecological and environmental balance. It makes research and visualization of research possible at the molecular assembly levels. It enables the evaluation of these processes as well as the discovery of self-assembly and molecular recognition patterns (Ball et al., 2019). A potential biotechnological method for producing NMs, microbial-mediated biosynthesis offers a "green" substitute for physical and chemical methods of nanosynthesis (Khan et al., 2018b). Many benefits and properties, such as the following, have been demonstrated by the broad exploration of microbial-mediated biosynthesis of NMs:

1. Chemical composition, size, and shape of synthesized NPs are well known.
2. Biosynthesis takes place in relatively moderate physicochemical environments.
3. Microbial cells can be grown and handled with ease, and cell culture can potentially be scaled up.
4. Potential to modify important aspects of the cell culture operational setup *in vivo* or through genetic engineering with respect to customize the properties of NMs (Prasad et al., 2016).

Reliable and environmentally benign nanotechnologies for NM synthesis must be developed in order to take advantage of future wide-impact nanostructured-based technologies and implementation, such as new optical and electrochemical (bio) sensoristic devices and therapeutic and diagnostic uses of nanostructured materials for the creation of antibacterial and antitumoral medications, drug administration, and *in vivo* and *in vitro* imaging (Kiessling et al., 2014). Utilizing various microbes and their enzymes, plant materials, and animal extracts, biological synthesis approaches have evolved as the biological ways of NM innovation (Akintayo et al., 2020). The development of novel nano-based goods and processes for various medicinal, industrial, agricultural, and environmental applications would be ushered in by these engagements, which would introduce microorganisms as new "nanofactories."

10.5.1 BIOSYNTHESIS OF NANOMATERIALS FROM MICROORGANISMS

NMs are currently the subject of extensive research for potential commercial uses. It is a new era of examination in the realm of advanced nanotechnology and nanorobotics. The application of nanoscale structures to disease detection, medical care, and mitigation with the goal of enhancing human health is known as nanomedicine (Patil et al., 2008). NMs can be utilized to adapt sites without interfering with other cellular machinery as they are akin to the size of cellular organelles, including nano-sized proteins (Salata 2004). NMs' characteristics differ significantly from those of macro- and micro-sized materials, which are useful in human health and medicine. In order to develop novel drug delivery systems, fast and extremely sensitive diagnostic tools like biosensors, biopharmaceutics, surgical aids, implantable biomaterials, etc., as well as groundbreaking medications for disease treatment and healing of tissues, nanomedicine sought to combine modern nanotechnology with traditional molecular tools and biotechnology (Karunaratne, 2010). Microbial-mediated production of NMs is a potential biotechnological method of producing nanoscopic vectors, offering a greener alternative to physical and chemical methods (Li et al., 2011; Khan et al., 2018b). Numerous microbial strains of bacteria, yeast, molds, and microalgae have been shown to be capable of producing metallic, nonmetallic, or metal oxide NPs, exopolysaccharide NPs (Nwodo et al., 2012; Giri et al., 2023), and bacterial nanocellulose (Sharma and Bhardwaj, 2019) through microbial-mediated biosynthesis (Hulkoti and Taranath, 2014). This part of the chapter focuses on the microbial-mediated biosynthesis of NMs for biomedical and sensoristic applications (Table 10.1). An overview is as follows:

10.5.1.1 BACTERIA

For over a decade, bacteria have been exploited to synthesize a variety of NMs, like metal and metal oxide NPs with intriguing capabilities for biofilm formation (Suresh et al., 2011), enabling the development of

TABLE 10.1 Microbes-Mediated Biosynthesis of Nanomaterials

Microbe	Microbial Source	Type of Nanoparticle	Characterization	Application	References
Bacteria	*Bacillus subtilis*	Selenium	Size: 50–400 nm; spherical in shape	H_2O_2 sensoristic device	Wang et al. (2010)
	Bacillus subtilis	Titanium dioxide	Size: 10–30 nm	Photocatalytic effect on aquatic biofilm	Dhandapani et al. (2012)
	Alcaligenes faecalis	Silver	Size: 30–50 nm; spherical in shape	Antimicrobial and antibiofilm activity	Divya et al. (2019)
	Idiomarina sp. strain PR58–8	Lead (IV) sulfide	Size: 6–10 nm	Bioimaging	Srivastava and Kowshik (2017)
	Paracoccus haeundaensis BC74171	Gold	Size: 20.93 ± 3.46 nm	Antioxidant activity and antiproliferative effect	Patil et al. (2019)
	Micrococcus yunnanensis	Gold	Size: 53.8 nm	Antibacterial, anticancer	Jafari et al. (2018)
	Shewanella loihica	Copper	Size: 10–16 nm	Antibacterial activity	Lv et al. (2018)
Fungi	*Penicillium oxalicum*	Silver	Size: 60–80 nm	Antibacterial activity	Feroze et al. (2020)
	Cladosporium perangustum	Silver	Size: 30–40 nm	Antioxidant, anticancer, and nano-toxicological study	Govindappa et al. (2020)
	Morchella esculenta	Gold	Size: 16.51 nm	Antimicrobial activity and cytotoxic activity	Acay (2020)
Yeast	*Yarrowia lipolytica* DSM 3286	Silver	Size: 12.4 ± 5.22 nm	Antibacterial activity	Bolbanabad et al. (2020)
	Candida lusitaniae	Silver and silver chloride	Size: 2–10 nm	Antiproliferative and microbicidal activity	Eugenio et al. (2016)
Virus	Potato virus X	Nanoconjugates	Size: 12 nm; Filamentous rod-shaped	Herceptin drug delivery in breast cancer therapy	Esfandiari et al. (2016)
	M13 virus	Titanium dioxide	Size: 20–40 nm; mesoporous nanowires	Photo-electrochemical properties	Chen et al. (2015)

third-generation biosensors (Du et al., 2007), biolabeling, cell imaging (Bao et al., 2010), sensoristic devices (Wang et al., 2010), and diagnostics (Ramya et al., 2015). Furthermore, the antibacterial (Manivasagan et al., 2015; Roychoudhury et al., 2016), antioxidant (Torres et al., 2012), antiproliferative, antimigration (Kalishwaralal et al., 2009), anticoagulant (Kalishwaralal et al., 2010), and anticancer (Shao et al., 2015; Al-Dhabi et al., 2018) properties of bacterially derived NPs demonstrated promising applications. Bacteria are favored over other microbes for the development of NPs because they can be effectively grown in artificial conditions. Due to their rapid growth rates and ease of handling, bacteria are the most desirable options for the synthesis of NPs due to their unique capacity to reduce metallic ions into NPs (Gahlawat and Choudhury 2019).

According to studies, bacteria's extracellular polymeric substances can be used to effectively encapsulate and bioreduce materials when synthesizing NPs from metal ions (Gahlawat et al., 2016; Raj et al., 2016). For example, Mehta et al. (2014) biosynthesized silver nanoparticles (AgNPs) using extracellular polymeric substances that were isolated from the marine bacteria *Alteromonas macleodii*. According to recently published research on the various processes involved in the production of NPs by bacterial cells, the intracellular or extracellular biosynthesis of NPs is thought to be a component of the bacterial cells' cellular detoxification mechanism through an enzymatic reduction that produces confirmatory changes in the solubility of metal ions (Koul et al., 2021). There are unique bacterial species that can biofabricate certain organic nanostructures. In contrast to nanofibrillated and nanocrystalline cellulose, bacterial nanocellulose (3D network of cellulose nanofibrils) was efficiently biosynthesized by aerobic acetic bacteria belonging to the genus *Gluconacetobacter* and was more crystalline, mechanically stable, and pure. Therefore, because of its unique qualities, bacterial nanocellulose can be applied as an antibacterial agent in biomedical utilization, as a scaffold for tissue engineering and drug delivery systems, and as a nanocomposite in biosensoristic uses (Morales-Narvaez et al., 2015; Pourreza et al., 2015). Microbial extracellular biopolymers called exopolysaccharides play a wide range of roles in bacterial biofilm adherence and as antimicrobial agents. For the bacteria *Lactobacillus plantarum*-605, a unique self-assembled and spherical nanosized nonglucan exopolysaccharide has been reported in a recent work. According to Li et al. (2017), the results indicate that the substance has the capacity to reduce the amount of gold (Au) NPs and AgNPs that biosynthesize quickly without requiring any pretreatment or modification. Intracellular Fe_3O_4 and/or Fe_3S_4 nanocrystals with an organic coating, known as bacterial magnetosomes, are produced by both magnetotactic and non-magnetotactic bacteria. The bacterial Fe_3O_4 magnetosomes exhibit stable single-magnetic domains that remain magnetic at room temperature. They are distinguished by their consistent crystal shape, narrow size range, and great chemical purity (Vargas et al., 2018). Molecular imaging (Boucher et al., 2017), cancer therapy (Alphandery et al., 2011), and the manufacturing of a chip-based whole-cell biosensor for toxicity study (Roda et al., 2013) are a few examples of present applications.

10.5.1.2 FUNGI

The word "myconanotechnology" emerged to describe a recently developing field of nanotechnology based on studies on the production of NMs by fungi, such as yeasts and molds. Using fungus for biofabrication is an additional biological approach toward NPs production. Compared to bacterial cells, fungi can produce more NPs due to their stronger potential to withstand metal concentrations and their high cell wall binding potential with metal ions (Singh et al., 2016). Fungi can be used for extracellular or intracellular nanosynthesis, similar to bacteria and cyanobacteria. According to Molnár et al. (2018) and Rajeshkumar and Sivapriya (2020), fungi can utilize metal salts in their mycelia, which undergo a transformation into a less harmful form *via* the intracellular pathway. The utilization of fungal extracts entails extracellular biosynthesis (Zhao et al., 2018a; Rajeshkumar and Sivapriya, 2020). Fungi are considerably more unique than bacteria in the development of NPs owing to their high aggregation, various bioactive metabolites, and enhanced production (Castro-Longoria et al., 2011; Alghuthaymi et al., 2015). The Bismarck brown dye had also been destroyed by up to 90%, and zinc oxide NPs mediated by *Aspergillus niger* showed strong antibacterial activity (Kalpana et al., 2018).

According to Hulkoti and Taranath (2014), yeasts are unicellular fungi that are primarily recognized for using multiple methods for the manufacture of NPs, which leads to important variations in size, particle position, monodispersity, and other attributes. Yeast cells exposed to harmful metals can often convert the absorbed metal ions into complex polymer molecules that are nontoxic to the cell as a resistance mechanism. According to Dameron et al. (1989), these NPs made in yeast are commonly referred to as "semiconductor crystals" or "quantum semiconductor crystals." Yeast cells are highly acknowledged for their capacity to produce semiconductor NPs, namely those containing cadmium sulfide (CdS) (Ghosh et al., 2021). The model organism yeast *Saccharomyces cerevisiae* has been described by researchers to be able to biosynthesize high water-soluble and biocompatible cadmium telluride quantum dots. These quantum dots of cadmium telluride have demonstrated intriguing properties such as size-tunable emission and photoluminescence quantum yield, which can be adjusted based on temperature and culture time. These qualities make them a promising option for bio-imaging and bio-labeling applications (Luo et al., 2014). According to Zheng et al. (2010) and Wei (2017), *S. cerevisiae* has also been utilized in the biosynthesis of Au–Ag alloy NPs for the development of electrochemical sensors. These NPs are intended to measure the amount of paracetamol in pill samples and vanillin in samples of vanilla beans and vanilla tea, respectively. According to Shah et al. (2015), yeasts possess the capacity to endure in environments with elevated metal ion concentrations and may also leave behind large amounts of metal ions. A study by Apte et al. (2013) reported that melanin, a brown pigment present in yeast, was linked to the green synthesis of AgNPs using the marine yeast *Yarrowia lipolytica* for AgNPs biosynthesis.

A wide variety of small filamentous fungi, including *Penicillium*, *Aspergillus*, and *Fusarium*, are grouped together as molds. Over a decade, a number of investigations have explored the biosynthesis of quantum dots (lead sulfide, zinc sulfide with gadolinium, and zinc sulfide) and NPs (silver, gold, and tellurium) using molds. In addition to their potential use in optical detection of heavy metals and arsenic in water (Priyanka et al., 2017; Elsoud et al., 2018; Uddandarao et al., 2019), these NPs have demonstrated both antibacterial activity (Dhillon et al., 2012; Saravanakumar et al., 2018) and antitumoral activity (Mishra et al., 2011; Syed et al., 2013; Husseiny et al., 2015).

10.5.1.3 VIRUS

In view of their biocompatibility, biodegradability, mass production capability, programmable scaffolds, and ease of genetic manipulation for desired traits, viruses have emerged as intriguing prospects as NPs for medicinal applications. Applications in biomedicine have taken advantage of their resilience and capacity to sense environmental changes and release genetic material. Vaccines and immunotherapeutics, imaging, theranostics, medication administration, and gene transfer have been the primary applications of viral NPs. Capsid proteins, which have nanoscale structures ranging from 20 to 500 nm, coat viruses and give metallic ions the right conditions to engage with their machinery (Kobayashi et al., 2012). Through the application of genetic engineering, the capsid protein can be altered to develop NMs for tailored drug delivery and cancer treatment, like nanocomposites and nanoconjugates of metal NPs (Gahlawat and Choudhury, 2019). Viruses have been effectively utilized to produce NPs, according to numerous reports.

With their enormous rotational correlation times and strong relaxivity resulting from their rigid structures, viral NPs are also used as MRI contrast agents. They can also be chelated to their interior or exterior surfaces by a large number of contrast agents, like gadolinium, due to their polyvalent nature. Researchers have also examined the utilization of these NPs in the development of vaccines against viruses like HIV, hepatitis B, and *Neospora caninum* (Oh and Han 2020). CdS and zinc sulfide semiconductor NPs, for example, have been effectively developed with the M13 bacteriophage as a model (Mao et al., 2003). Likewise, Czapar et al. (2016) exploited the tobacco mosaic virus (TMV) to develop hollow nanotubes with a polyanionic inner surface that were intended to be used for the targeted delivery of the anticancer medication phenanthriplatin. In this investigation, phenanthriplatin loading and delivery *via* TMV nanotubes were strongly exhibited in a mouse model using a one-step process. Chen et al. (2018) stated in a different study that the hepatitis E virus capsule was utilized in the biosynthesis of the hepatitis E virus nanoparticle (HEVNP). In this investigation, the HEVNP was combined with the cell-specific ligand LXY30 and a labeled near-infrared fluorescent dye. It was determined that these biosynthesized HEVNPs might be used as multipurpose delivery vehicles for tissue targeting, tumor imaging, and medication administration.

10.5.2 PATHOGEN DETECTION THROUGH NANOTECHNOLOGY

A significant scientific issue for the global health care system is the emergence and re-emergence of infections. Acute infections, severe illnesses, and potentially fatal situations are mostly caused by rapidly spreading infections caused by bacteria, viruses, fungi, protozoa, and other microbes. In particular, rapid and correct identification is necessary for conditions similar to sepsis, which have a roughly 30% fatality rate (Dey et al., 2019). The World Health Organization (WHO) stated in a 2017 report that the yearly number of fatalities caused by tainted food can reach around 600 million, or 1 in 10 individuals who would become ill (Ferone et al., 2020). The tiniest and most common parasites, viruses may alter the physiological behavior of their hosts—bacteria, plants, people, and animals—when they enter, multiply, and infect them. Many fatalities are happening worldwide as a result of their different modalities of action (Chippa and Suyarna 2021). The worldwide public health has been severely threatened by pathogenic microbial illnesses in recent times, particularly with the current COVID-19 epidemic (Udugama et al., 2020). Although other pathogens, such as fungi and protozoa, have distinct modes of contamination, they all have the ability to produce poisons when exposed to the extracellular biological milieu (Bolon et al., 2023). It is essential to find these biomolecules quickly since poisons lead to disease. Identification of secreted markers, or antigens and antibodies generated by the host, as well as surface indicators such as lipoproteins, lipids, glycoproteins, glycopeptides, and carbohydrates, is crucial in addition to toxin detection (Hussain, 2022).

Most pathogens, including bacteria, fungi, protozoa, and worms, are traditionally detected under a microscope, typically following growth in pure culture. Usually, a sample from the afflicted person is obtained, and the pathogen's existence is checked under a microscope. Additional biochemical testing and growth patterns in different media are used to confirm the presence of bacteria or fungus, with a few drawbacks despite their extreme specificity (Hailu and Hailu, 2020).

- Initially, high pathogen content is used in samples when using microscopy-based techniques.
- Second, in order for growth pattern approaches to provide results, the pathogen must typically grow in a specific medium and then be incubated for at least 24 hours.
- Third, the identification of certain microorganisms is made more difficult by the fact that they are difficult to develop in culture.

Numerous established techniques, such as blood culture, colony-forming unit counts, immunological tests, matrix-assisted laser desorption ionization time-of-flight mass spectrometry, microscopy, polymerase chain reaction (PCR), etc., are still used to test samples. While these techniques have a great degree of sensitivity, they have a number of disadvantages, including the need for expensive equipment, highly specialized labor, and additional time. Of these, immunological techniques take less time and are widely employed to identify poisons, viruses, and bacteria. They have several drawbacks, including poorer sensitivity, selectivity, specificity, affinity, and real-time pathogen detection. There is a need for quicker, less expensive, and maybe decentralized means of detection because, regrettably, there are still an infinite number of fatalities and morbidities that can be attributed to these delays. Numerous effective techniques have been developed in recent years for the immunoreaction-based detection of pathogens, including quartz crystal microbalance, colorimetry, PCR, fluorescence, electrogenerated chemiluminescence, enzyme-linked immunosorbent assay, time-resolved fluorescence assay, chemiluminescence immunoassay, bioluminescent immunoassay, and electrochemical immunoassay (Pirinçci et al., 2018; Alafeef et al., 2020). Many of these techniques have the drawbacks of being too costly, time-consuming, or nonselective. Furthermore, because these are subjective assessments, the interpretation of the results is constrained by the availability of specialized equipment (computer and software) and access to qualified professionals. Moreover, employing these methods to identify biofilm growth is difficult (Xu et al., 2020). In order to surmount the lack of available traditional methods, a variety of peptides, functionalized polymers, graphene-based polymer composites (Khan et al., 2018a), CRISPR-based probes (Shen et al., 2020), and NMs have been utilized to identify bacteria (Chen et al., 2018; Rajapaksha et al., 2019).

New ground has been made in the area of nanotechnology and the creation of the next generation of diagnostic instruments for pathogen detection with the development of unique and inventive NMs. In the field of biosensing, NMs such as nanotubes, nanowires, NPs, and nanosheets, along with porous nanostructures like anodic alumina, mesoporous silicon, porous silicon, and polystyrene nanochannels, have gained prominence recently due to their unique properties, which include small size (1–100 nm) and large surface area, which lead to reformed surface reactivity, quantum confinement effects, improved electrical conductivity, and magnetic properties (Reta et al., 2018). Gold nanoparticles (AuNPs), gold nanorods, quantum dots, silica NPs, and magnetic NPs are the ones garnering the most attention among all the NMs that provide optical sensing (Yin et al., 2019). Out of all of these materials, NPs have gained a lot of interest as a starting point for the creation of biosensors and as a nanoprobe for *in vivo* imaging to assess bacterial infections (Mustafa et al., 2017). A variety of NPs have been employed to create bacterial-responsive nanoprobes, including metallic NPs, metal oxide NPs, carbon NPs (CNPs), and other types of nanocomposites (Ostadhossein et al., 2018; Tang et al., 2019). This is because of its advantageous features, which include a sizable surface area, morphology that can be controlled, specialized and adjustable optical qualities, and remarkable mechanical, electromagnetic, and chemical properties (Fathi et al., 2019; Srivastava et al., 2019). CNPs are a new class of NPs designed for imaging and sensing agents because of their photobleaching resistance, which sets them apart from traditional fluorophores, as well as their low cost, biocompatibility, low toxicity, sensitivity to external stimuli, and scalable manufacture (Cui et al., 2020). Other kinds of NPs, such as metallic and metal oxide NPs, have special qualities like surface plasmon resonance (SPR), which makes them a viable option for identifying and imaging bacterial infections. CNPs are not among these classes of NPs (Peng and Chen, 2019). The creation of nanoprobes based on local SPR has received a great deal of interest. The creation of colorimetric, fluorescent, and nonlinear optical sensors for bacterial detection is made possible by the use of SPR (Zhao et al., 2018b).

NPs have shown to be very promising in the development of bacterial detection sensors (Table 10.2). Both *in vivo* and *in vitro* methods of microbe sensing are possible: *in vivo* involves monitoring living organisms in real time, while *in vitro* uses tissue samples for testing. Wireless exchange of personal health information is made possible by the increasing use of wireless internet (Han et al., 2018) and across all smartphones (Grossi et al., 2019). Detecting and monitoring infections in real time with a smartphone and sharing data with other locations through an internet server are made possible in large part by the Internet of Things (IoT). The Internet of Nano-Things, a network of nanoscale devices that are networked and link to the IoT, is the direction that the IoT is taking (Nayyar et al., 2017). Nanotechnology and artificial intelligence, a subset of machine learning, are working together to develop microbe detection techniques and bring humanity's goal of a sensor that fully satisfies the aforementioned requirements closer to reality (Hadoush et al., 2019).

TABLE 10.2 Various Nanoparticles-Enabled Methods for Bacterial Identification

Nanoparticles Material	Detection Approach	Pathogen Model	References
AuNP–polythiophene nanocomposite	Fluorescence	*P. acidilactici* *L. plantarum* *E. faecalis* *E. coli* *E. aerogenes* *P. aeruginosa*	Panda et al. (2008)
PDMS silver nanorod arrays	Surface-enhanced Raman scattering (SERS)	*P. aeruginosa*	Kumar et al. (2015)
Amphiphilic carbon dots	Fluorescence spectroscopy and microscopy	*E. coli* *S. typhimurium* *P. aeruginosa* *B. cereus*	Nandi et al. (2015)
Silver nanoparticle	Anodic particle coulometry technique	*E. coli*	Sepunaru et al. (2015)
Cysteine gold nanoparticles	Colorimetric	*E. coli*	Raj et al. (2015)
Silver nanoclusters	Visual inspection of the fluorescence output	*E. coli*	Xiong et al. (2016)
Au-coated magnetic nanoparticles conjugated with antibody	SERS detection method	*S. aureus*	Wang et al. (2016)
Polyethylenimine(PEI)-modified Au-coated magnetic microspheres and concentrated Au–Ag nanoparticles	SERS detection method	*E. coli* *S. aureus*	Wang et al. (2016)
CdS nanoparticles	Fluorescence microscopy	*D. caledoiensis* *P. aeruginosa* *E. coli* *S. aureus* *V. alginolyticus*	Qi et al. (2016)

TABLE 10.2 *(Continued)*

Nanoparticles Material	Detection Approach	Pathogen Model	References
Carbon dot nanoparticles	Nucleic acid detection	*K. pneumoniae*	Lee et al. (2017)
Carbon dots in alginate hydrogels	Fluorescence	*E. coli* (normal vs antibiotic resistant)	Chandra and Singh (2018)
HfO_2 NPs	*In vivo* imaging of bacteria using X-ray/CT	*S. mutans*	Ostadhossein et al. (2018)
Graphene nanoplatelet polymer composite	Electrochemical	*E. coli* *B. subtilis* *S. mutans*	Khan et al. (2018a)
Carbon dots encapsulated breakable organosilica nanocapsules	Immunofluorescence	*S. aureus*	Yang et al. (2018)
Au nanorods	Surface plasmon resonance response	*E. coli* *S. aureus*	Chen et al. (2018)
SiNPs-Ce6 nanocomposite	*In vivo* fluorescence imaging of bacteria	*P. aeruginosa* *S. aureus*	Tang et al. (2019)
Yttrium-doped carbon nanoparticles	Fluorescence	*E. coli* *B. subtilis* *S. mutans*	Alafeef et al. (2019)
Flower-based Au NPs	Colorimetric sensor	*S. typhimurium*, *L. monocytogenes*, *E. Coli*	Du et al. (2020)
Silver nanorod	SERS	*S. typhimurium*, *E. coli*, *B. Subtilis*	Prakash et al. (2019)

10.5.3 MICROBIAL NANOTECHNOLOGY AND DRUG DEVELOPMENT

Finding new drugs can be greatly aided by studying the seemingly limitless supply of unique bioactive chemicals found in nature. Natural products are the term used to describe these bioactive compounds. Plants, animals, and microbes are examples of living things that produce metabolites and/or by-products that are known as natural products. According to the WHO, about 60% of the world's population rely upon traditional medicine for their health care (El-Naggar et al., 2020; El-Sayed et al., 2020). Microbes are essential to the advancement of medicinal therapy and the chemistry of natural products. Since the discovery of penicillin, they have been regarded as a rich source of distinct bioactive chemicals. Although most polysaccharides come from plants, microorganism-derived polysaccharides have lately become important biopolymers. Today, microbe-derived polysaccharides are beginning to economically challenge other synthetic and natural polymers. The synthesis and utilization of microbial polysaccharides for a variety of purposes has several benefits (Table 10.3) (Abdel et al., 2020).

A handful of the polysaccharides derived from microorganisms that are used in nanoformulation for nutraceutical delivery for drug development have been highlighted in Table 10.4. The utilization of microbes in bio-mediated synthesis has surfaced as a viable preference to conventional techniques for synthesizing NPs. Microbial synthesis is a green, environmentally friendly method that produces NPs by using living organisms, including bacteria, actinomycetes, fungi, algae, viruses, and yeast. A safe, affordable, and sturdy method for synthesizing NPs with a range of sizes, shapes, compositions, and physicochemical characteristics is by the microbial approach. The synthesis of NPs in an aqueous environment with minimal expenses and energy requirements is made possible by this "green" approach, which is a practice that is appealing and can be readily expanded to a higher level. These microbiological agents also have the critical characteristic of being able to act as templates for the synthesis and organization of NPs into well-defined structures (Gahlawat and Choudhury 2019).

Nanotechnology may prove to be a ground-breaking invention for boosting the efficacy of nutraceuticals in numerous diseases by using their advantageous qualities, given their potential efficacy and limiting

TABLE 10.3 Microbial Polysaccharides and Its Application

Microbial Polysaccharides	Bacterial Source	Application	References
Alginate	Found in brown algae's cell walls, *Phyophyceae* included. Also, they come from a variety of bacterial sources, including *Macrocystis pyrifera*, *Laminaria*, *Ascophyllum nodosum*, *Azotobacter*, and *Pseudomonas*.	Due to their carboxyl and hydroxyl groups, they also have high mucoadhesive qualities, water solubility, thickening, and gelling characteristics, which make them useful for topical administration systems of nutraceuticals to boost their effectiveness and bioavailability.	Ahmad et al. (2022)
Curdlan	Isolated from *Rhizobium*, *Alcaligenes*, *Bacillus*, *Agrobacterium*, and *Cellulomonas*. This was seen in *Alcaligenes faecalis*.	Besides gelling, stabilizing, and thickening agents. Moreover, the pharmaceutical sector uses it to encapsulate medications. Phosphorylated and carboxymethylated derivatives of curdlan show great promise. Additionally, it has anti-inflammatory, anticancer, and immunomodulating qualities, all of which are beneficial when employing it as a medicinal delivery system.	Srivastava et al. (2022); Aquinas et al. (2022)
Dextran	Obtained from *Leuconostoc mesenteroides* and *Streptococcus*	It is the ideal biopolymer for creating nanoparticles for distribution since it is highly soluble, cytocompatible, biodegradable, and immunogenic. Furthermore, beginning April 2015, the World Health Organization (WHO) has recognized Dextran 70 as a necessary medication as a replacement for blood plasma. Nanocarriers made of highly water-soluble dextran can aid in drug dissolution and gastrointestinal membrane penetration. When artificial polymers build up as toxins and create negative effects, digestive enzymes metabolize dextran to a physiologically innocuous state. Prolonged retention duration, enhanced cargo molecule bioavailability, and colloidal stability against gastrointestinal tract enzyme degradation are critical for nanomaterials to maintain the integrity of delivery systems.	Hu et al. (2021)

TABLE 10.3 *(Continued)*

Microbial Polysaccharides	Bacterial Source	Application	References
Gellan	Found in *Sphingomonas elodea*	It is characterized by its quick gelation, mucoadhesiveness, biocompatibility, thermoresponsiveness, nontoxicity, elasticity, ease of derivatization, and resistance to heat and acid stress. In recent decades, there has been a significant increase in interest in pharmaceutical and biomedical research on this biopolymer, since it offers an ecologically sustainable alternative to synthetic polymers in drug delivery systems. For gellan, a variety of dose formulations are being investigated. Materials for coating, granulating agent, and tablet binder have been researched for traditional dosage forms.	Nayak et al. (2021); Costa and de la Torre (2022)
Levan	The first cultures that yield extremophilic levan were those of *Halomonas smyrnensis*. Levan has also been reported to be produced by *Bacillus, Acinetobacter, Acetobacter, Pseudomonas,* and *Zymomonas.*	It is an amphiphilic polymeric substance that is compatible with salts and surfactants and has the ability to create films with strong adhesion capabilities. Furthermore, it has great water retention capacity, biocompatibility, nontoxicity, and stability in hot, acidic, and alkaline conditions. One of levan's most appealing qualities is its ability to self-assemble into nanoparticles in water.	De et al. (2020)
Pullulan	Obtained from *Aureobasidium pullulans*	Because of its many qualities, including high solubility, structural flexibility, thickening, and encapsulating capacity, pullulan is widely employed in the food, biomedical, and pharmaceutical sectors. Pullulan is a flexible polymer with a high incidence of reactive hydroxyl groups. It may be conjugated with different bioactive substances or modified using different conjugation procedures to add more functional groups. Pullulan may be synthesized into a variety of shapes, such as nanospheres, nanogels, and nanoparticles, for effective bioactive chemical delivery. Several pullulan variants can be internalized by cells through integrin-mediated cell adhesion.	Rajalekshmy et al. (2021)
Xanthan	Found in *Xanthomonas campestris*	Xanthan is a perfect thickening, suspending, and stabilizing ingredient for the food, pharmaceutical, and cosmetics sectors because of its high viscosity, low pH, and resistance to salt.	Patel et al. (2021)

TABLE 10.4 Various Microbial Polysaccharide Nanoformulations

Polysaccharide Nutraceutical Encapsulation	Nanoformulation	References
Alginate/cashew gum *via* spray-drying method for *Lippia sidoides* essential oil encapsulation and delivery	Nanoparticles	Oliveira et al. (2014)
Curcumin water dispersibility and antioxidant activity using core–shell protein–polysaccharide	Nanoparticles	Huang et al. (2016)
Prebiotics enhance the antibacterial properties of *Lactobacillus plantarum*	Nanoparticles	Hong et al. (2019)
Resveratrol-loaded protein–polysaccharide–tea saponin complex	Nanoparticles	Wei et al. (2020)
Curcumin-casein-alginate-chitosan as a potential oral delivery system for cancer nutraceutical therapy	Nanoparticles	Elbialy and Mohamed (2022)
Effect of sodium alginate and different types of oil on the physical properties of ultrasound-assisted	Nanoemulsion	Branco et al. (2020)
Polysaccharide based like levan, fucoidan, alginate, guar gum , and κ-carrageenan, encapsulating curcumin	Nanoemulsion	Richa and Choudhury (2020)
Neorhizobiumurealyticum K1T sp. nov. exopolysaccharide astaxanthin to enhance the bioavailability	Nanoemulsion	Roychowdhury et al. (2021)
Developing natural, safe, and biocompatible nano-scale emulsions were prepared using γ-cyclodextrin (γ-CD), sodium caseinate (SC), and alginate (Alg) as emulsifiers	Nanoemulsion	Wang et al. (2022)
Curcumin is encapsulated in alginate aldehyde–gelatin (Alg Ald-Gel)	Nanogel	Sarika et al. (2016)
Preparation of protein/polysaccharide nanocomplexes for delivering environment-sensitive bioactive compounds is significant in the fields of functional foods and pharmaceuticals	Nanogel	Zeng et al. (2022)
Viscoelastic gels of xanthan gum-chitosan(X-Ch) in formic acid were electrospun to stabilize in aqueous media, for the encapsulation and release of curcumin (Cu)	Nanofibers	Shekarforoush et al. (2018)
Development of resveratrol-loaded chitosan-gellan, a novel gastrointestinal delivery system	Nanofibers	Rostami et al. (2019)
β-lactoglobulin (BLG) and four nutraceutical models, including β-carotene, folic acid, curcumin, and ergocalciferol	Nanocomplex	Hosseini et al. (2015)
Chitosan–Alginate nanocarrier for the encapsulation of essential oils as turmeric oil and lemongrass oil	Nanocapsule	Natrajan et al. (2015)
A novel delivery system was developed by coating dextran sulfate (DS) on the surface of amphiphilic chitosan derivative (DCMC-NL) through electrostatic interaction	Nanoliposomes	Zou et al. (2015)

features (Paolino et al., 2021). Bioactive molecules may be readily coupled with functional foods and beverages through the use of nanoencapsulation technologies, which preserve the product's beneficial qualities. The utilization of nanobiotechnology may allow nutraceuticals to be delivered directly to targeted organs in the human body, for instance, by crossing the blood–brain barrier to the brain (Figure 10.1) (Arshad et al., 2021).

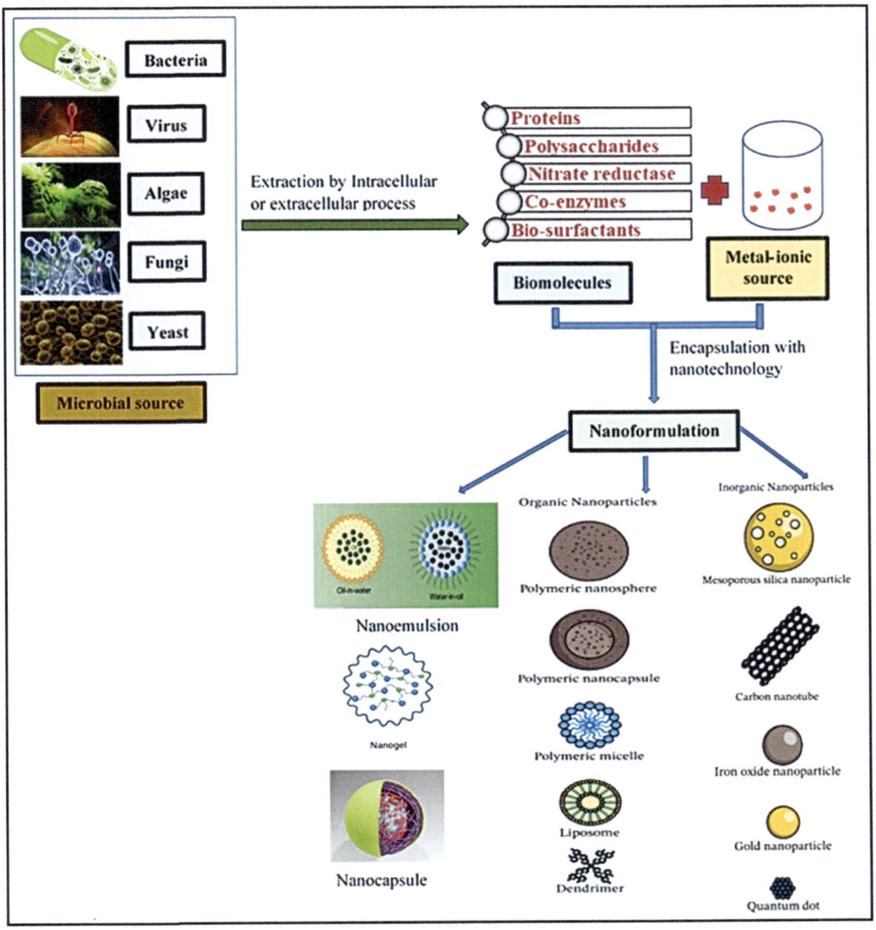

FIGURE 10.1 Various microbial-based nanoformulation.

10.5.3.1 MICROBIAL FORMULATION FOR CANCER THERAPY

At the molecular level, cancer is the second most common disease after cardiovascular-related diseases in terms of both death and morbidity. To treat diseases, numerous medications have been developed, produced, and/or separated from natural sources. A nano drug delivery system is a vital and substitute method of delivering chemotherapy drugs to the appropriate site at the appropriate timing, dose, and controlled amount in order to get the best possible therapeutic outcome with no or less toxicity. Due to improved permeability, retentive action, site-specific drug release, and accumulation, drug carriers at the nanoscale have less adverse pharmacological effects (Greish 2010; Shinde et al., 2012). Combining the actions of helpful bacteria with nanotechnology could provide a revolutionary therapeutic regimen for cancer treatments. Numerous advantageous microorganisms have demonstrated anticancer capabilities (Wu et al., 2016; Saxami et al., 2017; Chondrou et al., 2018), and combining them with nanotechnology can increase their efficacy. Table 10.5 provides an overview of the bacteria-based nanoformulation implemented in cancer treatment.

10.5.3.2 MICROBIAL FORMULATION FOR WOUND HEALING ACTIVITY

The process of healing wounds is intricate and necessitates the presence of multiple balanced microelements, antioxidants, matrix metalloproteins such as macrophage inflammatory protein 1 and chemoattractant protein 1, as well as growth factors. The cascade of wound healing may be impeded by deficiencies in copper, zinc, and calcium. Antimicrobial medicines are the best treatment for wound infection because they can stop the wound from becoming infected again. Antimicrobial drugs associated with NPs can address the wound-healing process (Ingle et al., 2017). A few of the microbes-based nanoformulation used for wound healing is discussed below:

An investigation reported the production of spherical-shaped AgNPs, AuNPs, and Ag/AuNPs utilizing the actinobacterium, *Streptomyces* sp., based on ointments *in vivo* wound model healing assessment revealed in Wistar rats 100% (after 19 and 21 days), correlated to the standard

TABLE 10.5 Bacteria-Based Nanoformulation in Cancer Treatment

Bacterial Source	Type of Cancer	Nanoformulation	Reference
Escherichia coli	HOS, MG63, and U2OS cancer cells	Polydopamine nanoparticles	Deng et al. (2021)
Shewanella oneidensis MR-1	CT26 tumor	Manganese dioxide nanoflowers	Chen et al. (2020)
Synechococcus 7942	4T1 tumor	Human serum albumin nanoparticles	Liu et al. (2020)
Salmonella typhimurium YB1	MB49 tumor	PLGA	Chen et al. (2019)
Escherichia coli MG1655	CT26 tumor	Magnetic Fe_3O_4 nanoparticle	Fan et al. (2019)
E. coli	4T1 and CT26 tumors	Carbon nitride (C_3N_4) semiconductor nanomaterials	Zheng et al. (2018)
S. typhimurium VNP20009	4T1 tumor	PLGA	Suh et al. (2019)
Bifidobacterium longum	MDA-MB-231 breast tumor	PLGA	Luo et al. (2019)

antibiotic nitrofurazone, 0.2% w/w ointment. In addition, the AuNPs produced by the bacteria demonstrated noteworthy antibacterial and anti-fungal properties against various strains of *Staphylococcus aureus* (NCIM 2079), *Escherichia coli* (NCIM 2256), *Pseudomonas aeruginosa* (NCIM 5031), *Klebsiella pneumoniae* (NCIM 2706), *Serratia marcescens* (NCIM 5246), *Candida albicans*, and *Candida glabrata*. The minimum inhibitory concentrations (MICs) of these strains were 25, 25, 6.25, 12.5, 12.5, 12.5, and 25 μg/mL, respectively (Shanmugasundaram et al., 2017). Alternatively, *Citrobacter braakii* microbial-developed AuNPs were further conjugated to polyethylene glycol (PEG) and polycaprolactone (PCL) and formed Au-PEG/PCL nanocomposites; wound healing was evaluated on the rats (Wang et al., 2018).

According to a study, the fungus *Fusarium oxysporum* mediated AgNPs showed considerable antibacterial activity against methicillin-resistant *S. aureus* (MRSA) and *S. aureus*, with MIC of 1.87 μg/mL for both bacterial strains. Additionally, AgNPs' ability to heal wounds was correlated to enoxaparin and AgNPs-enoxaparin conjugate on a rat model.

In one study, marine microalgae *Trichodesmium erythraeum* were used to create nanosized silver particles. These particles had an average particle size of 26.5 nm and shown outstanding antibacterial properties against clinical strains of *S. aureus* and *Proteus mirabilis*, with inhibition zones of 11 and 10 mm (Sathishkumar et al., 2019). As an alternative, an evaluation described the environmentally friendly production of selenium NPs (SeNPs) utilizing the probiotic bacteria *Lactobacillus acidophilus*, which had an average diameter of 2–15 nm. MIC90 values of 9.4, 1.2, 3.5, 6.5, and 4 μg/mL were recorded for the biogenic SeNPs against *E. coli*, *S. aureus*, *Bacillus subtilis*, *K. pneumoniae*, and *P. aeruginosa*, respectively, indicating their strong antibacterial properties.

On the other hand, AgNPs with an average hydrodynamic particle size of 86.38 nm were biofabricated using the cyanobacterium *Phormidium* sp. Following treatment, the wound contraction percentage was 26.67, 62.05, 86.45, and 100 at 3, 7, 14, and 21 days, respectively. The excision wound healing test demonstrated the wound healing activity of biogenic AgNPs at the concentration of 50 μg/kg of ointment (Younis et al., 2021).

In a related study, *Proteus vulgaris* was used to synthesize iron oxide NPs (IONPs) mediated by bacteria. The antibacterial activity of biogenic IONPs at a concentration of 40 μg/mL was assessed using the disc diffusion method against *Salmonella typhi*, *E. coli*, *S. aureus*, *Vibrio cholera*, and *Staphylococcus epidermidis*, with IZ values of 14, 13, 16, 11, and 12 mm, respectively (Majeed et al., 2021).

10.5.3.3 MICROBIAL FORMULATION FOR DIABETIC FOOT ULCER

One of the most dangerous and catastrophic effects of diabetes is diabetic foot ulcers (DFU), which cause a major reduction in life quality and high healthcare costs across the globe. This is one of the dominant causes of lower limb amputations and affects about 15% of diabetic individuals. Considering the delayed healing process and increased likelihood of microbial infections, which cause tissue damage, DFUs typically have poor clinical outcomes. Antimicrobial resistance is an increasing risk to world health these days, resulting in treating and caring for DFU being a challenge. Identifying more sustainable and less hazardous ways to combat these resistant microorganisms is of the utmost importance in consideration of the aforementioned fact. Antimicrobial peptides (AMPs) are tiny, naturally occurring compounds that are significant to the host's innate immune system. Certain molecules exhibit both wound-healing and broad-spectrum antibacterial traits, which make them prospective beneficial agents for the management of DFUs (Teixeira et al., 2023). Gram-positive strains such as *Corynebacterium striatum*, MRSA, and *S. aureus*, as well as Gram-negative strains like *P. aeruginosa* and *Alcaligenes faecalis*, constituted the majority of the bacteria discovered in DFU (Kalan and Brennan 2019). These findings were consistent with prior microbiological investigations that found *Proteus* species and *E. coli* to be the most common screened strains from DFU (Kalan and Brennan, 2019; Kareliya et al., 2019; Uivaraseanu et al., 2020). Moreover, a few anaerobes, such as *Peptostreptococcus* species, *Bacteroides* species, *Prevotella* species, and *Clostridium* species, have been detected in the deeper layers of tissue of diabetic wounds (Da Silva et al., 2021; Ramirez-Acuña et al., 2019; Kalan and Brennan 2019).

The discovery of novel alternative compounds and therapeutic techniques is unquestionably essential to address illnesses caused by bacteria that are resistant to many drugs. AMPs have received significant attention recently as a new group of antimicrobials with promising therapeutic applications (Browne et al., 2020). All living organisms include AMPs, sometimes referred to as host-defense peptides, which are effectors or molecules of the innate immune system (Browne et al., 2020; Uivaraseanu et al., 2020; Fry 2018). These tiny molecules have a variety of vital roles in the immune system's defense against infection, including immunomodulatory responses and other processes related to wound healing (Rademacher et al., 2021). The most prevalent manner that AMPs work is by targeting the membranes of bacteria (Da Silva et al., 2021; Browne et al., 2020). Marine organisms have evolved a broad range of bioactive compounds and defense mechanisms against viral and prokaryotic infections across their evolutionary history (Smith et al., 2010). In this regard, cyanobacteria and microalgae offer interesting sources of compounds with antibacterial properties. They can counter various environmental pressures and nutritional sources, and they can accustom to a broad range of environmental circumstances, including highly competitive ones, due to their flexible metabolism. They are also exposed to a variety of microbiological infections and predators (Rojas et al., 2020). These microbes have responded to these stimuli by developing an extensive spectrum of antimicrobial compounds that have a broad range of potential utilization in the domains of biotechnology, medicine, agriculture, and aquaculture (Falaise et al., 2016).

From Piti Bomb Holes in Guam, Montaser et al. discovered pitipeptolides C–F from the marine cyanobacterium *Lyngbya majuscula*. According to this investigation, the most effective substance against *Mycobacterium tuberculosis* in a disc diffusion test was pitipeptolides F (Montaser et al., 2011). Isolated from the cultivated cyanobacterium *Microcystis aeruginosa* (NIES-88), the cyclic undecapeptide Kawaguchipeptin B shows antibacterial activity against *S. aureus* (Ishida et al., 1997). A different investigation by Dussault et al. found that some cyanobacterial peptides (laxaphycins A, B, and C3) displayed antibacterial action against Gram-positive bacteria after investigating the impact of 10 cyanobacterial isolates on the proliferation of foodborne pathogens (Dussault et al., 2016). Peptides from the Lyngbyazothrins combination C/D and laxaphycin A, B, and B3 that were produced using environmentally sustainable methods also demonstrated efficacy against common infections associated with chronic DFUs. *P. aeruginosa, B. subtilis, E. coli*, and *S. marcescens* were all susceptible to the antibacterial action of the cyclic undecapeptides Lyngbyazothrins C/D. *Listeria monocytogenes, Bacillus cereus*, and *S. aureus* were all susceptible to the antibacterial activity of the cyanobacterial peptides laxaphycins A, B, and B3 (Dussault et al., 2016).

Since AMPs acquired from microorganisms are active against a variety of Gram-positive and Gram-negative bacteria, they represent a possible substitute for treating infected wounds. Furthermore, AMPs have the capacity to promote cell migration and proliferation, have angiogenic and immunomodulatory effects, and hasten the healing of wounds (Da Silva et al., 2021). While the AMPs mentioned above were produced by sustainable methods and may be useful as a treatment option for DFUs, several of their internal processes still require improvement in order to provide an entirely environmentally friendly regimen.

10.6 CONCLUSION

The unique properties and accurately calibrated biocompatible measurements of microbe-produced NMs make them intriguing for a broad spectrum of medicinal and biological applications. Since NMs are frequently enclosed with biomolecule entities or a lipid layer that offers physiological solubility and stability—two attributes that are essential for medical utilization and a drawback of other synthesis techniques—biosynthesis *via* extracellular and intracellular approaches is also advantageous. The current review discussed an array of eco-friendly NM synthesis, showing how different biomolecules and organisms can be used as nanofactories. This review has also demonstrated how inexpensive, easy to scale up, and sustainable these nanofactories are for the production of drugs by means of microbial nanoformulation. This review covers the use of diverse biogenic NMs in a broad spectrum of applications, with an emphasis on nanoformulation for drug development for wound healing, diabetic foot ulcer treatment, cancer therapy, and pathogen detection.

Microbial nanotechnology is an exciting and growing subject for potential breakthrough NM synthesis, as seen by the current findings covered here. Microbial nanotechnology has the potential to significantly advance nanomanufacturing innovation through a "green" and sustainable manner, with significant implications for sensoristics and biomedicine, among other domains.

KEYWORDS

- **nanomaterials**
- **nanoformulations**
- **microorganisms**
- **biomolecules**
- **drug development**
- **bacteria**
- **fungi**

REFERENCES

Abdulla, N. K., Siddiqui, S. I., Fatima, B., Sultana, R., Tara, N., Hashmi, A. A., Chaudhry, S. A. (2021). Silver based hybrid nanocomposite: A novel antibacterial material for water cleansing. *Journal of Cleaner Production*, *284*, 124746.

Ahmad, A., Gulraiz, Y., Ilyas, S., Bashir, S. (2022). Polysaccharide based nano materials: Health implications. *Food Hydrocolloids for Health*, *2*, 100075.

Ahmad, R., Srivastava, S., Ghosh, S., Khare, S. K. (2021). Phytochemical delivery through nanocarriers: A review. *Colloids and Surfaces B: Biointerfaces*, *197*, 111389.

Akintayo, G. O., Lateef, A., Azeez, M. A., Asafa, T. B., Oladipo, I. C., Badmus, J. A., Ojo, S. A., Elegbede, J. A., Gueguim-Kana, E. B., Beukes, L. S., Yekeen, T. A. (2020). Synthesis, bioactivities and cytogenotoxicity of animal fur-mediated silver nanoparticles. *IOP Conference Series: Materials Science and Engineering*, *805*(1), 012041.

Alafeef, M., Moitra, P., Pan, D. (2020). Nano-enabled sensing approaches for pathogenic bacterial detection. *Biosensors and Bioelectronics*, *165*, 112276.

Al-Dhabi, N. A., Mohammed Ghilan, A. K., Arasu, M. V. (2018). Characterization of silver nanomaterials derived from marine *Streptomyces* sp. al-dhabi-87 and it's in vitro application against multidrug resistant and extended-spectrum beta-lactamase clinical pathogens. *Nanomaterials*, *8*(5), 279.

Alghuthaymi, M. A., Almoammar, H., Rai, M., Said-Galiev, E., Abd-Elsalam, K. A. (2015). Myconanoparticles: Synthesis and their role in phytopathogens management. *Biotechnology and Biotechnological Equipment*, *29*(2), 221–236.

Alphandery, E., Faure, S., Seksek, O., Guyot, F., Chebbi, I. (2011). Chains of magnetosomes extracted from AMB-1 magnetotactic bacteria for application in alternative magnetic field cancer therapy. *ACS Nano*, *5*(8), 6279–6296.

Apte, M., Sambre, D., Gaikawad, S., Joshi, S., Bankar, A., Kumar, A. R., Zinjarde, S. (2013). Psychrotrophic yeast *Yarrowia lipolytica* NCYC 789 mediates the synthesis of antimicrobial silver nanoparticles via cell-associated melanin. *AMB Express*, *3*, 1–8.

Aquinas, N., Bhat, M. R., Selvaraj, S. (2022). A review presenting production, characterization, and applications of biopolymer curdlan in food and pharmaceutical sectors. *Polymer Bulletin*, *79*(9), 6905–6927.

Arshad, R., Gulshad, L., Haq, I. U., Farooq, M. A., Al-Farga, A., Siddique, R., Karrar, E. (2021). Nanotechnology: A novel tool to enhance the bioavailability of micronutrients. *Food Science and Nutrition*, *9*(6), 3354–3361.

Ball, A. S., Patil, S., Soni, S. (2019). Introduction into nanotechnology and microbiology. In: Gurtler, V., Ball, A. S., Soni, S. (Eds.), *Methods in Microbiology* (pp. 1–18, Vol. 46). Academic Press: Australia.

Balzani, V. (2005). Nanoscience and nanotechnology: A personal view of a chemist. *Small*, *1*(3), 278–283.

Bao, H., Lu, Z., Cui, X., Qiao, Y., Guo, J., Anderson, J. M., Li, C. M. (2010). Extracellular microbial synthesis of biocompatible CdTe quantum dots. *Acta Biomaterialia*, *6*(9), 3534–3541.

Bhushan, B. (2017). Introduction to nanotechnology. In: Bhushan, B. (Ed.), *Springer Handbook of Nanotechnology* (pp. 1–19). Springer: Berlin, Heidelberg.

Blanco, E., Shen, H., Ferrari, M. (2015). Principles of nanoparticle design for overcoming biological barriers to drug delivery. *Nature Biotechnology*, *33*(9), 941–951.

Bolon, B., Uzal, F. A., Schutten, M. (2023). Bacterial toxins. In: Haschek, W. M., Rousseaux, C. G., Wallig, M. A., Bolon, B. (Eds.), *Haschek and Rousseaux's Handbook of Toxicologic Pathology* (Vol. 3, pp. 629–678). Academic Press: San Diego.

Boucher, M., Geffroy, F., Prévéral, S., Bellanger, L., Selingue, E., Adryanczyk-Perrier, G., Pean, M., Lefevre, C. T., Pignol, D., Ginet, N., Mériaux, S. (2017). Genetically tailored magnetosomes used as MRI probe for molecular imaging of brain tumor. *Biomaterials*, *121*, 167–178.

Branco, I. G., Sen, K., Rinaldi, C. (2020). Effect of sodium alginate and different types of oil on the physical properties of ultrasound-assisted nanoemulsions. *Chemical Engineering and Processing-Process Intensification*, *153*, 107942.

Browne, K., Chakraborty, S., Chen, R., Willcox, M. D., Black, D. S., Walsh, W. R., Kumar, N. (2020). A new era of antibiotics: The clinical potential of antimicrobial peptides. *International Journal of Molecular Sciences*, *21*(19), 7047.

Casillo, A., Lanzetta, R., Parrilli, M., Corsaro, M. M. (2018). Exopolysaccharides from marine and marine extremophilic bacteria: Structures, properties, ecological roles and applications. *Marine Drugs*, *16*(2), 69.

Castro-Longoria, E., Vilchis-Nestor, A. R., Avalos-Borja, M. (2011). Biosynthesis of silver, gold and bimetallic nanoparticles using the filamentous fungus *Neurospora crassa. Colloids and Surfaces B: Biointerfaces*,, *83*(1), 42–48.

Chandra, A., Singh, N. (2018). Bacterial growth sensing in microgels using pH-dependent fluorescence emission. *Chemical Communications*, *54*(13), 1643–1646.

Chen, P. Y., Dang, X., Klug, M. T., Courchesne, N. M. D., Qi, J., Hyder, M. N., Belcher, A. M., Hammond, P. T. (2015). M13 virus-enabled synthesis of titanium dioxide nanowires for tunable mesoporous semiconducting networks. *Chemistry of Materials*, *27*(5), 1531–1540.

Chen, C. C., Stark, M., Baikoghli, M., Cheng, R. H. (2018). Surface functionalization of hepatitis E virus nanoparticles using chemical conjugation methods. *Journal of Visualized Experiments*, *135*, e57020.

Chen, F., Zang, Z., Chen, Z., Cui, L., Chang, Z., Ma, A., Yin, T., Han, Y., Wu, Z., Zheng, M., Liu, C., Cai, L. (2019). Nanophotosensitizer-engineered Salmonella bacteria with hypoxia targeting and photothermal-assisted mutual bioaccumulation for solid tumor therapy. *Biomaterials*, *214*, 119226.

Chen, Q. W., Wang, J. W., Wang, X. N., Fan, J. X., Liu, X. H., Li, B., Han, Z. Y., Cheng, S. X., Zhang, X. Z. (2020). Inhibition of tumor progression through the coupling of bacterial respiration with tumor metabolism. *Angewandte Chemie International Edition*, *59*(48), 21562–21570.

Chen, S., Li, Q., Wang, X., Yang, Y. W., Gao, H. (2018). Multifunctional bacterial imaging and therapy systems. *Journal of Materials Chemistry B*, *6*(32), 5198–5214.

Chippa, S., Suvarna, V. (2021). Nanotechnology for detection of diseases caused by viruses-current overview. *International Journal of Pharmacy and Pharmaceutical Sciences*, *13*, 1–7.

Chondrou, P., Karapetsas, A., Kiousi, D. E., Tsela, D., Tiptiri-Kourpeti, A., Anestopoulos, I., Kotsianidis, I., Bezirtzoglou, E., Pappa, A., Galanis, A. (2018). *Lactobacillus paracasei* K5 displays adhesion, anti-proliferative activity and apoptotic effects in human colon cancer cells. *Beneficial Microbes*, *9*(6), 975–983.

Costa, A. L. R., de la Torre, L. G. (2022). Gellan gum nanoparticles in drug delivery. In: Jana, S., Jana, S. (Eds.), *Micro- and Nanoengineered Gum-based Biomaterials for Drug Delivery and Biomedical Applications* (pp. 127–156). Elsevier.

Cui, F., Ye, Y., Ping, J., Sun, X. (2020). Carbon dots: Current advances in pathogenic bacteria monitoring and prospect applications. *Biosensors and Bioelectronics*, *156*, 112085.

Czapar, A. E., Zheng, Y. R., Riddell, I. A., Shukla, S., Awuah, S. G., Lippard, S. J., Steinmetz, N. F. (2016). Tobacco mosaic virus delivery of phenanthriplatin for cancer therapy. *ACS Nano*, *10*(4), 4119–4126.

Da Silva, J., Leal, E. C., Carvalho, E. (2021). Bioactive antimicrobial peptides as therapeutic agents for infected diabetic foot ulcers. *Biomolecules*, *11*(12), 1894.

Dameron, C. T., Reese, R. N., Mehra, R. K., Kortan, A. R., Carroll, P. J., Steigerwald, M. L., Brus, M. L., Winge, D. R. (1989). Biosynthesis of cadmium sulphide quantum semiconductor crystallites. *Nature*, *338*, 596–597.

de Oliveira, E. F., Paula, H. C., de Paula, R. C. (2014). Alginate/cashew gum nanoparticles for essential oil encapsulation. *Colloids and Surfaces B: Biointerfaces*, *113*, 146–151.

Demain, A. L. (2002). Prescription for an ailing pharmaceutical industry. *Nature Biotechnology*, *20*(4), 331–331.

Demain, A. L., Adrio, J. L. (2008). Contributions of microorganisms to industrial biology. *Molecular Biotechnology*, *38*, 41–55.

Deng, X., Yang, W., Shao, Z., Zhao, Y. (2021). Genetically modified bacteria for targeted phototherapy of tumor. *Biomaterials*, *272*, 120809.

Denyer, S. P., Hodges, N. A., Gorman, S. P. (2004). Introduction to pharmaceutical microbiology. In: Denyer, S. P., Hodges, N. A., Gorman, S. P. (Eds.), *Hugo and Russell's Pharmaceutical Microbiology* (pp. 220–232). Blackwell Science: UK.

Dey, P., Fabri-Faja, N., Calvo-Lozano, O., Terborg, R. A., Belushkin, A., Yesilkoy, F., Fabrega, A., Ruiz-Rodriguez, J. C., Ferrer, R., Gonzalez-Lopez, J. J., Estevez, M. C., Altug, H., Pruneri, V., Lechuga, L. M. (2019). Label-free bacteria quantification in blood plasma by a bioprinted microarray based interferometric point-of-care device. *ACS Sensors*, *4*(1), 52–60.

Dhandapani, P., Maruthamuthu, S., Rajagopal, G. (2012). Bio-mediated synthesis of TiO_2 nanoparticles and its photocatalytic effect on aquatic biofilm. *Journal of Photochemistry and Photobiology B: Biology*, *110*, 43–49.

Dhillon, G. S., Brar, S. K., Kaur, S., Verma, M. (2012). Green approach for nanoparticle biosynthesis by fungi: Current trends and applications. *Critical Reviews in Biotechnology*, *32*(1), 49–73.

Divya, M., Kiran, G. S., Hassan, S., Selvin, J. (2019). Biogenic synthesis and effect of silver nanoparticles (AgNPs) to combat catheter-related urinary tract infections. *Biocatalysis and Agricultural Biotechnology*, *18*, 101037.

Du, L., Jiang, H., Liu, X., Wang, E. (2007). Biosynthesis of gold nanoparticles assisted by *Escherichia coli* DH5α and its application on direct electrochemistry of hemoglobin. *Electrochemistry Communications*, *9*(5), 1165–1170.

Du, J., Wu, S., Niu, L., Li, J., Zhao, D., Bai, Y. (2020). A gold nanoparticles-assisted multiplex PCR assay for simultaneous detection of *Salmonella typhimurium*, *Listeria monocytogenes* and *Escherichia coli* O157: H7. *Analytical Methods*, *12*(2), 212–217.

Dussault, D., Vu, K. D., Vansach, T., Horgen, F. D., Lacroix, M. (2016). Antimicrobial effects of marine algal extracts and cyanobacterial pure compounds against five foodborne pathogens. *Food Chemistry*, *199*, 114–118.

Dykman, L., Khlebtsov, N. (2012). Gold nanoparticles in biomedical applications: Recent advances and perspectives. *Chemical Society Reviews*, *41*(6), 2256–2282.

Elbialy, N. S., Mohamed, N. (2022). Fabrication of the quaternary nanocomplex curcumin-casein-alginate-chitosan as a potential oral delivery system for cancer nutraceutical therapy. *Journal of Drug Delivery Science and Technology*, *70*, 103226.

Elegbede, J. A., Lateef, A., Azeez, M. A., Asafa, T. B., Yekeen, T. A., Oladipo, I. C., Aina, D. A., Beukes, L. S., Gueguim-Kana, E. B. (2020). Biofabrication of gold nanoparticles using xylanases through valorization of corncob by *Aspergillus niger* and *Trichoderma longibrachiatum*: Antimicrobial, antioxidant, anticoagulant and thrombolytic activities. *Waste and Biomass Valorization*, *11*, 781–791.

El-Naggar, M. E., Soliman, R. A., Morsy, O. M., Abdel-Aziz, M. S. (2020). Nanoemulsion of capsicum fruit extract as an eco-friendly antimicrobial agent for production of medical bandages. *Biocatalysis and Agricultural Biotechnology*, *23*, 101516.

El-Sayed, S. M., El-Naggar, M. E., Hussein, J., Medhat, D., El-Banna, M. (2019). Effect of *Ficus carica* L. leaves extract loaded gold nanoparticles against cisplatin-induced acute kidney injury. *Colloids and Surfaces B: Biointerfaces*, *184*, 110465.

Elsoud, M. M. A., Al-Hagar, O. E., Abdelkhalek, E. S., Sidkey, N. M. (2018). Synthesis and investigations on tellurium myconanoparticles. *Biotechnology Reports*, *18*, e00247.

Esfandiari, N., Arzanani, M. K., Soleimani, M., Kohi-Habibi, M., Svendsen, W. E. (2016). A new application of plant virus nanoparticles as drug delivery in breast cancer. *Tumor Biology*, *37*, 1229–1236.

Eugenio, M., Müller, N., Frases, S., Almeida-Paes, R., Lima, L. M. T., Lemgruber, L., Farina, M., de Souza, W., Sant'Anna, C. (2016). Yeast-derived biosynthesis of silver/silver chloride nanoparticles and their antiproliferative activity against bacteria. *RSC Advances*, *6*(12), 9893–9904.

Falaise, C., François, C., Travers, M. A., Morga, B., Haure, J., Tremblay, R., Turcotte, F., Pasetto, P., Gastineau, R, Hardivillier, Y., Leignel, V., Mouget, J. L. (2016). Antimicrobial compounds from eukaryotic microalgae against human pathogens and diseases in aquaculture. *Marine Drugs*, *14*(9), 159.

Fan, J. X., Peng, M. Y., Wang, H., Zheng, H. R., Liu, Z. L., Li, C. X., Wang, X. N., Liu, X. H., Cheng, S. X., Zhang, X. Z. (2019). Engineered bacterial bioreactor for tumor therapy via Fenton-like reaction with localized H_2O_2 generation. *Advanced Materials*, *31*(16), 1808278.

Fariq, A., Khan, T., Yasmin, A. (2017). Microbial synthesis of nanoparticles and their potential applications in biomedicine. *Journal of Applied Biomedicine*, *15*(4), 241–248.

Fathi, P., Khamo, J. S., Huang, X., Srivastava, I., Esch, M. B., Zhang, K., Pan, D. (2019). Bulk-state and single-particle imaging are central to understanding carbon dot photo-physics and elucidating the effects of precursor composition and reaction temperature. *Carbon*, *145*, 572–585.

Ferone, M., Gowen, A., Fanning, S., Scannell, A. G. (2020). Microbial detection and identification methods: Bench top assays to omics approaches. *Comprehensive Reviews in Food Science and Food Safety*, *19*(6), 3106–3129.

Fry, D. E. (2018). Antimicrobial peptides. *Surgical Infections*, *19*(8), 804–811.

Gahlawat, G., Choudhury, A. R. (2019). A review on the biosynthesis of metal and metal salt nanoparticles by microbes. *RSC Advances*, *9*(23), 12944–12967.

Gahlawat, G., Shikha, S., Chaddha, B. S., Chaudhuri, S. R., Mayilraj, S., Choudhury, A. R. (2016). Microbial glycolipoprotein-capped silver nanoparticles as emerging antibacterial agents against cholera. *Microbial Cell Factories*, *15*, 1–14.

Ghosh, S., Ahmad, R., Zeyaullah, M., Khare, S. K. (2021). Microbial nano-factories: Synthesis and biomedical applications. *Frontiers in Chemistry*, *9*, 626834.

Gilmore, B. F., Denyer, S. P. (Eds.). *Hugo and Russell's Pharmaceutical Microbiology*. John Wiley & Sons, 2023.

Giri, S., Markandeywar, T. S., Irfan, Z., Manna, S. (2023). Gellan gum and sodium alginate in-situ gel of monocaprin for effective corneal permeation. *Food Hydrocolloids for Health*, *4*, 100156.

Grasso, G., Zane, D., Dragone, R. (2019). Microbial nanotechnology: Challenges and prospects for green biocatalytic synthesis of nanoscale materials for sensoristic and biomedical applications. *Nanomaterials*, *10*(1), 11.

Greish, K. (2010). Enhanced permeability and retention (EPR) effect for anticancer nanomedicine drug targeting. In: Grobmyer, S., Moudgil, B. (Eds.), *Cancer Nanotechnology* (Vol. 624, pp. 25–37), Humana Press: Totowa, NJ, USA.

Grossi, M. (2019). A sensor-centric survey on the development of smartphone measurement and sensing systems. *Measurement*, *135*, 572–592.

Hadoush, H., Alafeef, M., Abdulhay, E. (2019). Automated identification for autism severity level: EEG analysis using empirical mode decomposition and second order difference plot. *Behavioural Brain Research*, *362*, 240–248.

Hailu, F. A., Hailu, Y. A. (2020). Agro-ecological importance of nematodes (round worms). *Acta Scientific Agriculture*, *4*(1), 156–162.

Han, S., Kim, J., Won, S. M., Ma, Y., Kang, D., Xie, Z., Lee, K.-T., Chung, H. U., Banks, A., Min, S., Heo, S. Y., Davies, C. R., Lee, J. W., Lee, C.-H., Kim, B. H., Li, K., Zhou, Y., Wei, C., Feng, X., Huang, Y., Rogers, J. A. (2018). Battery-free, wireless sensors for full-body pressure and temperature mapping. *Science Translational Medicine*, *10*, eaan4950.

Hasanin, M. S., Mostafa, A. M., Mwafy, E. A., Darwesh, O. M. (2018). Eco-friendly cellulose nano fibers via first reported egyptian *Humicolafuscoatra* Egyptia X4: Isolation and characterization. *Environmental Nanotechnology Monitoring and Management*, *10*, 409–418.

Hong, L., Kim, W. S., Lee, S. M., Kang, S. K., Choi, Y. J., Cho, C. S. (2019). Pullulan nanoparticles as prebiotics enhance the antibacterial properties of *Lactobacillus plantarum* through the induction of mild stress in probiotics. *Frontiers in Microbiology*, *10*, 142.

Hosseini, S. M. H., Emam-Djomeh, Z., Sabatino, P., Van der Meeren, P. (2015). Nanocomplexes arising from protein-polysaccharide electrostatic interaction as a promising carrier for nutraceutical compounds. *Food Hydrocolloids*, *50*, 16–26.

Hu, Q., Lu, Y., Luo, Y. (2021). Recent advances in dextran-based drug delivery systems: From fabrication strategies to applications. *Carbohydrate Polymers*, *264*, 117999.

Huang, X., Huang, X., Gong, Y., Xiao, H., McClements, D. J., Hu, K. (2016). Enhancement of curcumin water dispersibility and antioxidant activity using core–shell protein–polysaccharide nanoparticles. *Food Research International*, *87*, 1–9.

Hulkoti, N. I., Taranath, T. C. (2014). Biosynthesis of nanoparticles using microbes—a review. *Colloids and Surfaces B: Biointerfaces*, *121*, 474–483.

Hussain, C. M. (2022). *Handbook of Microbial Nanotechnology* (pp. 45–69). Academic Press.

Husseiny, S. M., Salah, T. A., Anter, H. A. (2015). Biosynthesis of size-controlled silver nanoparticles by *Fusarium oxysporum*, their antibacterial and antitumor activities. *Beni-Suef University Journal of Basic and Applied Sciences*, *4*(3), 225–231.

Ingle, A. P., Paralikar, P., Pandit, R., Anasane, N., Gupta, I., Rai, M., Chaud, M. V., Alves dos Santos, C. (2017). Nanoformulations for wound infections. In: Rai, M., dos Santos, C. A. (Eds.), *Nanotechnology Applied to Pharmaceutical Technology* (pp. 223–246). Springer: Cham.

Inshakova, E., Inshakov, O. (2017). World market for nanomaterials: Structure and trends. In: *MATEC Web of Conferences* (Vol. 129, p. 02013). EDP Sciences.

Ishida, K., Matsuda, H., Murakami, M., Yamaguchi, K. (1997). Kawaguchipeptin B, an antibacterial cyclic undecapeptide from the cyanobacterium *Microcystis aeruginosa*. *Journal of Natural Products*, *60*(7), 724–726.

Jafari, M., Rokhbakhsh-Zamin, F., Shakibaie, M., Moshafi, M. H., Ameri, A., Rahimi, H. R., Forootanfar, H. (2018). Cytotoxic and antibacterial activities of biologically synthesized gold nanoparticles assisted by *Micrococcus yunnanensis* strain J2. *Biocatalysis and Agricultural Biotechnology*, *15*, 245–253.

Jeevanandam, J., Chan, Y. S., Danquah, M. K. (2016). Biosynthesis of metal and metal oxide nanoparticles. *ChemBioEng Reviews*, *3*(2), 55–67.

Jeevanandam, J., Dable-Tupas, G., De Guzman, M. B. (2022). Applications of nanotechnology in pharmaceutical products. In: Egbuna, C., Gaman, M. A., Jeevanandam, J. (Eds.), *Applications of Nanotechnology in Drug Discovery and Delivery* (pp. 119–156). Elsevier.

Kalan, L. R., Brennan, M. B. (2019). The role of the microbiome in nonhealing diabetic wounds. *Annals of the New York Academy of Sciences*, *1435*(1), 79–92.

Kalishwaralal, K., Banumathi, E., Pandian, S. R. K., Deepak, V., Muniyandi, J., Eom, S. H., Gurunathan, S. (2009). Silver nanoparticles inhibit VEGF induced cell proliferation and migration in bovine retinal endothelial cells. *Colloids and Surfaces B: Biointerfaces*, *73*(1), 51–57.

Kalishwaralal, K., Deepak, V., Pandian, S. R. K., Kottaisamy, M., BarathManiKanth, S., Kartikeyan, B., Gurunathan, S. (2010). Biosynthesis of silver and gold nanoparticles using *Brevibacterium casei*. *Colloids and Surfaces B: Biointerfaces*, *77*(2), 257–262.

Kalpana, V. N., Kataru, B. A. S., Sravani, N., Vigneshwari, T., Panneerselvam, A., Rajeswari, V. D. (2018). Biosynthesis of zinc oxide nanoparticles using culture filtrates of *Aspergillus niger*: Antimicrobial textiles and dye degradation studies. *OpenNano*, *3*, 48–55.

Kapoor, D., Sharma, P., Sharma, M. M. M., Kumari, A., Kumar, R. (2020). Microbes in pharmaceutical industry. In Sharma, S. G., Sharma, N. R., Sharma, M. (Eds.), *Microbial Diversity, Interventions and Scope* (pp. 259–299). Springer: Singapore.

Kareliya, H., Bichile, L., Bal, A., Varaiya, A., Bhalekar, P. (2019). Fungal infection in diabetic foot a clinicomicrobiological study. *Acta Scientific Microbiology*, *2*, 49–55.

Karunaratne, D. N. (2010). Nanotechnology in medicine. *Journal of the National Science Foundation of Sri Lanka*, *35*, 149–152.

Khan, M. S., Misra, S. K., Dighe, K., Wang, Z., Schwartz-Duval, A. S., Sar, D., Pan, D. (2018a). Electrically-receptive and thermally-responsive paper-based sensor chip for rapid detection of bacterial cells. *Biosensors and Bioelectronics*, *110*, 132–140.

Khan, T., Abbas, S., Fariq, A., Yasmin, A. (2018b). Microbes: Nature's cell factories of nanoparticles synthesis. In: Prasad, R., Jha, A., Prasad, K. (Eds.), *Exploring the Realms of Nature for Nanosynthesis* (pp. 25–50). Springer: Cham.

Kiessling, F., Mertens, M. E., Grimm, J., Lammers, T. (2014). Nanoparticles for imaging: Top or flop? *Radiology*, *273*(1), 10–28.

Kobayashi, M., Tomita, S., Sawada, K., Shiba, K., Yanagi, H., Yamashita, I., Uraoka, Y. (2012). Chiral meta-molecules consisting of gold nanoparticles and genetically engineered tobacco mosaic virus. *Optics Express*, *20*(22), 24856–24863.

Koul, B., Poonia, A. K., Yadav, D., Jin, J. O. (2021). Microbe-mediated biosynthesis of nanoparticles: Applications and future prospects. *Biomolecules*, *11*(6), 886.

Kröger, N., Poulsen, N. (2008). Diatoms—from cell wall biogenesis to nanotechnology. *Annual Review of Genetics*, *42*, 83–107.

Kumar, S., Lodhi, D. K., Goel, P., Mishra, P., Singh, J. P. (2015). A facile method for fabrication of buckled PDMS silver nanorod arrays as active 3D SERS cages for bacterial sensing. *Chemical Communications*, *51*(62), 12411–12414.

Lambert, B. J., Hansen, J. M., Bryans, T. D., Lam, S. (2021). Sterility assurance across-sectors—new paradigms and tools. *Frontiers in Medical Technology*, *3*, 622710.

Lateef, A., Ojo, S. A., Elegbede, J. A., Akinola, P. O., Akanni, E. O. (2018). Nanomedical applications of nanoparticles for blood coagulation disorders. In: Dasgupta, N., Ranjan, S., Lichtfouse, E. (Eds.), *Environmental Nanotechnology* (pp. 243–277, Vol. 14). Springer: Cham, Switzerland.

Lee, H. N., Ryu, J. S., Shin, C., Chung, H. J. (2017). A Carbon-dot-based fluorescent nanosensor for simple visualization of bacterial nucleic acids. *Macromolecular Bioscience*, *17*(9), 1700086.

Li, C., Zhou, L., Yang, H., Lv, R., Tian, P., Li, X., Zhang, Y., Chen, Z., Lin, F. (2017). Self-assembled exopolysaccharide nanoparticles for bioremediation and green synthesis of noble metal nanoparticles. *ACS Applied Materials and Interfaces*, *9*(27), 22808–22818.

Li, X., Xu, H., Chen, Z. S., Chen, G. (2011). Biosynthesis of nanoparticles by microorganisms and their applications. *Journal of Nanomaterials*, *2011*, 1–16.

Liu, L., He, H., Luo, Z., Zhou, H., Liang, R., Pan, H., Ma, Y., Cai, L. (2020). In situ photocatalyzed oxygen generation with photosynthetic bacteria to enable robust immunogenic photodynamic therapy in triple-negative breast cancer. *Advanced Functional Materials*, *30*(10), 1910176.

Lorenzo, J. M., Munekata, P. E., Dominguez, R., Pateiro, M., Saraiva, J. A., Franco, D. (2018). Main groups of microorganisms of relevance for food safety and stability. In: Barba, F. J., Sant'Ana, A. S., Orlien, V., Koubaa, M. (Eds.), *Innovative Technologies for Food Preservation* (pp. 53–107). Academic Press, Elsevier.

Luo, Q. Y., Lin, Y., Li, Y., Xiong, L. H., Cui, R., Xie, Z. X., Pang, D. W. (2014). Nanomechanical analysis of yeast cells in CdSe quantum dot biosynthesis. *Small*, *10*(4), 699–704.

Luo, Y., Xu, D., Gao, X., Xiong, J., Jiang, B., Zhang, Y., Wang, Y., Tang, Y., Chen, C., Qiao, H., Zou, J. (2019). Nanoparticles conjugated with bacteria targeting tumors for precision imaging and therapy. *Biochemical and Biophysical Research Communications*, *514*(4), 1147–1153.

Lv, Q., Zhang, B., Xing, X., Zhao, Y., Cai, R., Wang, W., Gu, Q. (2018). Biosynthesis of copper nanoparticles using *Shewanella loihica* PV-4 with antibacterial activity: Novel approach and mechanisms investigation. *Journal of Hazardous Materials*, *347*, 141–149.

Magdy, M. (2014). Brief introduction to pharmaceutical microbiologist. *Journal of Microbiology and Experimentation*, *1*(5), 165–166.

Majeed, S., Danish, M., Mohamad Ibrahim, M. N., Sekeri, S. H., Ansari, M. T., Nanda, A., Ahmad, G. (2021). Bacteria mediated synthesis of iron oxide nanoparticles and their antibacterial, antioxidant, cytocompatibility properties. *Journal of Cluster Science*, *32*, 1083–1094.

Malik, S., Muhammad, K., Waheed, Y. (2023). Nanotechnology: A revolution in modern industry. *Molecules*, *28*(2), 661.

Malvankar, N. S., Lovley, D. R. (2012). Microbial nanowires: A new paradigm for biological electron transfer and bioelectronics. *ChemSusChem*, *5*(6), 1039–1046.

Manivasagan, P., Alam, M. S., Kang, K. H., Kwak, M., Kim, S. K. (2015). Extracellular synthesis of gold bionanoparticles by *Nocardiopsis* sp. and evaluation of its antimicrobial, antioxidant and cytotoxic activities. *Bioprocess and Biosystems Engineering*, *38*, 1167–1177.

Mao, C., Flynn, C. E., Hayhurst, A., Sweeney, R., Qi, J., Georgiou, G., Iverson, B., Belcher, A. M. (2003). Viral assembly of oriented quantum dot nanowires. *Proceedings of the National Academy of Sciences*, *100*(12), 6946–6951.

Maurya, D. K., Kumar, A., Chaurasiya, U., Hussain, T., Singh, S. K. (2021). Modern era of microbial biotechnology: Opportunities and future prospects. In: Solanki, M. K., Kashyap, P. L., Ansari, R. A., Kumari, B. (Eds.), *Microbiomes and Plant Health* (pp. 317–343). Academic Press, Elsevier.

Mehta, A., Sidhu, C., Pinnaka, A. K., Roy Choudhury, A. (2014). Extracellular polysaccharide production by a novel osmotolerant marine strain of *Alteromonas macleodii* and its application towards biomineralization of silver. *PLoS One*, *9*(6), e98798.

Miao, T., Wang, J., Zeng, Y., Liu, G., Chen, X. (2018). Polysaccharide-based controlled release systems for therapeutics delivery and tissue engineering: From bench to bedside. *Advanced Science*, *5*(4), 1700513.

Mishra, A., Tripathy, S. K., Wahab, R., Jeong, S. H., Hwang, I., Yang, Y. B., Kim, Y. S., Shin, H. S., Yun, S. I. (2011). Microbial synthesis of gold nanoparticles using the fungus *Penicillium brevicompactum* and their cytotoxic effects against mouse mayo blast cancer C_2C_{12} cells. *Applied Microbiology and Biotechnology*, *92*, 617–630.

Molnár, Z., Bódai, V., Szakacs, G., Erdélyi, B., Fogarassy, Z., Sáfrán, G., Varga, T., Konya, Z., Toth-Szeles, E., Szucs, R., Lagzi, I. (2018). Green synthesis of gold nanoparticles by thermophilic filamentous fungi. *Scientific Reports*, *8*(1), 3943.

Montaser, R., Paul, V. J., Luesch, H. (2011). Pitipeptolides C–F, antimycobacterial cyclodepsipeptides from the marine cyanobacterium *Lyngbya majuscula* from Guam. *Phytochemistry*, *72*(16), 2068–2074.

Morales-Narváez, E., Golmohammadi, H., Naghdi, T., Yousefi, H., Kostiv, U., Horák, D., Pourreza, N., Merkoçi, A. (2015). Nanopaper as an optical sensing platform. *ACS Nano*, *9*(7), 7296–7305.

Mustafa, F., Hassan, R. Y., Andreescu, S. (2017). Multifunctional nanotechnology-enabled sensors for rapid capture and detection of pathogens. *Sensors*, *17*(9), 2121.

Nandi, S., Ritenberg, M., Jelinek, R. (2015). Bacterial detection with amphiphilic carbon dots. *Analyst*, *140*(12), 4232–4237.

Nasrollahzadeh, M., Sajadi, S. M., Sajjadi, M., Issaabadi, Z. (2019). An introduction to nanotechnology. In: Nasrollahzadeh, M., Sajadi, S. M., Sajjadi, M., Issaabadi, Z., Atarod, M. (Eds.), *Interface Science and Technology* (pp. 1–27, Vol. 28). Elsevier.

Natrajan, D., Srinivasan, S., Sundar, K., Ravindran, A. (2015). Formulation of essential oil-loaded chitosan–alginate nanocapsules. *Journal of Food and Drug Analysis*, *23*(3), 560–568.

Navya, P. N., Daima, H. K. (2016). Rational engineering of physicochemical properties of nanomaterials for biomedical applications with nanotoxicological perspectives. *Nano Convergence*, *3*, 1–14.

Nayak, A. K., Bera, H., Hasnain, M. S., De, A., Pal, D., Samanta, A. (2021). Gellan gum-based nanomaterials in drug delivery applications. In: Bera, H., Hossain, C. M., Saha, S. (Eds.), *Biopolymer-based Nanomaterials in Drug Delivery and Biomedical Applications* (pp. 313–336). Academic Press, Elsevier.

Nayyar, A., Puri, V., Le, D. N. (2017). Internet of nano things (IoNT): Next evolutionary step in nanotechnology. *Nanoscience and Nanotechnology*, *7*(1), 4–8.

Nwodo, U. U., Green, E., Okoh, A. I. (2012). Bacterial exopolysaccharides: Functionality and prospects. *International Journal of Molecular Sciences*, *13*(11), 14002–14015.

Ostadhossein, F., Misra, S. K., Tripathi, I., Kravchuk, V., Vulugundam, G., LoBato, D., Pan, D. (2018). Dual purpose hafnium oxide nanoparticles offer imaging *Streptococcus mutans* dental biofilm and fight it in vivo via a drug free approach. *Biomatererials*, *181*, 252–267.

Panda, B. R., Singh, A. K., Ramesh, A., Chattopadhyay, A. (2008). Rapid estimation of bacteria by a fluorescent gold nanoparticle– polythiophene composite. *Langmuir*, *24*(20), 11995–12000.

Paolino, D., Mancuso, A., Cristiano, M. C., Froiio, F., Lammari, N., Celia, C., Fresta, M. (2021). Nanonutraceuticals: The new frontier of supplementary food. Nanomaterials, *11*(3), 792.

Pastorino, F., Brignole, C., Di Paolo, D., Perri, P., Curnis, F., Corti, A., Ponzoni, M. (2019). Overcoming biological barriers in neuroblastoma therapy: The vascular targeting approach with liposomal drug nanocarriers. *Small*, *15*(10), 1804591.

Patel, J., Maji, B., Moorthy, N. H. N., Maiti, S. (2020). Xanthan gum derivatives: Review of synthesis, properties and diverse applications. *RSC Advances*, *10*(45), 27103–27136.

Patil, M. P., Kang, M. J., Niyonizigiye, I., Singh, A., Kim, J. O., Seo, Y. B., Kim, G. D. (2019). Extracellular synthesis of gold nanoparticles using the marine bacterium *Paracoccus haeundaensis* BC74171T and evaluation of their antioxidant activity and antiproliferative effect on normal and cancer cell lines. *Colloids and Surfaces B: Biointerfaces*, *183*, 110455.

Patil, M., Mehta, D. S., Guvva, S. (2008). Future impact of nanotechnology on medicine and dentistry. *Journal of Indian Society of Periodontology*, *12*(2), 34–40.

Peng, H., Chen, I. A. (2018). Rapid colorimetric detection of bacterial species through the capture of gold nanoparticles by chimeric phages. *ACS Nano*, *13*(2), 1244–1252.

Pirinçci, Ş. Ş., Ertekin, Ö., Laguna, D. E., Özen, F. Ş., Öztürk, Z. Z., Öztürk, S. (2018). Label-free QCM immunosensor for the detection of ochratoxin A. *Sensors*, *18*(4), 1161.

Pourreza, N., Golmohammadi, H., Naghdi, T., Yousefi, H. (2015). Green in-situ synthesized silver nanoparticles embedded in bacterial cellulose nanopaper as a bionanocomposite plasmonic sensor. *Biosensors and Bioelectronics*, *74*, 353–359.

Prasad, R., Pandey, R., Barman, I. (2016). Engineering tailored nanoparticles with microbes: Quo vadis? *Wiley Interdisciplinary Reviews: Nanomedicine and Nanobiotechnology*, *8*(2), 316–330.

Prakash, O., Sil, S., Verma, T., Umapathy, S. (2019). Direct detection of bacteria using positively charged Ag/Au bimetallic nanoparticles: A label-free surface-enhanced Raman scattering study coupled with multivariate analysis. *Journal of Physical Chemistry* C, *124*(1), 861–869.

Priyanka, U., KM, A. G., Elisha, M. G., Nitish, N. (2017). Biologically synthesized PbS nanoparticles for the detection of arsenic in water. International *Biodeterioration and Biodegradation*, *119*, 78–86.

Qi, P., Zhang, D., Zeng, Y., Wan, Y. (2016). Biosynthesis of CdS nanoparticles: A fluorescent sensor for sulfate-reducing bacteria detection. *Talanta*, *147*, 142–146.

Rademacher, F., Gläser, R., Harder, J. (2021). Antimicrobial peptides and proteins: Interaction with the skin microbiota. *Experimental Dermatology*, *30*(10), 1496–1508.

Raj, R., Dalei, K., Chakraborty, J., Das, S. (2016). Extracellular polymeric substances of a marine bacterium mediated synthesis of CdS nanoparticles for removal of cadmium from aqueous solution. *Journal of Colloid and Interface Science*, *462*, 166–175.

Raj, V., Vijayan, A. N., Joseph, K. (2015). Cysteine capped gold nanoparticles for naked eye detection of *E. coli* bacteria in UTI patients. *Sensing and Bio-Sensing Research*, *5*, 33–36.

Rajalekshmy, G. P., Mariya, R. A., Rekha, M. R. (2021). Pullulan-based nanomaterials in drug delivery applications. In: Bera, H., Hossain, C. M., Saha, S. (Eds.), *Biopolymer-based Nanomaterials in Drug Delivery and Biomedical Applications* (pp. 383–404). Academic Press.

Rajapaksha, P., Elbourne, A., Gangadoo, S., Brown, R., Cozzolino, D., Chapman, J. (2019). A review of methods for the detection of pathogenic microorganisms. *Analyst*, *144*(2), 396–411.

Rajeshkumar, S., Sivapriya, D. (2020). Fungus-mediated nanoparticles: Characterization and biomedical advances. In: Shukla, A. (Ed.), *Nanoparticles in Medicine* (pp. 185–199). Springer: Singapore.

Rambaran, T., Schirhagl, R. (2022). Nanotechnology from lab to industry – a look at current trends. *Nanoscale Advances*, *4*(18), 3664–3675.

Ramirez-Acuña, J. M., Cardenas-Cadena, S. A., Marquez-Salas, P. A., Garza-Veloz, I., Perez-Favila, A., Cid-Baez, M. A., Flores-Morales, V., Martinez-Fierro, M. L. (2019). Diabetic foot ulcers: Current advances in antimicrobial therapies and emerging treatments. *Antibiotics*, *8*(4), 193.

Ramya, S., Shanmugasundaram, T., Balagurunathan, R. (2015). Biomedical potential of actinobacterially synthesized selenium nanoparticles with special reference to anti-biofilm, anti-oxidant, wound healing, cytotoxic and anti-viral activities. *Journal of Trace Elements in Medicine and Biology*, *32*, 30–39.

Reta, N., Saint, C. P., Michelmore, A., Prieto-Simon, B., Voelcker, N. H. (2018). Nanostructured electrochemical biosensors for label-free detection of water-and food-borne pathogens. *ACS Applied Materials and Interfaces*, *10*(7), 6055–6072.

Richa, R., Choudhury, A. R. (2020). Exploration of polysaccharide based nanoemulsions for stabilization and entrapment of curcumin. *International Journal of Biological Macromolecules*, *156*, 1287–1296.

Roda, A., Cevenini, L., Borg, S., Michelini, E., Calabretta, M. M., Schüler, D. (2013). Bioengineered bioluminescent magnetotactic bacteria as a powerful tool for chip-based whole-cell biosensors. *Lab on a Chip*, *13*(24), 4881–4889.

Rojas, V., Rivas, L., Cárdenas, C., Guzmán, F. (2020). Cyanobacteria and eukaryotic microalgae as emerging sources of antibacterial peptides. *Molecules*, *25*(24), 5804.

Rostami, M., Ghorbani, M., Delavar, M., Tabibiazar, M., Ramezani, S. (2019). Development of resveratrol loaded chitosan-gellan nanofiber as a novel gastrointestinal delivery system. *International Journal of Biological Macromolecules*, *135*, 698–705.

Roychoudhury, P., Gopal, P. K., Paul, S., Pal, R. (2016). Cyanobacteria assisted biosynthesis of silver nanoparticles—a potential antileukemic agent. *Journal of Applied Phycology*, *28*, 3387–3394.

Roychowdhury, R., Srivastava, N., Kumari, S., Pinnaka, A. K., Choudhury, A. R. (2021). Isolation of an exopolysaccharide from a novel marine bacterium *Neorhizobium urealyticum* sp. nov. and its utilization in nanoemulsion formation for encapsulation and stabilization of astaxanthin. *LWT*, *151*, 112105.

Salata, O. V. (2004). Applications of nanoparticles in biology and medicine. *Journal of Nanobiotechnology*, *2*(1), 1–6.

Sandle, T. (2016). Introduction to pharmaceutical microbiology. In: Sandle, T. (Ed.), *Pharmaceutical Microbiology* (pp. 1–14). Woodhead Publishing.

Saravanakumar, K., Chelliah, R., MubarakAli, D., Jeevithan, E., Oh, D. H., Kathiresan, K., Wang, M. H. (2018). Fungal enzyme-mediated synthesis of chitosan nanoparticles and its biocompatibility, antioxidant and bactericidal properties. *International Journal of Biological Macromolecules*, *118*, 1542–1549.

Sardar, M., Mishra, A., Ahmad, R. (2014). Biosynthesis of metal nanoparticles and their applications. In Tiwari, A., Turner, A. P. F. (Eds.), *Biosensors Nanotechnology* (pp. 239–266), John Wiley & Sons.

Sarika, P. R., James, N. R., Raj, D. K. (2016). Preparation, characterization and biological evaluation of curcumin loaded alginate aldehyde–gelatin nanogels. *Materials Science and Engineering: C*, *68*, 251–257.

Sathishkumar, R. S., Sundaramanickam, A., Srinath, R., Ramesh, T., Saranya, K., Meena, M., Surya, P. (2019). Green synthesis of silver nanoparticles by bloom forming marine microalgae *Trichodesmium erythraeum* and its applications in antioxidant, drug-resistant bacteria, and cytotoxicity activity. *Journal of Saudi Chemical Society*, *23*(8), 1180–1191.

Saxami, G., Karapetsas, A., Chondrou, P., Vasiliadis, S., Lamprianidou, E., Kotsianidis, I., Ypsilantis, P., Botaitis, S., Simopoulos, C., Galanis, A. (2017). Potentially probiotic *Lactobacillus* strains with anti-proliferative activity induce cytokine/chemokine production and neutrophil recruitment in mice. *Beneficial Microbes*, *8*(4), 615–623.

Sepunaru, L., Tschulik, K., Batchelor-McAuley, C., Gavish, R., Compton, R. G. (2015). Electrochemical detection of single *E. coli* bacteria labeled with silver nanoparticles. *Biomaterials Science*, *3*(6), 816–820.

Shah, M., Fawcett, D., Sharma, S., Tripathy, S. K., Poinern, G. E. J. (2015). Green synthesis of metallic nanoparticles via biological entities. *Materials*, *8*(11), 7278–7308.

Shanmugasundaram, T., Radhakrishnan, M., Gopikrishnan, V., Kadirvelu, K., Balagurunathan, R. (2017). In vitro antimicrobial and in vivo wound healing effect of actinobacterially synthesised nanoparticles of silver, gold and their alloy. *RSC Advances*, *7*(81), 51729–51743.

Shao, W., Liu, H., Liu, X., Sun, H., Wang, S., Zhang, R. (2015). pH-responsive release behavior and anti-bacterial activity of bacterial cellulose-silver nanocomposites. *International Journal of Biological Macromolecules*, *76*, 209–217.

Sharma, C., Bhardwaj, N. K. (2019). Bacterial nanocellulose: Present status, biomedical applications and future perspectives. *Materials Science and Engineering: C*, *104*, 109963.

Shekarforoush, E., Ajalloueian, F., Zeng, G., Mendes, A. C., Chronakis, I. S. (2018). Electrospun xanthan gum-chitosan nanofibers as delivery carrier of hydrophobic bioactives. *Materials Letters*, *228*, 322–326.

Shen, J., Zhou, X., Shan, Y., Yue, H., Huang, R., Hu, J., Xing, D. (2020). Sensitive detection of a bacterial pathogen using allosteric probe-initiated catalysis and CRISPR-Cas13a amplification reaction. *Nature Communications*, *11*(1), 267.

Shende, P., Mallick, C. (2020). Nanonutraceuticals: A way towards modern therapeutics in healthcare. *Journal of Drug Delivery Science and Technology*, *58*, 101838.

Shinde, N. C., Keskar, N. J., Argade, P. D. (2012). Nanoparticles: Advances in drug delivery systems. *International Journal of Advances in Pharmacy, Biology and Chemistry*, *3*(1), 922–929.

Singh, P., Kim, Y. J., Zhang, D., Yang, D. C. (2016). Biological synthesis of nanoparticles from plants and microorganisms. *Trends in Biotechnology*, *34*(7), 588–599.

Smith, V. J., Desbois, A. P., Dyrynda, E. A. (2010). Conventional and unconventional antimicrobials from fish, marine invertebrates and micro-algae. *Marine Drugs*, *8*(4), 1213–1262.

Srivastava, N., Choudhury, A. R. (2021). Recent advances in composite hydrogels prepared solely from polysaccharides. *Colloids and Surfaces B: Biointerfaces*, *205*, 111891.

Srivastava, I., Khamo, J. S., Pandit, S., Fathi, P., Huang, X., Cao, A., Haasch, R. T., Nie, S., Zhang, K., Pan, D. (2019). Influence of electron acceptor and electron donor on the photophysical properties of carbon dots: A comparative investigation at the bulk-state and single-particle level. *Advanced Functional Materials*, *29*(37), 1902466.

Srivastava, N., Kumari, S., Kurmi, S., Pinnaka, A. K., Choudhury, A. R. (2022). Isolation, purification, and characterization of a novel exopolysaccharide isolated from marine bacteria *Brevibacillus borstelensis* M42. *Archives of Microbiology*, *204*(7), 399.

Srivastava, P., Kowshik, M. (2017). Fluorescent lead (IV) sulfide nanoparticles synthesized by *Idiomarina* sp. strain PR58-8 for bioimaging applications. *Applied and Environmental Microbiology*, *83*(7), e03091–16.

Suh, S., Jo, A., Traore, M. A., Zhan, Y., Coutermarsh-Ott, S. L., Ringel-Scaia, V. M., Allen, I. C., Davis, R. M., Behkam, B. (2019). Nanoscale bacteria-enabled autonomous drug delivery system (NanoBEADS) enhances intratumoral transport of nanomedicine. *Advanced Science*, *6*(3), 1801309.

Suresh, A. K., Pelletier, D. A., Wang, W., Broich, M. L., Moon, J. W., Gu, B., Allison, D. P., Joy, D. C., Phelps, T. J., Doktycz, M. J. (2011). Biofabrication of discrete spherical gold nanoparticles using the metal-reducing bacterium *Shewanella oneidensis*. *Acta Biomaterialia*, *7*(5), 2148–2152.

Syed, A., Saraswati, S., Kundu, G. C., Ahmad, A. (2013). Biological synthesis of silver nanoparticles using the fungus *Humicola* sp. and evaluation of their cytoxicity using normal and cancer cell lines. *Spectrochimica Acta Part A: Molecular and Biomolecular Spectroscopy*, *114*, 144–147.

Tang, J., Chu, B., Wang, J., Song, B., Su, Y., Wang, H., He, Y. (2019). Multifunctional nanoagents for ultrasensitive imaging and photoactive killing of Gram-negative and Gram-positive bacteria. *Nature Communications*, *10*(1), 4057.

Teixeira, I. D., Carvalho, E., Leal, E. C. (2023). Green antimicrobials as therapeutic agents for diabetic foot ulcers. *Antibiotics*, *12*(3), 467.

Torres, S. K., Campos, V. L., León, C. G., Rodríguez-Llamazares, S. M., Rojas, S. M., Gonzalez, M., Smith, C., Mondaca, M. A. (2012). Biosynthesis of selenium nanoparticles by *Pantoea agglomerans* and their antioxidant activity. *Journal of Nanoparticle Research*, *14*, 1–9.

Uddandarao, P., Balakrishnan, R. M., Ashok, A., Swarup, S., Sinha, P. (2019). Bioinspired ZnS: Gd nanoparticles synthesized from an endophytic fungi *Aspergillus flavus* for fluorescence-based metal detection. *Biomimetics*, *4*(1), 11.

Uddin, T. M., Chakraborty, A. J., Khusro, A., Zidan, B. R. M., Mitra, S., Emran, T. B., Dhama, K., Ripon, M. K. H., Gajdács, M., Sahibzada, M. U. K., Hossain, M. J., Koirala, N. (2021). Antibiotic resistance in microbes: History, mechanisms, therapeutic strategies and future prospects. *Journal of Infection and Public Health*, *14*(12), 1750–1766.

Udugama, B., Kadhiresan, P., Kozlowski, H. N., Malekjahani, A., Osborne, M., Li, V. Y., Chen, H., Mubareka, S., Gubbay, J. B., Chan, W. C. (2020). Diagnosing COVID-19: The disease and tools for detection. *ACS Nano*, *14*(4), 3822–3835.

Uivaraseanu, B., Bungau, S., Tit, D. M., Fratila, O., Rus, M., Maghiar, T. A., Maghiar, O., Pantis, C., Vesa, C. M., Zaha, D. C. (2020). Clinical, pathological and microbiological evaluation of diabetic foot syndrome. *Medicina*, *56*(8), 380.

Vargas, G., Cypriano, J., Correa, T., Leão, P., Bazylinski, D. A., Abreu, F. (2018). Applications of magnetotactic bacteria, magnetosomes and magnetosome crystals in biotechnology and nanotechnology: Mini-review. *Molecules*, *23*(10), 2438.

von Woedtke, T., Kramer, A. (2008). The limits of sterility assurance. *GMS Krankenhhyg Interdisziplinar*, *3*(30), Doc19.

Wang, C., Li, X., Sang, S., McClements, D. J., Chen, L., Long, J., Jiao, A., Wang, J., Jin, Z., Qiu, C. (2022). Preparation, characterization and in vitro digestive behaviors of emulsions synergistically stabilized by γ-cyclodextrin/sodium caseinate/alginate. *Food Research International*, *160*, 111634.

Wang, F., Xu, Y., Lv, C., Han, C., Li, Y. (2018). Enhanced wound healing activity of PEG/PCL copolymer combined with bioactive nanoparticles in wound care after anorectal surgery: Via bio-inspired methodology. *Journal of Photochemistry and Photobiology B: Biology*, *187*, 54–60.

Wang, J., Wu, X., Wang, C., Rong, Z., Ding, H., Li, H., Li, S., Shao, N., Xaio, R., Wang, S. (2016). Facile synthesis of Au-coated magnetic nanoparticles and their application in bacteria detection via a SERS method. *ACS Applied Materials and Interfaces*, *8*(31), 19958–19967.

Wang, T., Yang, L., Zhang, B., Liu, J. (2010). Extracellular biosynthesis and transformation of selenium nanoparticles and application in H_2O_2 biosensor. *Colloids and Surfaces B: Biointerfaces*, *80*(1), 94–102.

Waters, A. L., Hill, R. T., Place, A. R., Hamann, M. T. (2010). The expanding role of marine microbes in pharmaceutical development. *Current Opinion in Biotechnology*, *21*(6), 780–786.

Wei, R. (2017). Biosynthesis of Au–Ag alloy nanoparticles for sensitive electrochemical determination of paracetamol. *International Journal of Electrochemical Science*, *12*(10), 9131–9140.

Wei, Y., Li, C., Dai, L., Zhang, L., Liu, J., Mao, L., Yuan, F., Gao, Y. (2020). The construction of resveratrol-loaded protein–polysaccharide–tea saponin complex nanoparticles for controlling physicochemical stability and in vitro digestion. *Food and Function*, *11*(11), 9973–9983.

Wu, Z., Wang, G., Pan, D., Guo, Y., Zeng, X., Sun, Y., Cao, J. (2016). Inflammation-related pro-apoptotic activity of exopolysaccharides isolated from *Lactococcus lactis* subsp. *lactis*. *Beneficial Microbes*, *7*(5), 761–768.

Xiong, H., Zheng, H., Wang, W., Liang, J., Wen, W., Zhang, X., Wang, S. (2016). A convenient purification method for silver nanoclusters and its applications in fluorescent pH sensors for bacterial monitoring. *Biosensors and Bioelectronics*, *86*, 164–168.

Xu, Y., Dhaouadi, Y., Stoodley, P., Ren, D. (2020). Sensing the unreachable: Challenges and opportunities in biofilm detection. *Current Opinion in Biotechnology*, *64*, 79–84.

Yan, L., Da, H., Zhang, S., López, V. M., Wang, W. (2017). Bacterial magnetosome and its potential application. *Microbiological Research*, *203*, 19–28.

Yang, L., Deng, W., Cheng, C., Tan, Y., Xie, Q., Yao, S. (2018). Fluorescent immunoassay for the detection of pathogenic bacteria at the single-cell level using carbon dots-encapsulated breakable organosilicananocapsule as labels. *ACS Applied Materials and Interfaces*, *10*(4), 3441–3448.

Yin, M., Wu, C., Li, H., Jia, Z., Deng, Q., Wang, S., Zhang, Y. (2019). Simultaneous sensing of seven pathogenic bacteria by guanidine-functionalized upconversion fluorescent nanoparticles. *ACS Omega*, *4*(5), 8953–8959.

Younis, N. S., El Semary, N. A., Mohamed, M. E. (2021). Silver nanoparticles green synthesis via cyanobacterium *Phormidium* sp.: Characterization, wound healing, antioxidant, antibacterial, and anti-inflammatory activities. *European Review for Medical and Pharmacological Sciences*, *25*(7), 3083–3096.

Zeng, Q., Zeng, W., Jin, Y., Sheng, L. (2022). Construction and evaluation of ovalbumin-pullulan nanogels as a potential delivery carrier for curcumin. *Food Chemistry*, *367*, 130716.

Zhao, X., Li, M., Xu, Z. (2018a). Detection of foodborne pathogens by surface enhanced Raman spectroscopy. *Frontiers in Microbiology*, *9*, 1236.

Zhao, X., Zhou, L., Riaz Rajoka, M. S., Yan, L., Jiang, C., Shao, D., Zhu, J., Shi, J., Huang, Q., Yang, H., Jin, M. (2018b). Fungal silver nanoparticles: Synthesis, application and challenges. *Critical Reviews in Biotechnology*, *38*(6), 817–835.

Zheng, D. W., Chen, Y., Li, Z. H., Xu, L., Li, C. X., Li, B., Fan, J. X., Cheng, S. X., Zhang, X. Z. (2018). Optically-controlled bacterial metabolite for cancer therapy. *Nature Communications*, *9*(1), 1680.

Zheng, D., Hu, C., Gan, T., Dang, X., Hu, S. (2010). Preparation and application of a novel vanillin sensor based on biosynthesis of Au–Ag alloy nanoparticles. *Sensors and Actuators B: Chemical*, *148*(1), 247–252.

Zou, L., Peng, S., Liu, W., Chen, X., Liu, C. (2015). A novel delivery system dextran sulfate coated amphiphilic chitosan derivatives-based nanoliposome: Capacity to improve in vitro digestion stability of (−)-epigallocatechin gallate. *Food Research International*, *69*, 114–120.

Index

T

U

V

W

X

Z

For Product Safety Concerns and Information please contact our EU representative GPSR@taylorandfrancis.com Taylor & Francis Verlag GmbH, Kaufingerstraße 24, 80331 München, Germany